BELLY FAT IN MIDLIFE

PRACTICAL STEPS TO REVITALIZE YOUR CHANGING BODY

ROSE M. KADENDE-KAISER, Ph.D.

Belly Fat in Midlife: Practical Steps to Revitalize Your Changing Body

The content of this book is for general instruction only. Each person's physical, emotional, and spiritual condition is unique. The information in this book is not intended to replace or interrupt the reader's relationship with a physician or other health or wellness professional. Please consult your doctor for matters pertaining to your specific health.

Published by Season of Health: https://www.seasonofhealth.net/ Burlington, North Carolina, USA
Edited by: Eileen Kinch
Cover and interior design by: Jana Rade

ISBN (Paperback): 978-0-9847099-2-2
ISBN (Ebook): 978-0-9847099-3-9

TABLE OF CONTENTS

DEDICATION

To my late mom, Marie Bayaga, I no longer take home-cooked meals for granted. Thank you!

To my late dad, Gervais Kadende, your capacity for resilience, your creative skills with both the spoken and the written word, and your happy nature are a legacy you passed on to more than one generation already. I honor you with each line of this book.

To all my siblings whose many stories we share, I hope to inspire each of you to make self-care a priority for your sake and the sake of the next generation.

To the women in midlife, the ones I know and those I will never meet, I hope this book will serve as a useful resource for you now and into the future.

To my husband Paul and to our two sons, Dylan and Delmar, you are the best gift I have in this life, a treasure without value.

ACKNOWLEDGEMENTS

Many people showed up as I reflected on what this book means to me and what it took to bring it to completion.

First and foremost, I thank my husband, Paul Kaiser, my best friend and life partner for being there for me and with me throughout the long journey of putting the manuscript together. When I started out, I knew very little about where it would take me as I took time to dig deep and sought to personalize it as best as I could. I still feel the joy and excitement that came out after you read one of the earlier chapters, saying "this is powerful stuff, keep writing!" Then and there, I knew you heard my voice. You connected with my narrative. You understood what I had previously tried to express when I shared about my intent to write a book, one of the many paths I have been on as I seek to build a life of purpose through wellness coaching and training. You held me accountable throughout the writing process, reminding me to stay consistent chapter after chapter. You reviewed each chapter multiple times. You provided what I needed to bring it to completion. Saying "thank you" does not seem like enough, but let me say it more than once, in another language you understand, to emphasize just how grateful I am for all the love and support you continue to give me. Asante saaana kwa kila kitu!

A special thank you goes to my teachers, trainers, mentors, and advisors, past and present. Because of them, I have been able to find my voice, and a style of writing that can appeal to a particular audience. Professor Beverly Stoeltje was the first among this list of former teachers to really have an impact on who I am today. I am grateful for your confidence in me, especially in those days and years when, as a graduate student, I lacked my own self-confidence. You encouraged me when I did not trust that my English language proficiency would enable me to make it through graduate school without too many hiccups. What you did then sowed the seed that is still bearing fruit. This book is one of the fruits of that seed. Thank you!

To Eric Thurman, a spiritual brother, a friend with a deep passion to bring head and heart in all that we do, thank you for encouraging me and providing me with numerous opportunities to pour my heart out, as I continued to put my writing skills to the test. With your guidance, I knew it was ok to be myself, express my thoughts most authentically, and to recognize that there was an audience out there that could connect with my voice and my heart and to be moved to action.

To Chris Fowles, with you as a trusted mentor, I had no choice but to push my writing skills to a new level. While you held my hands as you did with my other colleagues, you also held each of us accountable to learning, improving, and taking ownership of our respective roles and duties. You celebrated with us our successes. Thank you for your guidance during an important phase of my professional development. Thank you for providing critical feedback during my journey of putting important ideas to paper and doing so with unprecedented efficiency.

To all my trainers and instructors at Institute for Integrative Nutrition, including those who provided necessary guidance during the writing of this book, you provided me and thousands of others, with a sample roadmap for self-care, teaching us why we must prioritize it if we wanted to be authentic as change-makers. You encouraged us to believe that balance and healing are possible. This book is a small expression of one of the seeds you have planted in me.

To my siblings and other members of my family and to each of you my clients, whom I have had the privilege to coach, the changes you continue to make and share, following the suggestions and advice I provide, remain a source of encouragement for me. It makes my life purposeful beyond personal gains and instant gratification. Thank you for helping me to recognize the value of the work I do, as you share testimonials of the changes you see in your health, your lives. I know that many of you will relate to this part of my journey as well. Thank you for who you are in my life.

Two of my friends and colleagues deserve a special mention here. Nadine Ndeberi Wani, you knew about this project months before anyone else outside my immediate family. You were with me even before the project I was working on pivoted into a book. You worked with me, sharing ideas, challenging me by asking the right questions, and even helping me to confirm that a focus on belly fat, more than other topics I had in mind then, will appeal to women in midlife. Our focused conversations at the time, are what helped me to seal the topic in and move forward in a clearer direction. Thank you for your trust, friendship, and encouragement.

Pat Noonan, you may not know why you appear here but a conversation with you during our time in Rwanda helped me to start questioning many false assumptions I had about relationships and marriage and how to maintain healthy boundaries. You and Ron, who sadly left us way too soon (may he rest in eternal peace) became role models for what it means to remain true to who you are, while also working hard, making a difference in other people's lives and enjoying life together as a couple. Hearing you and observing both of you set me on a more balanced path, a healthier direction in my own life and triggered more serious thinking about this wellness journey I am on.

Two people have been consistently asking about this book. No phone call with either of you would end without you asking: when is the book coming out? I consider Susan Parker as one of my most trusted cheerleaders. Thank you. Joe Kaiser, my father-in-law may forget certain things, understandably so, as a 96-year-old great grandpa, but you never forget to ask about when my book is coming out. Thank you for being excited about my book project and for the value you attach to my work.

To my brother-in-law Kevan Olesen, thank you for your continued interest in my work and for your support as I moved the book towards the final stages of production. I am grateful to have you as a trusted member of the Season of Health technology team!

I would be remiss not to thank all the women in midlife who participated in one my surveys and many others who confirmed what I had suspected that there is a need for such a resource that focuses on this particular category of women. I hope that this book will inform and serve as a guide for you, so that you can keep self-care on your front burner.

Last, but not least, a special thank you goes to my children, Dylan and Delmar. In spite of the delays in seeing my business take off, you have never stopped believing in me and recognizing the value of the work I do. Thank you for your patience and understanding. Thank you also for trusting my counsel and doing what you can to take care of yourselves. Seeing you healthy makes all my efforts worthwhile. You rock! I'm proud.

INTRODUCTION

I entered the fitting room with a dress that I thought was my size. I tried it on and realized quickly that it was too small because it wouldn't even move past my shoulders. I went back and brought the next larger size. The dress felt tight, and it just did not look good on me. I told myself there is no way I could fit into a size bigger. I went back and got that next size up and *voila*. It worked! Somewhat. Because what was holding it in place was my belly. Protruding and giving me stretch marks while also putting pressure on my lower back. By the time I came to realize that I was wearing a size fourteen, I had been living in it for at least a couple of years. A decade before, I was wearing mostly size eight and that was okay with me, even though it also marked a significant shift from my younger adult years when I wore a size 4 or smaller. In that fitting room and subsequently looking through my closet with many outfits that no longer fit, a thought came. It was the idea that what led me to this point could easily lead to wearing even larger sizes, unless I took action to stop it.

I embarked on a long journey of learning about what happens that creates the right conditions for the belly to expand more and more once women reach midlife. The initial actions I took to lose weight did not help to shrink my belly effectively. So, I continued to learn and adjust my actions for nearly seven years to reach consistent results that I will share throughout this book. Each step of the way required a mindset shift. I had to align my thinking and my actions with my goals. This is what I will explore in the first chapter of this book. It is based on a recognition that we are individually responsible for making necessary changes that move us in the direction of our health goals.

Chapter 1, therefore, introduces the concept known as the stages of behavior change, a tool and a methodology that many psychoanalysts have found to be useful in supporting people willing to move through the change process effectively and in a sustainable manner. The process works the same way for self-changers, whether or not they are familiar with the stages of change. I will explain how applying the stages of change helps us recognize where we may be resisting change and what we can do to support ourselves to move gradually but effectively from an unwanted habit to a more desired behavior.

The second chapter focuses on the actions I had to take once I became aware of the impact that sugar had been having on my body and my weight and belly fat. You will also discover how deep I had to dig to understand my own sugar habits, how misinformed I was about where sugar hides, and how it is disguised under many different names, making it challenging to identify it and limit it in our diet. The journey to breaking my sugar habits took longer than I imagined because what it required was more than just staying away from sugary foods. I will share the detailed plan I implemented that helped me break free from the grip of sugar and how limiting sugar intake contributed to improving my health and to weight loss much more effectively.

In Chapter 3, I discuss the starches also commonly referred to as carbohydrates (carbs). I reflect on how challenging it was to make carbs work for me. Sugar is also a carbohydrate in its simplest form. I separated sugar from the other carbohydrates because this was more in line with my own thinking and my behaviors regarding both. Even when I knew that I needed to limit my sugar intake, I was not aware that sugar and starchy foods often had similar impacts on the body. Therefore, the steps I took to manage each came in two distinct phases.

I will discuss how I was able to make carbs work better for me and support my efforts to maintain a healthy weight once I had finally reached it.

Therefore, understanding the effects of sugar and starchy foods on blood sugar and insulin is one of the most important lessons that I hope anyone reading this book needs to walk away with. For many of us, without managing insulin and preventing insulin resistance, losing weight and keeping a healthy weight is nearly impossible.

So much has been written that links carb consumption to weight gain or a resistance to weight loss. If you listen to Mark Hyman, Michael R. Eades and Mary Dan Eades, Robert C. Atkins, or pay attention to the points that Gary Taubes makes regarding *Why We Get Fat*, you will hopefully come away convinced that if we manage our carb intake carefully, we are better able to conquer blood sugar problems as well. As we do, we have a higher chance of preventing weight gain and diabetes. I will summarize what I learned from these health experts and others that I refer to throughout the chapter. You will come away knowing which among your carb choices are least impactful and which are most harmful when it comes to their effects on blood sugar, insulin and your weight.

In the context of the changes I adopted related to my diet, the biggest learning curve came when I was introduced to the health benefits of fermented vegetables and other fermented foods and drinks. Chapter 4 is about my experiences with fermentation and the benefits of ferments for keeping the gut healthy. With more of our immune cells located in the gut than in other parts of our body, it is nearly impossible to imagine any level of healing and restoring balance without healing the gut. Therefore, adding fermented foods to my diet reached deeper inside my body, restoring a level of balance that I never thought was possible. Among the many benefits of a healthy gut is a healthy weight. If you are not familiar with fermented vegetables, I hope that what you will learn from Chapter 4 will convince you to give them a try. If you are already consuming store-bought fermented vegetables, I hope you will try making your own, following the instructions I share. If you already make your own, I hope what I share resonates with you and reinforces your practices in this area.

Chapter 5 is focused on dietary fats. I admit that fats were among the food groups I shunned the most, associating most sources with weight gain and other health issues we most want to avoid, particularly heart disease and high cholesterol. In this chapter, you will get acquainted with my long journey and how I was able to clear my misconceptions about fat by learning to separate the good, from the not-so good and the bad sources of fat. I explain which sources of fat I rely on these days and the many benefits I have gained from reintroducing healthy fats into my diet after nearly fifteen years of limiting all fats. Learning about the health benefits of dietary fat was truly an eye opener, and perhaps it will be for you as well.

The last three chapters of this book focus on what I call the "lifestyle trio," namely exercise, stress, and sleep, and their impact on weight and belly fat. I start with exercise in Chapter 6. While there almost never was a time when I was not aware of the importance of regular exercise for health, there were still a few barriers to my success in making exercise work best for me. One of the barriers was tied to a mindset that I did not have time when I was too busy with other priorities. Eventually, when I finally recognized that without exercise I was not going to lose the excess weight that I had accumulated, I still faced the challenge of understanding which types of exercises would enable me to reach the results I most wanted. I was aiming for losing weight, assuming that weight loss would also result in shrinking belly fat.

You will get a clear picture about where I got it wrong, what types of exercises actually shrink belly fat, and why in exercise, like in diet, there is no one-size-fits-all. You will also come away with an understanding that what might have worked for you in your younger and perhaps more fit years will not continue to work for you in midlife, especially if your waistline has expanded out of control. Fortunately, there are different choices to fit your needs, and with practice, you can always improve. As you build strength and stamina gradually but with persistence, the right types of exercises will support your efforts to shrink belly fat as well.

This chapter recognizes also that taking exercise as a standalone, beneficial activity under all circumstances we find ourselves in, can be misleading. Many women, in midlife or in other phases, push themselves too hard at the gym, with high hopes that the harder they work, the better the results they will achieve in terms of weight and fat loss. Exercise can work in your favor, when done properly, based on individual physiological and emotional needs. Eric Berg writes that "[t]he goal is to use exercise strategically to maximize and keep your body in fat burning and minimize fat-making stress hormones" (241). When you work out, you will want to maximize the effectiveness of exercise. Being informed and strategic keeps the wrong types of exercises from setting you up for failure in achieving your fat-burning goals. You will learn more how to achieve the best exercise results in Chapter 6.

Chapter 7 is dedicated to the importance of recognizing your stressors, as well as the impact of stress on your health, your weight, and belly fat. Some of the stressors are short-lived while other stressors can last a lifetime, if not managed carefully. New stressors emerge as women enter midlife, and we must be equipped to deal with each of them consistently, if we want to maintain a level of balance and prevent stress from contributing to belly fat. I will show you the stressors I failed to manage when my weight was not an issue, and how stress controlled me and kept me from focusing on self-care as my weight started gradually getting out of my control. As you go on this journey with me, you will perhaps relate to where I have been and be inspired to take the steps to recognize your own stressors and to deal with them one by one. I include the various steps and strategies I rely on to continue to manage stress better.

Stress-induced belly fat is real and must be dealt with as such. Recognizing the impact of stress on your weight will hopefully convince you that you must manage it better and keep yourself from allowing it to control what happens to your health.

Belly fat is not just about aesthetics and fitting into the cute little dress that looked so good on you in your younger and more fit years. It is a health risk and a key to several chronic diseases, including diabetes that unfortunately runs in my family line.

The last chapter of this book focuses on sleep. I will summarize what I learned from some of the top sleep experts regarding the importance of sleep and its link to weight gain and belly fat. I have adopted many of these expert recommendations. I am happy to share what has worked for me, bringing improvements both in the amount and the quality of sleep I get, following a phase of midlife insomnia that honestly caught me by surprise. In fact, I did not worry much about midlife until I was in the thick of it with health struggles, particularly insomnia. Through personal experiences, I came to realize that midlife is a unique phase with its own sets of challenges that we, as women, must learn to and be prepared to overcome if we want to keep ourselves grounded and in balance. This will help us to succeed in other areas of our lives, in work, in relationships, in our parenting roles, or even in our desires to live a life of purpose.

I hope that the sleep habits I have adopted, and that I include in Chapter 8, will inform and inspire you to take similar actions to improve the quality of your sleep. You will get to know what your sleep robbers are and where they may be hiding as well. You will need to look over and beyond where you would normally think to look as many of the sleep robbers are actually outside your bedroom. You will also be happy to know that you can control many of them. It is a matter of increasing your awareness of where they are, as well as your knowledge of how they affect your sleep, and from there, you must make a promise to yourself that you must kick these sleep robbers out of your life. And you must do so sooner rather than later. Action is required because insomnia is dangerous to your survival.

I discuss sleep also in the context of the lifestyle trio. It is hard to feel motivated to get out of bed and go to the gym when you did not sleep well the night before. Lack of sleep therefore acts as an exercise de-motivator. Not exercising in turn keeps all the weight on. You will also appreciate how sleep lowers cortisol, and lack of sleep therefore does the opposite. In turn, elevated cortisol increases insulin output. In her book *The Hormone Cure*, Sara Gottfried states that "[w]hen you make too much cortisol, you raise your blood sugar excessively. This may lead to prediabetes (as measured by a fasting glucose level between 100 and 125 mg/dL) or diabetes (fasting glucose > 125). Newer data suggest you should keep fasting glucose less than 87 mg/dL" (79). You will understand how insulin works, why anything you do that keeps it turned on is bad news for shrinking belly fat. Poor quality sleep keeps it on. Stress turns it on. Lack of exercise and the weight gain that tends to follow builds on an increase in insulin. Therefore, lack of sleep, stress, and lack of exercise often act as co-factors that affect your fat-storage hormones and keep you from reaching your goals of shrinking belly fat.

As you will see throughout each chapter of this book, I apply a similar approach. I start with a reflection, which can be a personal story that relates to the problem I identified and that I needed to address in order to lose weight and shrink belly fat in midlife. Then I review existing research that establishes the link between the identified problem area and weight gain and/or belly fat. From there, I explain how I was able to make the necessary changes and overcome the challenges related to that particular area. I include the results I achieved that brought me closer to my goal of shrinking belly fat in midlife.

Formal training through the Institute for Integrative Nutrition provided the knowledge base and direction, and introduced me to experts such as Mark Hyman, Donna Gates, Walter Willett, Andrew Weil, and many others that I refer to throughout this book. I relied on other resources, both online articles and blog posts as well as printed material, as I built my own library of books that supported my knowledge base and enabled me to focus on the main areas that I needed to deal with in order to shrink my own waistline when it became the most visible change of my physique in midlife.

If you are like me and want to age gracefully, you will agree that we must question some of our assumptions regarding the root causes of imbalances that manifest themselves most prominently in midlife. Fat accumulation around the waistline is one such manifestations. We must recognize that regardless of how far we have gone out of balance and how big our middle is, we are not going to lose it if we do not take action to maintain or restore this balance.

And since what leads to fat accumulation is not something that happens overnight, it may also take time for us to notice. Our moments of ignorance or the times when we're too busy to do anything about it, is the time when things get out of control inside our bodies and around our bellies in particular.

WHY DID I GET MYSELF INTO THIS?

I will get more personal throughout this book and bring you along with me on this journey. What keeps me motivated to shrink belly fat is more than the aesthetic value I would normally attach to a smaller waistline. If you are like me and the cluster of diseases known as the metabolic syndrome that include diabetes, heart disease, high blood pressure, and high cholesterol levels, run in your family, then taking action to shrink your waistline also contributes to preventing these diseases. You will perhaps relate to some of my stories, and I hope you will feel motivated to take action knowing that the efforts you make will yield worthwhile results.

We rarely know enough to think in terms of disease progression, from a point where we can safely apply natural mechanisms to return to homeostasis, to a different point where treatment with pharmaceuticals is the only option we are left with. I don't want you to prepare for midlife or to go through it with the level of ignorance I had when I came into it.

Throughout this journey, I continued to search for targeted knowledge and practical tools I could use to help me reach the goals I indicate in each chapter. Now, I want to be a resource for others, particularly those who are searching for answers that I have already found. Naturally, women in midlife fit my profile. I know that I am not alone in this search for ways to stop weight gain and how to shrink belly fat as our bodies change in midlife. There is no school that teaches us what to expect during this phase, or at least I have not attended any. I want to create a life of purpose out of the lessons learned along this journey. What I share in this book is part of a learning process and the application of what I have learned that brought me the results I consider worth sharing with you. My goal continues to be about staying healthy through midlife and beyond. It is based on an understanding that reaching a healthy weight and a smaller waistline contribute to this goal. My goal also became about developing expertise that would benefit you, my readers, along with others I am able to reach through health coaching, convening workshops, or holding live and online events. I hope to keep women from making the mistakes I made.

My goal is also about preparing you to better appreciate midlife as a time of freedom, as many others do. When I posted a survey on my social media network about what women associate midlife with, freedom was what showed up the most. Although in hindsight, I can understand their point of view, I must be honest that freedom is not what I would have intuitively associated with midlife. You have the opportunity to experience it, though, if you take action now and follow the guidance in this book. I want you to live inside your skin with the freedom you so much deserve.

Taking charge of your health is freeing.

The steps you will take following the guidelines I share in each chapter will support you on this journey to your freedom, with better health and a few inches off your waistline. This book is meant as a resource to help answer questions I used to have but that I now have answers for. It took me at least seven years to find these answers. You don't have to wait this long.

If you are younger and not yet in midlife, I hope that this book will also leave you feeling empowered. Know that when you keep an open mind and take a proactive approach, you can avoid making many of the assumptions and mistakes that rob us of a life of balance both physically and emotionally in midlife. What if we could start believing that it is still possible to feel healthier in our senior years than we did when we entered midlife or even years before? What if we could avoid the health issues that befell our mothers? What if we could manage the various symptoms of aging in a more proactive and informed manner? It seems like a worthwhile goal, but it requires keeping your belly fat in check and maintaining a healthy weight and waistline. You will learn how to throughout this book.

Therefore, this book is a call to action as it recognizes that it's never too late to support the body to rebalance itself. Action is crucial because belly fat will not go away by simply wishing it away, nor by doing more of the same thing. Belly fat is the most dangerous fat, hovering around our most vital organs, and gradually preventing the organs from performing their key functions and eventually destroying them. Mary Dan Eades and Michael Eades write that "[v]isceral fat is not just a passive repository of extra calories as was once believed; it is a metabolically active organ that responds to neurotransmitters and hormones and sends out chemical messages of its own to the brain and other tissues. When its accumulation reaches a critical mass, it begins to behave more like a tumor than a storage reservoir, infiltrating the organs and muscles - most importantly the liver - and, at least to some degree, wresting metabolic control from them" (21). The choice is ours. We can shrink visceral fat and protect our liver and other organs from the damage belly fat causes. I am happy to share what I do to keep it in check.

PART ONE

CHANGE YOUR MINDSET

CHAPTER 1

ALIGN YOUR ACTIONS WITH YOUR GOALS

"It isn't that they can't see the solution. It is that they can't see the problem"
G.K. Chesterton in James O. Prochaska et. al., *Changing for Good* (40).

This same idea has been expressed a bit differently by others. Lewis Carroll said, "If you don't know where you're going, any road will get you there." Yogi Berra put it, slightly differently: "If you don't know where you're going, you'll end up some place else." The different actions outlined in each of the chapters of this book aim to prevent you from getting lost and ending up some place else. They provide guidance on what to do to shrink belly fat. But you have to do the work. You have to take action. If you follow through, you will experience positive results no matter how far out of shape your waistline has become. Not knowing where you are going increases your chances of getting lost and wasting your time when a roadmap would have served you better. This book is a roadmap that will give you the tools you need to shrink your midlife middle. It includes guidelines on mindset, diet, and lifestyle habits that helped me to conquer belly fat and reclaim my waistline. It worked for me and it can work for you, too.

I am sharing this knowledge because I find it useful to follow the lead of someone who has already gone where I need to go. This underscores the importance of making sure you set a goal (or goals) and knowing where you want to go first and foremost, before starting on your journey. Once this is clear, then every action you take must lead in the direction of your goal or else you will get lost and, at best, you will delay achieving intended results. This chapter is about what it took for me to understand what my goal should have been all along and how re-defining it helped me to move more efficiently towards where I wanted to go.

Knowing what your goal is and making sure that the steps you take and your behaviors align with that particular goal, is key to your success. The goal of this book is to serve as a guide for anyone who wants to shrink their waistline and revitalize their changing body in midlife. Each chapter invites you to join me on the journey I took to shrink my waistline, and they offer a roadmap that can help you shrink yours. This chapter will introduce you to a tool that can help you check in with yourself as you move forward to implement what you learn in each chapter. According to psychoanalysts and experts in behavior change, this tool is known as the "six stages of change," also referred to as the "six stages of behavior change."

These stages fall along a continuum that moves from "pre-contemplation," which is the first stage, to "termination" which is the last stage. Pre-contemplation is a place where the person who needs to change lacks total awareness that she needs to change, even if others around her see that need and may even hint to her that she needs to consider changing in a particular area. The last stage of change referred to as "termination" is a place of total security and safety, where temptations will never again trigger a relapse into old undesired behaviors. There are four other stages in between the two ends of the spectrum in this order: contemplation, preparation, action, and maintenance. We all experience the stages of change more than once in our lifetime. The idea here is that with each of the changes required to succeed at shrinking belly fat, as with all other major changes we have to make in life, we go through all of the stages of behavior change.

I present this information in the first chapter of this book because I believe that making important changes in life, especially moving in a positive direction that we want to go, involves increased awareness of a problem and the need to find a solution for it. We must know what the problem is before we take action and work to maintain those helpful actions. We may start out at the pre-contemplation or any other stage, but ultimately, we will not see change until we take actions that help us achieve the ultimate goal, which in my case was shrinking my waistline and improving my overall health. It is important for us to continue checking in with ourselves to be sure that we are not standing in our own way, resisting necessary change in the direction of positive change. In his book, *The Power of Positive Thinking*, Norman Vincent Peale writes that "[t]he world in which you live is not primarily determined by outward conditions and circumstances but by thoughts that habitually occupy your mind" (327).

Making a shift in our thinking opens us up to a whole new world of possibilities.

This shift in thinking, however, requires noticing and increasing awareness of where the problem lies, which allows us to free ourselves from the grip of inaction, and instead we move ourselves towards positive change.

Paraphrasing what's commonly known as the Zen theory of change, Rick Carson writes in his book, *Taming Your Gremlin*: "I free myself not by trying to be free, but by simply noticing how I am imprisoning myself in the very moment I am imprisoning myself" (10). Taking action in the right direction is freeing. It moves us towards a goal that enables us to feel satisfied and enjoy the fullness of life. Taking action is an individual responsibility. It is the self-responsibility for our own health and wellness that Donald B. Ardell refers to in his book, *High Level Wellness*. This is how Ardell calls us to action: "Without an active sense of accountability for your own well-being, you won't have the necessary motivation to lead a health-enhancing lifestyle .... So, in the sense that you will not grow in other areas if you neglect this dimension, self-responsibility represents your keystone to a life of high level wellness" (94).

I hope this book will serve as a resource, a guide and a roadmap for anyone who wants to shrink belly fat in midlife, an important step in improving your overall wellness. Some of the changes are going to be easy. Others will be challenging. All are important and required as a part of the big picture that together can keep your waistline under control and yourself in better health. This chapter underscores the importance of embracing change, and recognizing, that the actions you will take, by following the guidelines laid out for you, will help you lose those excess inches around your waistline. The more of those inches you hang on to, the greater your risks of serious health issues, including diabetes, heart disease and hypertension. Many changes take place as we enter midlife. Some are irreversible, but there are some that can be prevented or reversed. We must own the actions needed to reclaim a healthier body and mind in midlife. From here, we can reclaim a healthy spirit, as well.

While this is based on my personal journey, I have relied on various sources, and triangulated the information I reviewed, to come to the conclusion that belly fat in midlife is not insurmountable and that we can take action to shrink it. The results you achieve will depend on how consistent you are with your actions. This book reveals key actions required to revitalize your changing body and melt inches off your waistline. Each chapter establishes goals, pieces of a puzzle that highlight specific steps needed to shrink belly fat in midlife. By implementing the tasks and activities in the next seven chapters, you will lose one, two or more inches around your waistline. The more consistent you are with the actions, the greater your chances of success at reaching your ideal waistline. If you are inconsistent with your actions, you will set yourself up for failure or take longer to see the results you want. Without a guide, you will get lost or take a long and winding road. With a guide, your path is clear.

To succeed requires a mindset shift. As you open yourself up for new ways of thinking about foods and lifestyle habits, you will give up behaviors that don't work and embrace new actions and steps that will empower you to shrink your waistline. Not everyone will move at the same pace, but anyone who follows through will achieve positive results. The pace at which each person will move will depend on the stage of change where she is. Look at the stages of change as a tool that can help us understand ourselves and our openness or resistance to new behaviors, new ways of living our lives. Not taking action, either because we think there is nothing that can help or because of other self-limiting messages in our heads, our "very own personal gremlin" (Carson 118) precludes us from the very steps needed to move ourselves forward.

I will walk you through the stages of behavior change and remind you that a mindset shift was required at each stage in order for me to embrace the foods and lifestyle habits that would lead me to my ultimate goal of shrinking belly fat. As a reminder, these stages are pre-contemplation in the first stage, followed by contemplation, preparation, action, maintenance and termination, which is the last of the six stages of change. Let me share how each stage brought me to a different level of awareness and a set of actions that led me eventually to a place of clarity regarding what my goal, shrinking belly fat, should have been all along.

1. PRE-CONTEMPLATION

At this stage, the person who needs to take action, does not know that different behaviors, different actions, or different habits, even exist, and she is not looking for them. Being in this stage keeps the pre-contemplator in disbelief, denial, or ignorance that there is a problem that needs to be changed. In fact, in the pre-contemplator's mind, it may be that those who see the problem are the ones who need to change, which leaves the pre-contemplator stuck, focusing neither on the problem nor on the solution.

This is where I was when my weight moved gradually from a size 8 to a size 14, and it was at this point that I no longer felt good inside my own body. Up to that point, I never felt unease with the distribution of my weight nor questioned what my ideal size should be. I had become used to a size 8—and then a size 10. In fact, I continued to believe that size 10 was my actual size even when it stopped fitting me. I lacked awareness and information that would have helped me to make an informed decision about how to get myself out of the trajectory of weight gain I was on. I was not even looking for a way out of what was becoming my status quo. This type of behavior pattern can take years before the pre-contemplator is able to shift her thinking and develop a level of awareness that prompts her to move towards change.

I lived in total ignorance that I had become overweight. No one around me seemed to be concerned enough to say anything about it, which reinforced my pre-contemplation routine. What I was doing, however, was focusing on the one thing I knew everyone needs: healthy foods. I expected the "healthy" food choices I was making, as a general rule for my family, would take care of all the other health needs, including keeping my weight under control. Perhaps this is why I made assumptions in my head that my weight did not change and that it did not need to change.

What I eventually discovered when I moved to later stages of behavior change, was that this way of thinking only reinforced my level of ignorance around what it means to eat healthy as opposed to eating right based on one's specific needs and health goals. I also was aware that exercise is good for everyone, whether or not they need to lose weight. But my time was limited, so I put off exercising. Putting off necessary actions because the time is not ideal is an excuse that leaves every pre-contemplator stuck in the rut. I was stuck as I justified my sedentary lifestyle. Between work, taking care of my kids, cooking, cleaning, laundry and everything else, the thought of adding another activity to my schedule seemed unrealistic at best. My priorities were justified, and they came from a good place in my heart. I had more important responsibilities to keep me busy day in and day out. Prioritizing myself would have been selfish given that my problem did not bother anyone else. It never occurred to me that people will notice a problem only when they're looking for it or recognize it as such. Hence, I continued to take no action because I lacked awareness around my weight problem. I did not believe there was anything I could do to stop aging, and I considered some weight gain as one of its manifestations. How much weight gain is a normal and safe as we age was not a question on my mind yet.

With this way of thinking, I stayed in the pre-contemplation for most of my 40s. I was not your typical pre-contemplator, however, because in conventional pre-contemplation those around the one who needs to change are aware of the problem and have even suggested ways to overcome the problem. That no one around me seemed to be concerned about my weight gain, not my husband, or my kids (perhaps they were too young to be thinking about this), or my siblings or my friends, made it easier for me to accept myself as I was, overweight and settled there. At one point, when my level of awareness had increased, I confronted my husband about it. He must have noticed, because when we met, I was a slim girl. So, I asked him, "Why didn't you tell me that I had become overweight?" His answer was very telling. "I thought you knew, and it didn't bother me." He was right. I should have known. After all, was I not the one living inside that body of mine, and did we not have mirrors all around the house for me to see myself clearly? "For those who have eyes, let them see" reads the title of the first chapter of *Change your brain. Change your life* by Daniel G. Amen (16).

I had eyes to see, but I failed to see what I needed to see, and my blinders kept me from moving myself out of the weight gain trajectory I was on. Clearly, I could not count on my closest partner, my husband. Who was he to judge? He, too, had put on a few more pounds than was ideal for him. How could he have known where to start to get me out of where I was—and where I was heading? I have seen, especially in the United States, that the body has an incredible ability to expand as it builds layers upon layers of fat around it. With all the excess weight around my body, I started feeling heavy, tired, and unable to move fast enough to keep up with others, especially when we had to walk uphill. It was embarrassing because in my head, my weight was normal. I was just out of shape because I didn't have time to exercise. I had been adding to my wardrobe and was buying dresses that were bigger each time. It never registered that somehow that meant I was getting bigger. Looking inside my closet, I must have worn a size 10 for a while as many of my outfits were this size. I literally cannot remember when I started wearing a size 12 or 14, but there I was, almost in disbelief that I had gone that far. With total lack of awareness of the shift in my weight, I could not set any goal aimed at shrinking my waistline. I could not align my behaviors with a goal that was not clear in my head.

2. CONTEMPLATION

My level of awareness increased and got me out of pre-contemplation when I went shopping for the perfect dress to wear to a friend's wedding. I liked a size 8 the best, and in my head, I thought that should have been my size. Of course, it did not fit me. Not even a bit! That trip to the store precipitated my mindset shift. It raised my level of self-awareness around my weight and caused me to rethink my position and ignorance of how much weight I had gained over the years. I ended up buying a size 12. When

I returned home, I pulled out of my closet some of my favorite dresses that no longer fit, and I was reminded that I needed to lose weight. When that reality became clear in my head, I knew I had to take action. With this mindset shift, I entered contemplation, the second phase in the process of behavior change. Contemplation is a time of reflection and recognition that one has a problem, and getting ready to deal with it is an important next step.

In contemplation, an increased level of self-awareness makes it uncomfortable for us to stay where we are. We no longer feel good about refusing to change. This phase is marked by an openness to considering change not just as necessary but also as beneficial. Contemplation is the stage where one starts looking to increase knowledge that is necessary before taking informed action. At this time, my focus was on two main areas, diet and exercise. I knew that these two mattered for anyone who needed to lose weight and stay healthy. I was not thinking about losing weight as a woman in midlife, and I was not looking for ways to lose belly fat. My assumption then was that by staying on a healthy diet and exercising more regularly, I would not only lose excess weight, but the weight would melt away gradually from all parts of the body where the excess had settled. It would take much longer before I would reach a higher level of awareness, recognizing that actually losing weight might be the easier part.

Belly fat is a whole different beast and to lose it requires major tweaks in the actions required for losing weight.

I started reading whatever I could lay my hands on. I bought a few books on nutrition. I even inherited a few that were given to me as gifts by those who knew about my interest in healthy diets. In my mind, I still lacked the time, knowledge and guidance necessary to help me define my actual goals and point me in the direction I needed to take, to align my behaviors with clear goals. Work and family responsibilities continued to take precedence. The competing interests at the time did not allow me to even believe that I could take action and succeed. However, I knew that it was a matter of time before I had to move through the next stage and get ready for action and change. I was no longer ignorant that my weight was problematic. I knew that even if my actions would not allow me to reach my ideal weight, losing some of the weight would still benefit me. I was certain that I did not want any more weight gain. The excess weight I had, already was putting me on the trajectory of developing health issues linked to being overweight, namely hypertension and diabetes. Preventing or delaying the onset of diabetes remains a motivation for action to this day. What I was to change and how I was going to do it remained among the questions I had to address in my next phase of the behavior change process.

Until then, I could no longer shut off the small voice inside of me as it got louder and louder telling me, "Do something now! You know what happened to your parents. You know that with them, diabetes is in your line. You don't want the same thing to happen to you!" No, I did not want to die at 70. In fact, I wanted to be healthier and stronger in my 70s than I felt in my 40s. That was a long-term goal. But I had shorter-term goals, as well, and they too kept me motivated. I want to feel and look strong and healthy. I wanted to fit into that cute size 8 red dress I had kept in my closet for years. I stayed in contemplation for at least a year, unable to find the time for consistent exercise, the one action I was convinced held the key to the results I wanted to see. I took this time to reflect on what would be the ideal time for me to exercise. I was in my mid-forties then, not caring that I was entering the last stretch before menopause hit.

So, I proceeded through the stages of change with a skewed understanding of what I wanted to achieve. Then, evidence of change would have been to lose a size or two off my dresses. Then, getting back to size 10 would have been good enough for me. Reaching size 6 would have been a dream come true. My assumption was that once I was finally able to take action, I would not only feel lighter, but I would also feel overall healthier, in good physical shape, and happier. As I gained more knowledge about the relationship between foods, health and balance, my confidence in making the next steps in the process of change increased. At the same time, however, the more I learned, the more I realized how confusing the whole field of nutrition and weight management is. It seemed like everybody had an opinion and theirs was the best. But my increased awareness that I did not like the sizes 12 and 14 that I was wearing kept me motivated to stay engaged and keep searching with an open mind. In this regard, I was similar to many other contemplators who "struggle to understand their problem, to see its causes, and to wonder about possible solutions" (Prochaska 42). Contemplation for me required gaining additional knowledge and achieving a better understanding of what it is that had been causing me to keep gaining weight and what I needed to do to stop it. I was inquiring more and more, reading what I could find on the topic of weight loss.

Eventually, I discovered that certain foods, including the healthy ones that I had been eating regularly, do not support weight loss. Carbohydrates are a specific target. Perhaps no other food group has been under so much scrutiny as carbs have. So, I had to take the time to understand how carbs make us fat and what carbs I had been consuming that did not support my efforts to keep my weight (and belly fat) in check. I needed to know what foods I could eat to replace the ones I was to give up. My resources were many, but when it comes to diets, those that supported my efforts the most, converged on the idea that carbs are the primary culprit for our weigh problem, while also refuting the idea that fat makes us fat.

During this time of contemplation and through the phase of preparation, I did not know enough to focus my attention on lifestyle factors beyond exercise that impact weight and belly fat. And I was not yet focusing on the types of exercises that work best to support fat-burning. I proceeded with incomplete knowledge as I sought to apply new knowledge to support myself to lose weight. I relied on my own sense of discernment to prevent myself from being discouraged by other women around my age who had given up trying because they had come to believe that being round is part of the territory of aging. Perhaps their point of view is what kept me from taking action earlier.

Each chapter of this book summarizes what I learned during the contemplation and preparation stages, as well as how I put learning into action with the aim of losing weight, before I eventually sought to target belly fat in particular. Separating my weight problem from excess fat required paying attention to where in the body it was located. Subcutaneous fat is not as dangerous as the fat that settles around the middle, and that is wrapped around major organs inside the abdomen. This fat known as visceral fat is the one that is hardest to lose. I had to revisit the question of weight management when I internalized the importance of focusing on the waistline more than excess weight gain associated with strong muscles and distributed around other parts of the body.

3. PREPARATION

Good preparation involves "planning carefully, developing a firm, detailed scheme for action, and making sure that you have learned the change processes you need to carry you through to maintenance and termination" (Prochaska 43). Preparation is a time when people start "making the final adjustments before they begin to change their behavior .... Awareness is high and anticipation is palpable" (Prochaska 43).

As you can imagine, preparation involved tremendous growth in my knowledge as I gradually shifted my attention to focus on developing a level of expertise around women in midlife. I moved pretty quickly through the preparation stage, the third stage of change when one takes necessary steps to remove real and potential obstacles to change. To lose weight, for example, I prepared by reorganizing my food pantry and refrigerator and removed unhealthy foods that are tempting when they were around.

I stopped making *mandazis*, deep-fried African donuts that are made with white or whole wheat flour (though our preference was white), yeast, eggs, and large amounts of sugar. It used to make me happy watching my kids enjoy biting into freshly made hot donuts. They were a treat I shared at parties with friends, students and colleagues for many years. I took further actions as well. I continued to look for ways to limit the amount of fat and oil I consumed, stir-frying vegetables with as little oil as possible. I replaced whole milk or full-fat yogurt with low-fat or fat-free versions. I continued to keep butter in the fridge for the kids, because I did not want to impose my new low-fat diet on them.

As for exercise, walking seemed to be the simplest and easiest plan to implement, especially when I have an exercise buddy to keep me motivated. I enlisted my husband. Preparation for us meant that we would find a time slot on our busy schedule and dedicate it to our regular walk. We looked at our schedule and agreed that we could go for a walk immediately after work, and earlier on weekends. My husband agreed that losing 20 pounds would not hurt him either. It also meant knowing our neighborhood better and finding the right pathway that would make it easier for us to enjoy our walk, without too many car fumes and too much noise as we walked. We were then based in Lilongwe, Malawi. We had to take into account other duties that could not fall off our plates because we had added daily walk to our schedule. Preparing dinner, for example, was mostly my duty, and we agreed that pushing dinner back by a few minutes would still work for us, given that we were in the habit of eating between 6:30 and 7 p.m. We planned to go for a walk as many times during the week as possible, even if we only had 20 minutes to spare.

4. ACTION

"We must remember we are not the sum of our intentions but of our actions", Brendon Burchard, *The Motivation Manifesto: 9 Declarations to Claim Your Personal Power* (xiv).

There will never be change without action to bring it to fruition. Taking action to change ingrained behavior requires a level of boldness that can feel uncomfortable at first, but it is out of this discomfort that we begin to see the fruits of our labor. Any action in the right direction will bring us closer to the results we desire. But sometimes, the wrong action, or one that is less than ideal, will delay the sought-after results. Being less than clear on the change I needed to make for best results, I proceeded into the action stage, the fourth stage of behavior change. The action stage is the most visible to others and therefore receives the most recognition by those around the self-changer. "The danger in this is that many people ... often erroneously equate action with change, overlooking not only the critical work that prepares people for successful action but the equally important (and often more challenging) efforts to maintain the changes following action" (Prochaska 44).

I remained focused on making changes around exercise and diet for the next couple of years. Going for a walk four to five times a week helped me lose some weight and all the size 14 dresses had to go. Within a year, I lost 10 pounds which brought me down to 147 pounds from my highest weight of 157 pounds. I was happy with the progress I had made but needed to lose more weight to feel healthier overall. The challenge for me was to stay motivated when my husband was travelling. It was also challenging to get back into the routine when we experienced anything that disrupted our routine, even for one week at a time.

But once I got myself going again, I was able to quickly get back into the routine and I would say that today, more than ten years later, walking remains one of our exercise habits. In addition to walking more regularly, I continued to restrict my intake of fat, not using butter on toast or when I did, using as little as possible. I knew, thanks to my husband, that margarine is bad and had given that up years before. So, I used either real butter or no butter. I drank low fat or no fat milk with my morning cereal. And I limited my intake of foods with added sugar, as much as I knew how to identify them. I ate less meat and eggs and almost no nuts or seeds, ignoring that they provide specific health benefits. I preferred a vegan diet, albeit one based on uninformed choices. I could not imagine there could be other dietary changes I needed to make. My actions failed to bring me intended results. This left me feeling frustrated. Why did I stall after losing only 10 pounds? My goal was to lose another 20 pounds.

We got off dairy, for example, something we had tried to avoid when we learned from a relative that dairy could be a trigger in my son's asthma flare ups. It seemed to help when we got him off dairy. We switched to soy, almond, or rice milk. I don't remember how we returned to dairy. Perhaps we did when we moved and no longer could find alternatives to dairy that we could trust. When we had this choice after we moved back to the United States, getting off dairy again relieved us of sensitivities we did not know were attributed to this staple in our home.

We made a few other additional dietary changes that I will discuss in detail in chapters two through five. At that time, the only additional change I could think of was to make my walks longer and I tried that as often as I could. As time went by, with continued commitment to figuring out the best course of action, I learned that the actions I had taken were causing some good and some harm. My exercise and dietary choices were part of the problem, as well as part of the solution. I had to understand better which parts were serving me and reinforce them and which were hurting me and remove them.

5. MAINTENANCE (AND TERMINATION)

Maintenance is before termination, which is the very last stage of the behavior change spectrum. At the maintenance stage, the person who needs to change has taken action and these actions, habits and behaviors have been repeated so many times that they have become second nature. This is what I did with walking as the main type of exercise that I engaged in consistently. Choosing longer walks did not necessarily help me improve results. However, walking until I sweat made me feel good. So, I was able to keep up with it, and it did help me keep the weight I had lost off. "For it is during maintenance that you must work to consolidate the gains attained during the action and other stages, and struggle to prevent lapses and relapses" (Prochaska 45). Maintenance is therefore not a passive stage, but rather an ongoing process, one in which we consciously and consistently repeat the action that is meant to bring us closer to our intended goal.

Failure to maintain the right actions can, in fact, take us backwards in the cycle of behavior change, leaving us to contemplate the best course of action, when we already had found it.

Maintenance is the key to the success of all previous stages. Maintenance is the stage when repeated actions are combined for cumulative results. Over the last seven years, I have tried many types of actions, as I explain in the rest of the chapters, to get my weight gradually down to around 130 pounds. I did not know how long this journey would take before I would reach this goal. Even today, I continue to hone in on my own habits and the actions that enable me to sustain my goals. I have come too far to feel tempted to give up what I have achieved. With each change and adjustment, there is increased awareness and increased knowledge that help me stay on track, which means that I am able to prevent my waistline from taking over not just my physical appearance but also my overall health.

I continue aiming to prevent the health risks associated with belly fat, including diabetes that runs in my family. "Curiosity is a shit-starter. But that's okay. Sometimes we have to rumble with a story to find the truth," exclaims Brené Brown in her book, *Rising Strong* (44). I hope you are as curious as I am to understand what it takes to reach a healthy middle in midlife. I hope that knowing the actions that brought me to a healthy waistline will motivate you to get yourself going to achieve similar results, if not more. I hope reaching a healthier middle will compel you to keep it that way for the rest of your life. It is a worthwhile goal. And the changes we make that are aligned with this goal will only lay the foundation for a healthier future.

"We can learn and we can grow and we must begin now for destiny favors the bold", Brendan Burchard, *The Motivation Manifesto: 9 Declarations to Claim Your Personal Power* (47).

Termination

Once the self-changer has reached a point where the fear of a relapse, of being tempted to return to undesirable behaviors no longer exists, we are in the very last stage of change known as termination. This is the ideal, the gold standard of behaviors. Have I reached it? Not exactly. To avoid the risk of rushing myself towards termination, I have decided that it is safer to enroll in a lifetime of maintenance. As I cannot predict what the future holds, maintenance protects me from the guilt I would feel even with a short relapse to one of the previous stages, which should not represent failure. I believe that success is about maintaining positive change. It is about maintaining the habits we adopt that continue to serve us well.

Ultimately, isn't maintaining positive change through one's lifetime the same as termination? In maintenance, I continue to focus on the quality of foods, choosing organic whenever possible, and walking and doing other forms of exercise as many times a week as I can. Throughout this process, I also have increased my awareness that our nutritional needs change as we age. Those foods that might have been right for me in my younger years no longer serve me in midlife. During this phase, we need to know our nutritional gaps and fill them as best as we can, as well.

As you will see throughout the rest of the book, I could not succeed until I understood better the changes that women experience in midlife and how these changes play a role in weight gain and the accumulation of fat around the belly. I could not succeed until I was clear about my overall goal and the specific goals as outlined in each chapter. I could not succeed until I took actions that were in line with my specific goals and with my overall goal. And I could not succeed until my combined actions were aligned with the combined goals. I learned then that the process of change will require a constant back and forth effort that involves the phase of preparation and improved actions to yield better results.

LOOKING BACK: THE STORY BEHIND MY WEIGHT GAIN

If I were to guess, the quick shift from a size 8 to 10 came following the birth of my two boys in my 30s. I was clearly not too concerned about this change then. I was still active and felt generally as agile as I was in my younger years. Nonetheless, similar to many new mothers, I rationalized my weight gain then because I associated it with the pregnancy stretch and the strong appetite that follows. However, this type of reasoning cannot explain why for many other women—those who have gone through pregnancy and those who have not—the fat around the waistline increases in midlife. For those who attribute it to pregnancy, we accept it as we do the weight gain that we associate with midlife and aging. But blame can only get us so far. In fact, "blame keeps us stuck in the past. Responsibility paves the path for a better future" (Adams 84). Taking responsibility to not allow that stretch and appetite stay where it left us when we delivered that bundle of joy is an important step in post-partum recovery.

Also, as I look at an old picture, I probably gained more weight between my late 20s and my early 30s when I fully embraced a Western diet, having moved to the United States during that time. My weight probably shifted from a size 4 to a size 8, which is much more then than it did following the birth of my two boys, shifting my dress size to a size 10. I must have been happy with whatever weight I added to my previously slim body, as a slender figure is not something valued in many African cultures. In my thinking, I was still years away from midlife and I had no reason to worry about becoming overweight given that I was not genetically pre-disposed to it.

Undoubtedly, I can attribute the significant weight gain in midlife to a career switch that took place as I entered my 40s. Around this time, I left a full-time academic job to take an international development position, something I had desired even years prior to that point. Over time in my new career, I started a more sedentary lifestyle. I was sitting down at my cubicle analyzing documents, writing reports, and discussing projects with colleagues, instead of moving from a classroom in one building to another in a different building, the routine of my days as an academic. Previously, the teaching position required standing while I taught, several days a week. I also lost the long summer breaks, a great privilege I never took for granted. This was the time when I would give my body the rest it needed, spend more time with my kids, and do academic research and write to keep advancing my career. My kids were much younger, around 4 and 6, when I embarked on the international development career path. I loved my job and really felt this was where I would make a bigger impact, learning alongside colleagues how to best support many community organizations through our work, and helping them lay a stronger foundation for their success. It was going to be win-win. Or so I thought.

Consequently, for at least the first five years of my 40s, I lived in total ignorance that my lifestyle habits were causing me to put on weight. Pressing career demands distracted me from noticing how much my weight had shifted from the small to average sizes of my younger adult years to about three times this size in my mid to late 40s. By this time, others did notice that I was not the small size I thought I was in my head. I remember vividly when my friends and I gathered for lunch at one of our church member's home in 2007. Our host, who had just returned from a trip to visit her family in South Asia, brought back souvenirs for all of us. I was not expecting anything because I was relatively new to the group and I had only recently met her. But she had enough gifts to go around. Some of them were these cute small size T-shirts. As she looked around for who they may fit, she passed them on to two other women in the group. Not me! I got a size larger. I was like, *What? Am I not their size?* The truth is I was not! In fact, the larger size she gave me was a bit too tight and I ended up giving it away to one of my smaller sisters. I registered this, but did not do much with what I was hearing. I must have been somewhere between pre-contemplation and contemplation in my own process to behavior change.

This attitude also prevented me from recognizing that my feelings of anxiety and stress were not normal and that I needed to do something to manage them better. Could these feelings have played a role in my ever-expanding body? I will address this question in Chapter 7 of this book. For now, let me bring you further along my journey of what increased my awareness that belly fat was the most obvious aspect of my physique, especially to those around me.

A BABY ON THE WAY?

Early in 2012, three years after my family had moved from Malawi and settled in Rwanda, I was attending a community outreach event organized by a colleague. While standing and watching community members dance in celebration of our visit, one of the participants, naturally unaware of my ignorance around the unhealthy distribution of my excess weight, motioned to me that there was an empty seat and that I should take it, assuming I was pregnant. I did not say anything to her. I took the seat, feeling a bit embarrassed because I ignored how big my midsection had become. Could I deny the fact that I was in bad shape and that the first thing people noticed when they saw me was my big belly?

To add insult to injury, towards the end of 2012, after my family had moved back to the United States, I met another woman at a local store in Silver Spring, Maryland, who looked like someone I knew. She looked at me as if she knew me, as well. So, we stopped and greeted each other. After chatting for a little bit, we realized that we had some things in common. The main one was that we shared the same background, which in our small part of the world that includes Rwanda and Burundi, meant that we could understand each other speaking our native languages. She literally asked when the baby was coming, kindly promising she would come and visit as we lived not far from each other.

This was the straw that broke the camel's back. Somehow, I told her that it was the baby belly that had refused to shrink back. A big fat lie, I know! Kindly again, she commented that a baby belly can take some time to shrink. What baby? I wondered. My younger son was already a teenager and much of my baby belly shrunk back within a year after he was born. Pregnancy did not leave me with the flat belly I once had, but I continued to fit into some of my size 8 dresses and only shifted my weight a little bit to a size 10 which I maintained for a few years as my wardrobe revealed later on.

I recorded all these encounters, determined to search harder for the answer to my ever-expanding waistline. My goal was clear. It was no longer about losing weight for the sake of it, although this remained an important goal. This time, I shifted my attention to losing belly fat and needed informed action that supports this goal before I could reach intended results. This took me back to the contemplation and preparation stages of change.

What was I missing? And what could I do to get my waistline to shrink? Why did eating healthy foods not keep my weight under control in the first place? Why did the weight loss I achieved, not target my belly? The training I received through the Institute for Integrative Nutrition helped me to build a knowledge base that would have been impossible to achieve on my own. Once I had the time to revisit the training modules and read many more books and articles on foods and lifestyle that impact belly fat, I was able to focus my attention on this area and gain a better grasp of the mystery around the midlife middle. This continuous learning increased my awareness that losing weight is one thing, losing belly fat is another, and losing belly fat in midlife is a completely different game with its own targeted set of actions.

Understanding midlife better was a part of the quest for a solution for my midlife belly.

What I share in this book is based on this cumulative knowledge and how I applied it to bring my waistline to healthy proportions.

CONCLUSION

I used the behavior change tool to walk you through the process I followed to move myself from a place where I ignored that I was heavier than I thought, to a different place where the focus of my actions was very clear. Prior to setting a clear goal regarding what in my excess weight was the real problem, I set the wrong goal and followed an inadequate set of actions even when I was involved in behavior change. Without knowing what the real problem was and getting to the root of it, I could not start looking for appropriate solutions. Setting behavior change goals requires a level of awareness and clarity of what needs to change. The real issue for me was belly fat. The real goal should have been about shrinking belly fat more so than losing weight.

Knowing that belly fat in midlife is preventable and can be brought back to healthy proportions is important. Acting on this knowledge is even more important, giving our body the support it needs to return to its homeostasis or to its most achievable level of balance. With consistent action, we can enjoy a healthy and balanced midlife and the ability to age gracefully. It requires shifting our mindset to reclaim our power to do what we can, to experience the amazing ability of the body to respond to the actions we take.

When it comes to the accumulation of fat around the belly in midlife, we have two choices: we can either let it be, and it will expand more and more, or we can take informed action to bring it to a halt, and begin to shrink it to a healthy size that we will be happy with. By choosing the later, I have shrunk my waistline and improved other health outcomes. I invite you to take similar actions. As you shrink your waistline, you too will achieve other positive health results. Aligning your actions with your goals is about laying the foundation for behavior change success, helping you achieve healthier outcomes that you will want to keep through midlife and the rest of your life. Ready for action? Read on as I share with you what to do for best results!

PART TWO

EAT RIGHT FOR YOUR MIDLIFE BODY

CHAPTER 2:

BREAK YOUR SUGAR HABITS

"Over the past two centuries, we have literally shocked our bodily systems with outrageous and ever-growing amounts of nutrient-robbing sugar" Anne Louise Gittleman in Jordan Rubin with Bernard Bulwer, *Perfect Weight: Change Your Diet. Change Your Life. Change Your World* (76).

It must have been in the fall of 1992 when I visited my boyfriend, who is now my husband, to celebrate his housemate's birthday. We made a nice middle Eastern dinner, a specialty of the birthday guy. We were in for an even more special after-dinner treat: a variety of ice cream choices, in the place of a birthday cake! We decided to pig out, and ate as much ice cream as we wanted, with hot fudge and fresh strawberries as toppings. My mouth waters even as I write! Ben & Jerry's, New York Super Fudge Chunk and other flavors were our way of celebrating a special friend's birthday. We had our first large serving. Then we went back for seconds, indulging until we consumed almost all the ice cream. Then we were full. Really full.

Not just full, but bloated. I felt sick. I had a stomachache. I was nauseated. The next day, we all admitted we had overdone it. No one wanted to see ice cream for a long time. We learned our lesson.

What was that lesson? That too much ice cream will make us sick? That in too much ice cream, there is too much sugar? That if we had stopped ourselves after we had had just enough, we would not have gotten sick? And what does "just enough" mean? One serving? How big or how small? Would a serving for me at around 120 pounds with a height of 5 feet 4 inches have been the same as a serving for my husband, 6 feet 1.5 inches tall and weighing around 190 pounds? And if ice cream was the culprit, would cookies or cake have been better?

We all have our own individual thresholds when it comes to sugar tolerance. Even for people who think they can handle more than the rest of us, there is a point at which sugar starts damaging our insides, with symptoms that show on the outside, as well. Those around us may not always notice when we have gone overboard with a food that creates sometimes immediate, but other times delayed, side effects. Sugar creates both. It is a winding road, and it is not always so obvious that we will be able to determine the point at which we crossed the line that broke the inner harmony, linking the symptoms we eventually feel or see, back to sugar overconsumption.

Symptoms often evolve gradually as part of the compounding effect of repeat doses of sugar at each meal or with each drink that contains natural or artificial sugar. Among the long-term side effects of this sugar overdose is consistent weight gain and belly fat especially as we reach midlife. Below, I provide more details on some of the side effects of a regular sugar overdose on the body and the mind.

The good news is that we can take steps to break our sugar habit, which will improve our physical appearance and boost our mental health as well.

We all desire to look and feel good about ourselves. Knowing what to do to break our sugar habit and taking action can bring us to a place of internal balance and happiness. When we fail to act on what we know, we achieve neither and when others notice what we already know to be the truth, this only compounds our frustration. To succeed requires knowing where sugar hides among our many food choices and preferences. It requires knowing how much sugar is enough and knowing how often we can eat it and still keep the right balance in the body to protect us from the damages that it causes when we overdo it. And there are many signs of this inner disharmony. Weight gain is often one of these signs. The culprits? There are quite a few we will discuss throughout this book but for now, let's focus on one of them, sugar. In obvious or hidden form, sugar is a major contributor to body systems imbalances.

Some people may develop such imbalances while still in the womb with mothers who consumed a regular dose of sugar. Unless someone breaks this cycle, we continue to see more and more children who start out with inherited imbalances caused by sugar, along with other dietary and environmental factors (Gates with Schatz 147-148; 186-187). Sugar creates a cascade of reactions that even children (or perhaps, especially children) cannot escape. Most of us have been around children who have indulged in cakes, cookies, and other sweets. I am not letting myself off the hook, either. I too did overindulge at least once, on ice cream. The aftershock taught me a lesson that I am now revisiting as I write.

Much has been written on the impact of sugar in creating inner disharmony and various weaknesses in the body. Sometimes the symptoms we feel show up gradually, and we often ignore the hint that something wrong is happening on the inside. Other times, signs hit us hard, like a brick wall, and we know we must act if we want to survive. One clear sign of sugar overconsumption is the accumulation of fat around the middle, especially as we age. It comes gradually and even when we fail to notice it, others will and eventually, we too will. The impact is not just external, its manifestations are felt on the outside as well. In fact, our health and wellness is at stake whenever we continue to overdo it on sugar.

"We also know that sugar is partly to blame for challenges with our waistlines, appetites, blood sugar control, obesity, type 2 diabetes, and insulin resistance", David Perlmutter, *Grain Brain: The Surprising Truth About Wheat, Carbs, and Sugar – Your Brain's Silent Killers* (103).

Understanding sugar and breaking my sugar habits was what I needed to do, first and foremost, if I was to conquer the initial symptoms I noticed. Taking informed action would enable me to reach a point in my journey where I would start healing, inside and out. This required going deeper and embarking on an extended period of sugar detoxification. It meant understanding more how sugar affects the blood, the skin, and in fact the whole body. As you read on, you will get a picture of what I did to increase my awareness of how sugar affected my health. Some symptoms showed up much earlier than I would have known to admit. My hope then was that those symptoms would naturally recede with time. And if they were going to continue, I would eventually resign myself to what I believed to be forces of nature at work, engrained in my genetic make-up, something I could not change, even if I wanted to.

Therefore, without the necessary competence, I spent several years, unable to connect the dots between my diet and the symptoms I saw or felt. I had no reason to assume that the initial symptoms would evolve into other challenges for my long-term health. No one around me knew enough to say anything about the impact of sugar on health so that we could even consider alternative choices that would limit our sugar intake. Eventually, monitoring my sugar consumption became one of the most important steps I had to take to begin shrinking my waistline, when in midlife, it had become the most obvious part of my changing physique. It was by embracing a healthier diet which carefully controlled my sugar intake that I could begin to welcome a healthier version of myself.

WHY SHOULD WE MONITOR OUR SUGAR INTAKE?

Understanding sugar, in all its broadness and its impact on the body has been one of the biggest learning curves and the most important journey I had to undertake to acquire the knowledge and skills I needed to eat right to achieve a healthier balance in midlife. What I share below will perhaps open your eyes to how far reaching sugar is and what you can do to take control over it, instead of allowing it to rule over your health. If you are on this journey already, I hope that this information will reinforce what you are doing and encourage you along your journey.

Sugar is in the foods and drinks we put in our body, but what tips the sugar balance is when these foods and drinks shift the dynamics of our blood sugar and insulin. Once I reached this level of awareness, I knew I could no longer take sugar for granted. I knew that keeping blood sugar stable and protecting myself from dysfunctional insulin were key to preventing type 2 diabetes, a disease that I am predisposed to because of family history.

Even if diabetes is not in your family line, there are many more reasons why you too should monitor your sugar intake and your blood sugar, because of the many other ways that it harms the body, mind and emotions. A March 14, 2018 article on the Harvard Medical School website states that blood sugar "levels above normal are toxic and can cause blindness, kidney failure or increase cardiovascular risk." High blood sugar levels are also linked to an inflamed liver, and an expanded waistline. Below, I discuss specifically eight reasons why we should pay attention to sugar in the blood, starting with a careful look at the foods we eat that bring it to toxic levels.

Sugar in foods has a direct impact on blood sugar and insulin

Harvard professor Walter Willett, in his book *Eat, Drink and Be Healthy*, illustrates how sugar in foods impacts blood sugar in everyone regardless of age or gender:

> "Every time you eat, the level of glucose in your blood rises. How much it rises depends on what you eat, how much you eat, and how much insulin your body produces in response to sugar loads. Pure glucose and white bread trigger large, rapid increases in blood sugar (glucose), while whole grains, beans, and most fruits and vegetables generate smaller, slower increases. Easily digested foods that trigger rapid spikes in blood sugar also stimulate a matching production of insulin, leading to rapid removal of glucose from the blood. The sudden drop in glucose, along with other hormonal changes, generates new hunger signals" (47).

To explain further how sugar is released from the foods we eat (or what we drink) to affect blood sugar, there are two broad categories into which foods are often divided: Low glycemic index (LGI) and high glycemic index (HGI) foods. I will provide further details on these glycemic index (GI) tools in the next chapter on carbs, but to give you an idea here, the glycemic index is a physiologic measurement tool used to determine the rate at which foods affect blood sugar levels, either raising it too fast on one end, or raising it evenly and gradually over time, with less of an impact on the host blood sugar, on the other end. Glucose is often used as the base, at a glycemic index (GI) of around 100. All other types of sugar and starchy foods are measured against this base and the closer a food's GI is to that of glucose, the higher the GI. Sugars in the form of sucrose, glucose and honey are high GI foods.

Because foods and drinks with high amounts of sugar are also the ones that quickly raise blood sugar levels fast when they have dropped below safe ranges, sugar is therefore known for its ability to make us feel good. Perhaps you have been around a loved one during a hypoglycemia comatose. We are advised to shove sugar into their system, either in pure form or in a drink, to help them recover their consciousness before the shock to the system becomes fatal. I saw this quick infusion of sugar work for my dad. It scared me! I heard it worked for my mom. It worried me!

While I have never required a quick sugar fix, I do remember suddenly feeling irritable when I was hungry. Irritability when hungry and fatigue when full can be a warning sign for pre-diabetes, which evolves into insulin resistance and diabetes. Every time the body experiences a rapid blood sugar drop, it sees this as life-threatening. It sees this as an emergency that requires quick action. Impulsively, we go looking for the next sugar fix, which leaves us trapped in a vicious cycle, as we continue playing yoyo with insulin levels and ... you guessed it, persistent fat storage. This is because consistent high blood sugar levels lead to insulin resistance which is linked to belly fat, depression, prediabetes, and type 2 diabetes, as Magdalena Wszelaki writes in her book, *Cooking for Hormonal Balance* (59). Wszelaki also links high blood sugar levels to systemic inflammation, high testosterone levels in women (and low testosterone levels in men), estrogen dominance and adrenal fatigue. These hormonal imbalances are, in large measure, triggered by a diet loaded with sugar, fructose and refined carbs.

With a family history of diabetes, understanding that sugar in the food - and in the blood - are at the heart of insulin resistance, left me with few options. Not taking action was not one of them. I saw a diet that caused consistent sugar spikes as one of the most straightforward ways of welcoming, sooner or later, diabetes into my life.

For people who are not at high risk for diabetes, a high-sugar diet can still trigger significant weight gain that is linked to other metabolic syndrome diseases, including hypertension and heart disease. I now know that a quick infusion of sugar is the answer only when we have allowed the body to go too far out of balance, with its supply having plummeted to dangerous levels. The better way would be to keep blood sugar stable, instead of waiting until it has fallen dangerously too low.

There is a safer way to eat that releases sugar gradually so the feeling of extreme hunger that diabetics and pre-diabetics often experience does not have to become so debilitating. Continuing to eat in a way that keeps blood sugar unregulated is self-defeating. Unfortunately, what triggers insulin is not just sugar, as we will learn throughout this book. The good news however is that most cases of insulin resistance can be prevented and/or reversed.

"... [P]eople with a genetic predisposition to insulin resistance can beat the condition by staying lean, being physically active, and eating the right diet" Walter Willett, *Eat, Drink, and Be Healthy* (89).

Sugar is addictive

Sugar stimulates the brain in distinct ways. It activates an area of the brain called the nucleus accumbens, which lights up whenever stimulated by sugar. The nucleus accumbens plays a role in activating dopamine, which is why it can trigger addictive behaviors. "When you continue to 'use' sugar and processed foods, your dopamine receptors are decreased. That means you need more and more of the addictive substance to generate the same amount of pleasure. This dynamic is called tolerance" (Mark Hyman 31).

A June 13, 2014 article titled, "Know Your Brain: Nucleus Accumbens" further explains this process: "When we do anything that is considered rewarding (e.g., eat food, have sex, take drugs), dopamine neurons (along with other types of neurons) in an area of the brain called the ventral tegmented area (VTA) are activated. These neurons project to the nucleus accumbens, and when they are activated it results in an increase in dopamine levels in the nucleus accumbens." In reality, as further research reveals, "dopamine levels in the nucleus accumbens rise in response to both rewarding and aversive stimuli," the article states. This may be how we remember the feeling we had after eating a food (or engaged in any other activity) that stimulated a feeling of pleasure and reward. At the same time, it explains why we seek to avoid aversive behaviors.

We enjoy sugar because of the feeling of pleasure we experience with it. And this is real, and a point of struggle for many people as one of my clients admitted at least once. It was a few years ago. I suggested to her that she replaced Coca-Cola with water, at least half the time, as a step to reduce her intake of sugar. She was severely over-weight and I worried about her. Her response was: "But it makes me feel good!" She was addicted to it. If making us feel good was all that the sugar in cola and other sweetened drinks did, I would not need any convincing to continue drinking it. Unfortunately, the added sugar in soft drinks has other side effects. We experience not just its short-term feel-good sensation, but also longer-term side effects on the brain, the kidneys, the liver, the pancreas, and other organs and body systems. Sugar contributes to gradual and persistent weight gain, even if we may initially feel good with a quick surge of dopamine.

Because of its addictive nature, it takes more than good intentions to stop our sugar habit, which piles any excess in fat cells. As in a vicious cycle, the more fat we hold onto, the greater our cravings for sweets (and carbs in general). Studies show correlations between excess body-fat and a reduced number of dopamine receptors, as well as an increased likelihood of craving sweets for some, or drugs including heroin, opium, or morphine, for others. These are the ones known to boost dopamine levels. Mark Hyman highlights the super-addictive nature of sugar, stating that it is "eight times as addictive as cocaine" in an interview with the *New York Daily News*. He explains this further in his book, *The Blood Sugar Solution, 10-Day Detox Diet* (29) as well. The fact that people who are suddenly cut off from sugar experience withdrawal symptoms is a clear indication that sugar is indeed addictive. Over time, the only way to feel normal is with a quick infusion of sugar, a reactive response. Addiction can be broken, fortunately.

"To break the addiction cycle, we need to shut down insulin production as much as possible" Mark Hyman, *The Blood Sugar Solution, 10-Day Detox Diet* (78).

Sugar harms the gut

Sugar is the best feed for harmful bacteria in the gut, which results in an imbalance between the good and the bad bacteria. This is what allows yeast fungi to take over different bodily systems as well. Authors Donna Gates and Linda Schatz comment on the importance of giving your body a break from all sources of sugar and other sources of nourishment for *candida* if the goal is to restore gut balance. They write that *candida* "thrives on some of the body's by-products: dead tissue and sugars from food. Unless its source of food is eliminated, it quickly monopolizes entire bodily systems, such as the digestive tract" (17-8). They even put it more bluntly: "Never eat sugar if you want to remain healthy and free of yeast" (66). In the chapter on ferments, I will provide more details on the importance of a healthy gut for a healthy weight, and why sugar does not belong to the equation.

Sugar is a nutrient-robber

When we eat foods with more added sugar than our body can handle, the body must use its store of minerals and enzymes to absorb it properly, hence creating the potential for nutrient deficiencies. This is what makes our body acidic, a fertile environment for yeast and other pathogens to grow and thrive. An acidic body lacks the necessary enzymes for proper food digestion and absorption of nutrients, which are both central to health and healing (Gates with Schatz 24). Willett agrees. His emphasis is on the importance of reducing our intake of high-sugar foods and all foods made with refined flour as these foods lack the necessary nutrients found naturally in whole, unprocessed foods. For these reasons, he recommends whole wheat, and other whole grains and unprocessed carbs as part of a healthy diet. The chapter on carbs (beyond sugar) will provide further clarity on how to make these starchy foods work for you if your goal is to shrink belly fat.

Sugar lowers serotonin

Sarah Gottfried recommends reducing daily intake of sugar to improve serotonin, the feel-good neurotransmitter. The other dietary culprits, in Gottfried's opinion, are refined carbohydrates and caffeine. She writes that "[a]ll these foods make you feel good in the short term - they give you a quick boost, but then your serotonin levels will begin to drop just as quickly" (368). Note that serotonin is "the brain chemical that helps ... mood, sleep, and appetite", Gottfried adds (368). We will learn more about the importance of sleep for losing belly fat, in the last chapter of this book.

Fructose is linked to non-alcoholic fatty liver disease (NAFLD)

One of the most harmful types of sugar added to popular foods and drinks is high fructose corn syrup (HFCS). High fructose corn syrup is a very cheap sweetener made from corn starch, and it is known to contribute to weight gain. It is sweeter than table sugar, making it a cheaper choice for food manufacturers. It is a significant ingredient in many highly processed foods including sodas, candy, store-bought cakes and cookies, some brands of sweetened yogurt, many low-calorie, fat-free salad dressings, frozen convenience foods, breads, canned fruit, and some juices (that may even contain more sugar than soda). Even some energy bars and coffee creamers and of course ice-cream contain HFCS. It is used by the food industry as a browning agent on steak, as well. The list of its uses goes on and on.

What's different about fructose and high fructose corn syrup in particular is that, unlike glucose, HFCS bypasses insulin's control mechanism and goes straight to the liver, turning sugar directly into fat. How does that work? According to Gary Taubes, this happens through a process known as *lipogenesis*, also referred to as hepatic *de novo lipogenesis* (DNL). This is the biochemical process of synthesizing fatty acids within the cells, through the most common pathway which is the metabolism of carbohydrates. The same mechanism applies to metabolizing alcohol, which is done mostly in the liver as well (137-139).

In reality, both glucose and fructose can drive DNL. "In the context of disease progression, DNL is considered to contribute to the pathogenesis of non-alcoholic fatty liver disease, a common condition often associated with the metabolic syndrome and consequent insulin resistance," write Francis W. B. Sanders and Julian L. Griffin in March 4, 2015 article on the National Institutes of Health website. HFCS is also associated with other health risks including hyperactivity, exhaustion, emotional ups and downs, excess acidity, belly fat, heart disease and nutrient deficiencies.

Sugar disrupts leptin

This neurotransmitter that signals to the brain that we are full and should stop eating (Gottfried 179; Wszelaki 13; 59) must function properly if we want to avoid overeating. Without a well-functioning leptin, much of this excess food turns to fat that settles around the belly. Insulin and leptin work closely together with the actions of one affecting the reactions of the other. Sugar and other processed carbs that are high GI foods signal to the brain that you need more food sooner than you would if you ate whole, unprocessed low-GI foods. These low-GI foods are the ones that keep blood sugar stable, a key requirement for losing belly fat. In the next chapter, we will learn more about how to make the most sense of carbs and how to know which affect blood sugar and belly fat the most, so that you can avoid them.

Sugar is linked to weight gain and fat storage

This is because sugar impacts your gut and there is growing evidence that link gut bacteria with one's ability to gain or lose weight.

"... [W]eight is not just a matter of calories consumed and calories burned in physical activity - the gut microflora also belongs in the equation", Gary Huffnagle with Sarah Wernick, *The Probiotic Revolution* (191).

The potential link between gut microbiome and weight loss is in fact what prompted the National Institutes of Health (NIH) to launch the Human Microbiome Project in 2007 with the goal to "identify and characterize microbial communities living inside and on us" write Fred Pescatore and Karolyn A. Gazella in *Boost Your Health with Bacteria* (30, 32). On the cover of this book, Pescatore and Gazella place losing weight on top of the list of six benefits that beneficial bacteria can offer us. Yeast infections are a sign of imbalance with the bad gut bacteria controlling the direction of your health and your weight. A healthy balance between the good and the bad keeps yeasts in check. Pescatore and Gazella promise further on the front cover of their book that supporting the good bacteria and helping them to thrive will not only boost your health, but it will also help to:

- Relieve digestive problems;
- Decrease inflammation;
- Increase energy;
- Combat allergies; and
- Enhance immunity.

William G. Crook writes in his book *The Yeast Connection: A Medical Breakthrough* provides anecdotal evidence that many of his overweight patients lost weight and kept it off when they followed his anti-*candida* protocol. In fact, one of them shares a testimony that is worth including here: "My weight had fluctuated between 200 and 250 for years. I tried diets of many types. Although I'd lose weight for a month or two, it would always come back. I also suffered from headaches, hives, recurrent vaginal yeast infection and PMS. Since taking nystatin, following the anti-*candida* diet and taking nutritional supplements, my life has been changed. I've lost 70 pounds, my sugar cravings have disappeared and I feel like a new person" (393). Furthermore, in a May 12, 2017 article Christopher Mohr writes that "[t]hese bacteria [the beneficial ones] help 'regulate our body weight'. For a healthy balance, the ratio between the good and the bad bacteria should be "85 percent to 15 percent" note Pescatore and Gazella (74).

Others, including Anthony Komaroff, editor-in-chief of Harvard Health Letter, link a diverse gut microbiome to a healthy weight. Komaroff offers an interesting response to the question: "To lose weight, should I focus more on my calorie count or the amount of time I spend exercising?". How he responds draws our attention to the workings of these gut microbiome, which may "profoundly affect our ability to achieve a healthy weight." Noting that the microbiome has "250 to 800 times more genes than there are human genes ... these microbial genes make natural chemicals that can enter our bloodstream and affect our body chemistry ... and the microbiome likely affects our weight." The mechanism through which this is done is based on how we absorb calories from foods into our blood, around the body, and even in fat cells.

For some people, these calories are excreted with waste products. What is interesting is that "there are people whose gut microbiome appears to cause them to absorb a lot more of the calories that they consume before the calories leave as waste," writes Komaroff. As with overeating, calories do add up. Therefore, it makes sense that if more calories are retained in some than in others, those who hold onto a lot more of these calories will also gain weight faster and hold onto the extra pounds longer.

Obviously, losing weight is a much more complex process and requires actions beyond what you need to do to rebalance your gut bacteria. Nonetheless, recurrent yeasts infections cannot be overlooked if you want to be successful at managing your weight and losing those excess pounds. Other important factors include overall "caloric intake, physical activity, stress, sleep patterns, medications, and other lifestyle-related influences on energy metabolism" writes Gerard E. Mullin and Kathie Madonna Swift in their book, *The Inside Tract: Your Good Gut Guide to Great Digestive Health* (208).

In Chapter 4, I will discuss further the steps I took to effectively build the supply of beneficial bacteria in my gut including practicing the art of fermentation, which helped me to control yeasts better. Adding fermented vegetables, a new food that had never entered my kitchen before 2013, as well as reintroducing probiotic supplements, helped to correct the shortcomings in my diet and to control yeast infections, while also supporting my efforts to reach and maintain a healthy weight.

Overeating high-sugar foods naturally creates a surplus that must be stored somewhere. All the excess calories are stored in the fat cells, turning into the type of fat we were meant to count on in times of food shortage. Artificial sugar is even worse than regular sugar. "Artificial sweeteners trick your metabolism into thinking sugar is on its way. This causes your body to pump out insulin, the fat-storage hormone, which leads to more belly fat" (Mark Hyman 35). Insulin's role is to remove excess sugar and send it to the muscles, fat, and other cells where it can be used as a source of energy. Unfortunately, the time of scarcity during which we would dip into stored fat rarely comes because sweetened foods, sugar, and highly processed carbs are often the cheapest and most easily accessible, in most countries today.

Easy access to processed and sugary foods makes it harder to resist them. The more we consume them, the more we train our body to rely on them as the main source of energy. And the more of these foods we eat, the more fat we store. Interestingly, the more body fat we hold onto, the more we crave sugar and other types of carb. Reducing sugar consumption and perhaps sometimes even taking a break from it completely, will give a much-needed break to your pancreas, the organ that is overtaxed by sending insulin to work when forced to handle a consistent supply of sugar. It is this overtaxing of the pancreas that leads, eventually, to insulin resistance.

Therefore, keeping blood sugar stable and insulin working properly is one of the most important actions you must take if losing weight and reducing your waistline are your main goals. This was my goal as well. I had to re-learn how to eat properly to keep blood sugar levels stable. I was able to get myself back on track eating right, limiting sugar intake as much as possible (along with other changes) to support hormonal balance and prevent diabetes. My actions, in turn, helped me to lose both overall weight and inches off my belly. The different strategies I apply even today, are informed by many experts, including Donna Gates, Mark Hyman, Sarah Gottfried, Walter Willett and Eric Berg, who shed light on what I needed to do to reach the fat inside my belly better.

"Obviously, if a woman is going to ever feel well, she must break the sugar habit", Donna Gates with Linda Schatz, *The Body Ecology Diet: Recovering Your Health and Rebuilding Your Immunity* (151).

THE SYMPTOMS THAT TRIGGERED ACTION

Fungal skin rash

Sometime in my teen years, I started developing a recurring fungal skin infection. At the time, people around me who had had similar skin rashes or knew others who had, recommended natural plant remedies that seemed to help. These ointments, however, did not get to the root of the problem, as the infection returned after a few months, sometimes spreading to a larger area, with spots on my neck and my back. While I cannot think of anything in particular that might have triggered this rash, I now know that eating sugar exacerbated the problem. Even with my limited knowledge then, I was aware that the rash was contagious, and, in fact, I stopped sharing clothes, as a preventive measure. I was ill-equipped to understand that my habits, including sugar consumption, were contributing to the rash, however.

Then, I did not have any reason to worry about what my health and my life would look like in midlife. Even if I had known that I would gain weight later, it would not have worried me given that gaining weight as we age was not something that was cause for concern for anyone else around me. In my culture, as in many others, it was in fact expected and appreciated. So, my only concern then was treating the symptoms, and keeping my skin smooth and clear. What I did to treat the visible signs on the outside was only masking the internal problem that only got worse as I got older. What I failed to do then laid a solid foundation for my sluggish midlife as well.

The rash continued to come and go and eventually I took it to a doctor who recommended a dose of antibiotics. These helped initially and the problem seemed to go away. However, within a year or so, the rash returned and after being on repeat antibiotics, I figured the medication was not the answer and I stopped going to the doctor for the rash. The problem for many of us is that, before we actually get sick we rarely know what to do that would allow the body to use its own defense mechanisms to recover and stay healthy. Often, many of the medications required to treat diseases, including preventable ones, contribute to other health problems. This is certainly true of antibiotics.

Gerard E. Mullin and Kathie Madonna Swift in their book *The Inside Tract* recognize that antibiotics have negative side effects and are especially not beneficial for anyone trying to keep a healthy gut. They count antibiotics, along with stress and excessive alcohol among the main contributors to the friendly bacteria die-off which "set[ting] the stage for evil invaders to get a foothold in the inside tract's microbial rainforest" (126). Repeat use of antibiotics eventually creates resistant strains. Rustam I. Aminov notes in his article, "A Brief History of the Antibiotics Era," that the problem may arise when no suitable antibiotic choice was made to treat the right symptom to begin with, or it may result from self-medication, when proper diagnosis was not done to match with the right antibiotic treatment. It also may be due to lack of monitoring practices to ensure "correct usage, compliance, and treatment efficiency," Aminov adds. The most effective solutions to prevent yeast overgrowth must therefore help to prevent their recurrence, as well as their side effects. Antibiotics may be required as part of the solution, but alone they are as problematic as they may offer temporary relief.

In my case, antibiotics exacerbated an underlying problem that had not come so clearly beyond the surface when I focused initially on the skin rash. Any sugar I consumed then only kept these evil invaders alive, helping them multiply further, while continuing to weaken my immune system. This is what allowed the bad bacteria in the gut to take over and also to allow yeasts to spread unencumbered.

My diet and other practices, including repeat doses of antibiotics, were inadequate for what I needed to get rid of the skin rash and potentially prevent yeast infections. In fact, even though antibiotics are recognized as one of the most important health discoveries of the twentieth century, known then as the "wonder drug," they might have contributed to weakening my immune system even further, continuing to make me a target for other infections and symptoms of poor health that followed.

Over time, antibiotics can exacerbate the condition they were meant to treat. Knowing that antibiotics were not offering long-term relief, I stopped relying on them but continued to look for different solutions. At one point, a different doctor recommended Selsun Blue, a dandruff shampoo that she said can be used to treat the same fungal infection I had on my skin. I applied it liberally and kept it in my medicine cabinet, ready to combat the rash whenever it re-emerged. Was there anything in the Selsun Blue that I should have been aware of? Could it have caused other problems that surfaced as my symptoms evolved? Was giving up antibiotics without a replacement to take care of the problem internally, a wise move? Were the antibiotics I was prescribed initially the most suitable choice of the options available? Were there safer and more natural ways to get rid of the fungus and prevent it from recurring?

Then was not the time for such questions. So, I moved on, feeling at least better that I could always find Selsun Blue at a grocery store or local pharmacy. I used Selsun Blue off and on for at least a decade, either as an anti-dandruff shampoo or as an ointment on my skin when the fungus resurfaced. It helped to mask the visible symptoms, but it did not get to the root cause of the problem. In fact, it eventually left shades of discoloration on my back.

What a shame that I did not know enough to protect my skin from further damage! What a shame that we are not taught preventive measures, to protect ourselves from recurring symptoms before they turn into debilitating diseases. What a shame that some of the diseases we face as we get older are preventable if we acted early enough. It is with the same level of ignorance that led me to walk over to a friend and neighbor's house to help massage her feet and rub off the fungus on her feet that seemed to have developed and quickly spread while undergoing cancer treatment. I used essential oils I had in my medicine cabinet, but I did this without protective gloves. What was I thinking? Having had relief for a number of years by that time, I thought the skin rash was something I had conquered for good. I was no longer thinking about it as a contagious disease, and I was not thinking about the rash I had years before as being related to the fungus that is associated with chemotherapy. How wrong was I?

This time, I started seeing the fungus on my neck again and it continued to spread behind my ears and on my back. This time, it seemed to have come back with a vengeance. It spread faster than before especially after we moved to hot and humid Liberia. Was it because I was in midlife and had other symptoms that perhaps together further weakened my immune system? Most likely. Humid environments allow the fungus to spread fast. I certainly experienced it first-hand.

I had become complacent. I did not know that when the immune system is challenged, with hormonal imbalances we tend to experience with the changes that hit us in midlife, symptoms that had laid dormant for years before can resurface. Massaging my friend and ignoring the fact that her fungus could spread to me, was clearly an act driven by the heart and not the intellect. By helping her, I focused on the worry I had that I may not have much time left with her. I wanted to offer support and express compassion. She lived for only six months from the time when I started massaging her. It was a tragic moment in our neighborhood.

Yeast infections

Yeast infections develop when the bacteria in our gut are out of balance. My first experience with yeast was when I felt this itchiness around my vaginal walls. It started sometime in my 20s. It would come and go and I left it alone. I never knew what gave me the relief so that I could repeat that action consistently. I did not know what yeasts were or what they meant in the context of my overall health. I did not know the long-term implications of leaving yeast infections untreated. I didn't know that the skin rash and yeasts belonged to the same family of fungi. I found vaginal itchiness to be a bit embarrassing to talk about, even when in consultation with my doctor.

This experience left me frustrated, as you can imagine. Why would they target this particular part of my body? The problem got especially worse during pregnancy in my 30s. The only reason I did not take treatment then was because, intuitively, I did not think that taking medications was safe for the baby. It was around the time of my second pregnancy, in particular, that my gynecologist highly recommended that I drink milk and other dairy products consistently for the extra calcium needed to build healthy bones in the baby and for the extra strength my body needed. I was never someone who enjoyed a glass of cold milk like others in my family. I could eat yogurt once in a while, and I even liked fresh, raw milk better, which I used to drink growing up on our family farm.

I asked the doctor if ice cream was fine, assuming that it would also count as part of this milk/dairy consumption requirement in pregnancy. He said it was fine in moderation. So, in addition to a little milk on my morning cereal, I had some ice cream in moderation, almost daily for weeks before the birth of my second son. We found it easily at a campus cafeteria where my husband and I met for lunch. We bought a small cup of ice cream and shared that after lunch. How much more in moderation can one go? And what exactly did the doctor mean when he said that eating a little bit of ice cream during pregnancy was OK? What did the doctor know about sugar's impact on the body in general? How safe was it for the fetus to be exposed to a daily dose (or an overdose) of sugar for weeks prior to birth?

We never got into the details of frequency of consumption. After all, I had received the answer I wanted. A little ice cream was OK for me and my developing baby and also my husband, who was always sure to pick up that cup of ice cream before we checked out to pay for our lunches. Were there any side effects from this habit? I did not know then, and it would take over a decade before I would revisit my issues with the skin rash and yeast infections and start connecting the dots that all led back to sugar overdose, a fact that is "bio-individual" as each person's level of tolerance is different. In other words, what sugar does to one person may be different from how it affects somebody else based on a number of factors, including overall dietary practices, gut flora, and state of your immune system in general.

Body Ecology Diet by Gates and Schatz was one of the most important resources that helped me make sense of these invaders to our bodily systems through yeasts overgrowth or candidiasis. Yeast overgrowth is a sign of gut imbalance. They write: "*candida albicans* is one of several yeast and fungal organisms present in our bodies. Normally, 'friendly bacteria' balance these organisms so they do not grow out of control, and a strong immune system overseas it all. But when we throw our body ecology out of balance due to stress and/or by ingesting sugar, antibiotics, or poor-quality air and water-- or compromise our health in other ways--the *candida* grows out of control and causes a variety of symptoms" (17).

The other symptoms that Gates and Schatz link to yeast overgrowth are food allergies, chronic fatigue syndrome, immune-system deficiencies, frequent digestive problems, as well constipation, PMS, headaches, muscle joint pains, and poor memory (xi-xii). The ones that bothered me, even as a kid, were digestive problems, in the form of frequent heartburn and constipation, as well as migraine headaches later on around my monthly cycles. While I could not link the recurring yeast infections to a known cause, it was a sign of a weak immune system, unable to protect me from other symptoms that emerged one at a time, and seemingly out of nowhere. I know now that these earlier symptoms were warning signs of what was to come. I did not know where to start to address them. So, I often did nothing or little to take better care of myself.

When I was introduced to the world of gut bacteria and the importance of supporting gut health, I read as much as I could lay my hands on to make sense of yeasts, but especially to familiarize myself with strategies for taking care of my gut. William G. Crook, in his book *The Yeast Connection: A Medical Breakthrough,* contributed significantly to my understanding of how an underlying yeast overgrowth works inside the body. Crook shows how yeast interacts with other factors, both internal and external to the body, and as yeast spreads, it makes us sick. He links *candida* to various modern-day ailments, affecting all body systems including the nervous, digestive, respiratory and other systems. He also highlights several factors that create a fertile environment for the harmful bacteria to outnumber the friendly ones. The first one is "twentieth century diets." Having spent more than half of my life in the 20th century, this diet was mine as well. Unfortunately, the twenty-first century diet is not getting any better. In fact, some would argue it's getting worse.

A top ingredient in modern-day diet is sugar. I never considered myself as having a special attachment to sugar. I never went food shopping looking for something sweet to boost my dopamine levels. You may be wondering, "If you didn't have an attachment to sugar, why did you inquire about ice cream at your visit with the gynecologist?" In my case, it was not as much about ice cream and the sugar in it, that led me to inquire about it. I was rather looking for a source of calcium that I could add to the limited options I was aware of at the time. I was looking for any other food I could add to my diet to support the growth and development of the skeletal structure of my baby. I was looking for ways for me to stay strong enough to carry the baby in my womb through full term. I was concerned that the little bit of milk I had with my morning cereal was not sufficient to supply the key nutrients milk and dairy products offer to keep me balanced while supporting the baby to develop well. Was ice cream a good supplement to the milk in my cereal? I'll let you guess!

After that experience, can I blame my son (or anyone else for that matter), for having a sweet tooth? To some degree, we all enjoy sweet foods because it's in our DNA. Think about it: Our very first food, mother's milk, is sweet! If a newborn baby naturally latches on and appreciates sweetness when it touches his/her unexperienced taste buds, can we blame ourselves for continuing along this path traced for us from the beginning? Breast milk offers sugar in its purest and most beneficial form. Breast milk sugar was "created for both the baby and its developing inner ecosystem [as] an expanding food, to help babies - who are contracted little beings - grow and expand," Gates and Schatz write. In fact, "if a healthy inner ecosystem has been established and maintained", we would not have to worry about a reasonable consumption of sugar in natural form, including the fructose in whole fruits (147-48). Eating naturally sweet foods such as carrots, fruits, sweet potatoes, winter squash, some of which are even given to infants as their first foods in pureed form, is not detrimental to our efforts to maintain this inner ecology balance. It is when the immune system is weakened that even a small amount of sugar can exacerbate existing imbalances.

Aside from diet, birth control pills, multiple pregnancies, and hormonal changes are among other factors that exacerbate a yeast condition, Crook writes. All of them can create fertile environments for yeast to grow unhindered. While I never took birth control pills, painful periods around my monthly cycles were a sure sign of hormonal imbalance as I understand it today. And I am not surprised that the more pregnancies, the greater the likelihood of yeast infections and overgrowth. In my case, I remember yeasts being particularly bothersome with my second child. Once yeasts have taken root inside, they create additional imbalances that get worse, if left uncontrolled. Yeasts create many additional side effects: They "release toxins," "weaken your immune system," make "enemies invade," causing "infections" that require treatment with "antibiotics" which only exacerbate yeasts, especially when taken repeatedly, Crook writes in the Preface to *The Yeast Connection*.

Like an invading army, these fungi use our body as a battlefield, with some there to defend while others are on the assault. What we eat and how we live our lives can determine which of these colonies win the war. In my case, getting to the root of the yeast problem required reflecting on what might have allowed it to surface in the first place, as well as what continued to feed it. For some, it may require going as far back as the time when one was still in the womb of her mother and knowing how one was delivered. Like being inoculated with breastmilk, the best first food any baby can ever have, vaginal birth has benefits that many mothers do not know about or consider worth advocating for. There is inoculation that benefits the baby passing through the birth canal rather than through a C-section across the abdomen. This is where kids are able to get an initial supply of friendly bacteria, assuming the mother has her own in sufficient supply (Fred Pescatore and Karolyn A. Gazella 36; Gates with Schatz 186). Where we take it from our very first experience of passing through the birth canal or a C-section, or with mother's breastmilk, if we had the privilege to be breastfed, is where it can get more complicated, unless our parents or guardians are sufficiently aware of the importance of a proper diet to keep the gut functioning properly. Keeping sugar out of the way, and especially preventing an overdose is an important step in this process. We all know that kids in general, and even many of us adults, do indulge when given the opportunity.

"The womb is a completely sterile environment. A baby's first exposure to beneficial bacteria is through vaginal birth and breastfeeding. Because of this, supplemental probiotics are vital to both mother and infant", Fred Pescatore and Karolyn A. Gazella, *Boost Your Health with Bacteria* (36).

On the positive side, I did benefit from both vaginal birth and I was breastfed for close to a year, I believe. However, my parents did not know enough about proper nutrition and diets that we needed to stay healthy. Fortunately, we could trust our diet at home, even though we were not intentional in making the right food choices most of the time. Aside from morning tea with sugar, my siblings and I had limited access to sweets at home, a plus for us as well.

Invisible symptom - my predisposition to diabetes

My genetic predisposition to diabetes remains my highest-level motivation, pushing me to continue doing whatever I can to prevent it or delay its onset. This has required learning more about how sugar triggers insulin to respond to any supply of it in the blood, and how, through a cascade of reactions, insulin fails to move sugar into the cells for use as a source of energy, marking the beginning of prediabetes, and eventually diabetes. Knowing that, with my own goodwill and a mindset shift, I could manage sugar intake and prevent insulin resistance, became a motivating factor for me to no longer allow sugar to take control over my health. This required adjusting my diet to focus on foods that would keep my blood sugar stable, while also minimizing sugar intake and the intake of foods that raise blood sugar too fast. I had to keep in mind that HGI foods overtax the pancreas, the organ that sends insulin to work when blood sugar is raised, which happens with each meal. Not so coincidentally, this same diet that keeps insulin working properly also helps to keep yeasts in check and the fungus at bay. This diet has also been key to reducing my weight and my waistline, bringing me in addition to a place that keep my A1C, a blood test that measures my average blood sugar over the previous two to three months, and fasting blood sugar test results in a safe zone, instead of showing an increased risk of diabetes. To work, such a diet has required breaking my sugar habits and paying attention to what I eat, one meal at a time.

WHAT I DID TO BREAK MY SUGAR HABITS

Breaking my sugar habits became priority No. 1 in my efforts to improve my diet and manage my symptoms while also preventing the onset of diabetes. I was not intending on targeting belly fat when I embarked on this part of my journey, not knowing enough to link any of the previous symptoms to their contribution to a sluggish midlife with an annoying belly. I embarked on a rather protracted sugar detoxification journey, making gradual changes based on what I knew to be the biggest suppliers of sugar to my body at the time. Some of my decisions were based on what I observed others do, and on my intuition, to make the best choices I could make, taking it, one step at the time. Gradually, my thinking evolved and I made better informed choices that started yielding results that to date, I remain pleased with.

My journey was protracted because, before I moved to the US in 1991, I was not aware that there was anything to worry about in the foods I ate that contained sugar in them. I did not grow up with all the sweets that many kids have access to in the West. We did not celebrate birthdays with cakes and cookies, either. We did, however, have fruits in season, sometimes less, sometimes more. However, for breakfast, growing up, we had black tea with milk and sugar and we had it with either *ibitumbura* or *mandazis* (African donuts), corn or wheat bread, or porridge made of wheat or other whole grains. We added sugar to our porridge. I would never have and still do not consider myself as having any particular attachment or addiction to sugar. My sources of it were limited in childhood, I thought. Could my typical breakfast have started me on an unhealthy supply of sugar to a body that perhaps, already lacked the immunity needed to protect it from recurring infections? Was what I considered to be a reasonable amount of sugar an overdose, considering the state of my immune system then? Was I born with those imbalances or did they develop gradually as I spent more and more time away from home, having gone to boarding school at age 13 and spent only school breaks and summer vacations at home since, up until I left home for the United States in my late 20s to never live there permanently again?

To recover from my symptoms required connecting all the dots, starting at least in my teens, up until my midlife years, when shrinking the fat around my waistline became my most visible symptom of imbalance, and a major motivating factor. I located all sources of sugar, some obvious others hidden, that contributed to my overall sugar intake and oftentimes, unknowingly, to overdose, given the state of my health and immune system. Continuously going past the threshold in terms of sugar intake is what keeps yeast alive and thriving. It is also why the fungus on my skin, and the fat around my belly continued to expand, which in turn, raised my risk of diabetes, by forcing insulin to overwork, instead of doing its job to protect me from all that was hijacking my metabolism.

Initial steps: A focus on healthy eating habits

Even before weight was an issue, I appreciated learning ways to keep myself healthy. Learning from housemates in my late 20s, I adopted the first step that became part of my efforts to control sugar intake.

Quit adding table sugar to tea and reduce sugar in other foods. This was the first and perhaps one of the easiest dietary changes I made. With this change, I also gave up caffeine in black tea, the one drink I was used to having every morning since as far back as elementary school, if not earlier. I never was a coffee drinker. Neither was anyone in my family, in general. When I gave up caffeinated black tea, I also stopped adding sugar to my tea, turning since to herbal teas. By this point, I was already living in the US. In addition to removing sugar from my tea, I reduced the amount of sugar I added to home-baked goods. I was never a regular baker of cakes, muffins, or brownies in my new home. When I embarked on the sugar detox, I made them even less frequently. Occasionally I bought cakes and cookies when we had guests and I needed a desert I thought they would enjoy. I did this especially when I had no time to make my own. Reducing or removing some processed sugar sources from my home was an important step aimed at successful sugar control. Fruits were my "go to" desert, just as they were the main snack or desert that my mom offered us (or our guests) at home.

When I stopped drinking regular black tea with sugar, I also gave up eating bread with butter and/or jam for breakfast. Boxed cereals became my replacement meal. I introduced cereals without adequate understanding of what to look for, to be sure the amount of added sugar was acceptable based on the limits I wanted to impose on myself, when this became my dietary focus. My choices were corn flakes, Rice Krispies, and Cheerios. They did not taste sweet but they were not bland either. I relied on my housemates to make recommendations. The one choice I did not care much about was Weetabix, which might have been the best choice if I had known what I needed most then. When I had it, which was only occasionally, I added slices of a banana to enhance its bland flavor a little bit. It took me years to reach a point of questioning my cereal choices. Until then, and for at least two decades, cereal for breakfast was part of my morning routines.

Give up soft drinks: Coke, sprite, and even Fanta orange, my favorite, were no longer a drink of choice at home or even at parties. By this time, I had stopped buying sodas for home consumption and we would have them around only for guests and if tempted, have a little bit with them, as well. Otherwise, I tried to stick to unsweetened drinks such as soda water or plain mineral water as much as possible. I do not think I have had any sweetened soda over the past ten years. As I understood more and more about how much sugar they contain, and especially that HFCS is the type of sugar added to most of these soft drinks, I know that there is nothing healthy I should pursue in them. I also know that I can never go wrong with good old water, especially when filtered properly.

Intermediate steps: Going deeper to manage skin rash and yeasts

The recurring skin rash and yeast infections were the two problems that forced me to find ways to limit sugar further. Below are some of the additional steps I took.

Give up ripe bananas. As healthy as they are, serving as good sources of potassium, fiber, and vitamin B6 especially, a medium size banana easily contains 14g of sugar, which is the equivalent of three and a half teaspoons of sugar. With this amount of sugar, bananas were not helpers in my efforts to uproot the skin rash and yeasts and even on a good day of healthy eating, they could easily push me over the limits of a sugar-controlled diet. I gave up bananas on the recommendation of my doctor treating my fungal infections, who said that they were high in sugar, which in turn feeds the fungus. I was more attached to bananas than any other fruit because then (not now), bananas helped me have regular bowel movements. I was willing to make the sacrifice though, because to take my health seriously, or so I thought, I had no choice but to respect my doctor's advice if I wanted to improve my skin and overall health. So, I left the doctor's office with a plan and high hopes that I would be able to get rid of the fungal infection once and for all. In my mind, I was doing a good job controlling sugar intake in my diet and I expected all the health benefits that this dietary change brings. I later realized I had more work to do.

Give up fruit juices: The label 100% fruit juice is misleading. Take Tropicana orange juice with pulp, for example. This used to be our favorite brand as a family. However, there are a few more details about this otherwise healthy orange juice that convinced me that it is not as healthful as it may seem on the package. According to the nutritiondata.self.com website, one serving (8oz) of Tropicana orange juice gives about 23g of sugar. This is nearly 6 teaspoons of sugar because one teaspoon is about 4g of sugar. You do the math and you realize this juice is a driver of sugar overdose. In the United States, the recommended daily allowance (RDA) for sugar, according to the Food and Drug Administration (FDA), is 25g of sugar daily (or not more than 32g according to some sources). When trying to control yeast infections, the amount should be much less.

What makes it misleading is that this "pure" orange juice has high amounts of vitamin C, an anti-oxidant that builds a strong immune system and plays a role in disease prevention. It is also high in folate and potassium, all of which are beneficial for our health. Orange juice was therefore my favorite juice until I learned that it, too, is loaded with sugar and too strong for my sensitive stomach, sometimes causing a stomachache and/or heartburn. It also was too strong for my teeth enamel as I learned once when I went to brush my teeth right after drinking a glass of orange juice, a definite no, no! While I have not had any soft drink, with the exception of soda water, for at least a decade now, I have had fruit juice occasionally at home, as we continued to buy it regularly for the kids. Even then, I have as little as possible, usually less than a serving, and I dilute it with water.

Our choice of this particular orange juice was based on an attempt to limit added ingredients that were found in some of the other juices or brands. We focused on its "purity," not realizing that sugar in fruit juices, even if it comes in its most natural form, has its limits when it comes to the benefits we can get from it. Indeed, even one serving can easily push us over the RDA for sugar. If you are one of those people who eat cereal, especially the sweetened kinds along with a glass of orange juice in the morning, regardless of how many nutrients you get from this combination, you will easily push yourself over the daily recommended limits by the time you are done with breakfast. If you eat more than one serving of cereal or get a refill of juice, then you might as well prepare for a nap first before you proceed with your daily routines.

Choosing a cereal that does not taste sweet can be misleading as well, and often, the tendency is to either add sugar, or to sweeten it naturally with fruits such as a banana. This is something I used to do often, as well. Remember that just because a cereal does not taste sweet, does not mean that it has no sugar in it or that it will have no impact on your blood sugar. Reading the nutrition facts label is a good habit, just to be sure. It is important to keep track of our sugar intake, because this is one of the easiest and quickest source of energy to burn and what is not used immediately is stored as fat, especially around the waistline. Because we all have our own specific nutritional needs and our tolerance of sugar varies from one person to the next, checking the nutrition facts label allows us to determine our own individual thresholds and keep our intake to an amount that we are comfortable with.

Fortunately, when I gave up orange juice, I did not feel the urge to replace it with any other fruit juice that I would drink on a regular basis. To date, I am not a regular fruit juice drinker. I am also no longer fooled by the "100% juice" or the "no sugar-added" labels. Had I known that in addition to an upset stomach, fruit juices contain much more sugar than the two teaspoons I had given up for my cup of black tea, I would have thought twice before getting in the habit of drinking it in the first place. The point is: fruit juices are very high in sugar and are not a good choice for anyone with weight, yeast infections, or blood sugar problems! On the positive side, during this time of sugar detoxification, I did get some relief from the fungus and for nearly two years, I did not see any visible signs of the problem on my back or my neck. Nonetheless, I was always on alert, making sure that if it resurfaced, it did not spread before I took action. In spite of all these changes, my weight was still far from ideal.

Choosing organic whenever possible: When I started learning about the benefits of organic foods, we decided as a family to look for organic brands. With such choices, rather than worry about sugar that was not highlighted on cereal boxes for example, I paid more attention to the healthy ingredients that stood out on the cereal box for example, ingredients such as "organic flax" or "organic pumpkin seeds," "all natural," and the long list of vitamins and minerals that we all need for good health. I assumed that the benefits of these would outweigh the risks of consuming a little bit of sugar (if any), especially when it was also organic. I assumed that those who valued organic food choices also lived according to higher dietary standards.

While this may be true when it comes to many unprocessed organic foods, the standards are questionable for processed food choices. Oh, how difficult it is to manage sugar in a typical Western diet, even when your choices are primarily organic! With more in-depth knowledge, I eventually stopped eating boxed cereal and made my own plain oatmeal, sometimes adding a little bit of berries (not bananas). When I started going on a gluten-free diet mostly, I switched to seed-like grains such as quinoa and amaranth and this step seemed to work better for me. Adding ground flax or chia seeds, or almond butter helped, as well. I used unsweetened almond milk with it, whenever I could find it.

Advanced steps: A focus on controlling yeasts and weight

I took the advanced steps when I increased my awareness that without controlling yeasts, I may also lose my battle to reach a healthy weight.

Getting a more accurate read of the nutrition facts label: Since I did not know enough to pay attention to the nutrition facts label and get a sense of how much sugar or HFCS was actually included in a serving of whatever food or drink I was consuming, I might as well stick with what was wrongly assumed that fat was the problem all along. In fact, if anyone had any weight and other health issues to worry about, fat was assumed to be the culprit. So, low-fat and fat-free, not low-sugar or sugar-free, featured prominently in the food choices I made for many years. That was the standard I lived by. Getting an accurate read of the nutrition facts label required knowing what counts as sugar in the list of ingredients, as well. Often on the box or other food packages, ingredients are more than meets the eye, especially when it comes to sugar. This is what continues to make managing sugar intake one of the hardest tasks in modern day eating, even for a keen eye like mine, nowadays.

Sugar is rarely highlighted as a key ingredient in packaged foods, and it is almost never highlighted on the menu at restaurants. When food shopping, it is rare to reach the checkout point without a packaged food, in a glass, box or can, inside the cart. These processed and packaged foods are where sugar tends to hide. Sugar is in everything including where you least expect it: not just in cakes, cookies and ice cream, but also in tomato sauces, plain yogurt, ketchup, peanut butter, salad dressings, bread, and many pre-cooked and packaged frozen meals. It can be easy to miss, especially when sugar is disguised under different names we do not recognize as sugar.

How was I supposed to know that corn syrup, dextrose, caramel, galactose, fruit juice concentrate, mannitol, sorbitol, fructose, molasses, maltose, diatase, refiner's syrup, or maltodextrin were all sugar in disguise?

Many of these are the same as high fructose corn syrup (HFCS) I had been trying to avoid when I could identify it. Like many, I missed it often.

Minimize consumption of all fruits: Until the doctor recommended I give up bananas, I never suspected fruits were something to worry about. So, I used to eat them liberally, when cheap and in season. Sometimes, I would buy fruits and have them for lunch instead of pizza, a sandwich, or a full meal, when I was too busy to go out and take a lunch break. For a long time, I believed I was holding good standards in healthy eating, managing added sugar in a rather restrictive way. Eating fruits is healthier than relying on refined sugar or even drinking it in a pure juice form, there is no doubt about that. But some fruits are as sweet as a piece of cake. Fruits were not supporting me on my journey to keep blood sugar stable, however. This is when I took another action aimed at going deeper in sugar detoxification. With more knowledge, I started paying attention to the types of fruits I consumed as well as serving sizes, even with the "safer" fruits such as green apples, raspberries, cranberries, blueberries and blackberries, as well as kiwi. I know to limit myself to a serving or less, because sugar does add up with each additional serving. These safer fruits are my "go to" choices when I know that yeast is in check. Otherwise, I take a break completely from all fruits for a couple of weeks at a time until I have restored some gut balance. My thinking and actions around fruits therefore evolved over time, as I explain further below.

* All fruits are healthy: For years, before I took initial and even intermediate steps, mangoes, bananas, pineapples, papayas, oranges, tangerines, golden berries, raspberries, were fruits I consumed in large amounts when they

were in season. This is what I did when I was still living at home before I left for the United States. I did the same when I returned to work at home in my late 40's.

* Some fruits don't agree with me in one way or another: These included Japanese prunes, for example. When I had them on an empty stomach, they seemed to cause heartburn or give me a stomachache. Both are signs of an acidic body, which creates fertile ground for yeast to thrive. Pineapples also leave a stingy feeling on my lips and my skin irritated. For this reason, I avoid slicing pineapples. However, I do not have any reaction when I eat already peeled and sliced pieces or drink freshly squeezed pineapple juice. I never paid attention to the amount of sugar in a serving of sliced pineapples, until a few years ago, when out of curiosity, one of my clients who had been complaining about her inability to lose weight asked what she could do about it. As I usually do with all my clients, I gave her a form to fill out, and one of the questions that helps me give targeted coaching asks about the foods that the client eats on a regular basis. When she returned the form, I realized that she was starting her day with a big bowl of fruits, including several slices of oranges, bananas, grapes, strawberries, and sometimes pineapples and others. When I estimated how much sugar they might add up to, based on a tool I found on the nutritiondata.self. com website, we were both shocked to find out that she was consuming nearly 60 grams of sugar for breakfast (around 15 teaspoons).

Knowing that she, like me, was concerned about her genetic predisposition to diabetes, we agreed that she would reduce the amount of sugar she consumed in her first meal of the day. She cut her fruits to less than half and started replacing fruits with a different breakfast that would keep blood sugar stable at least throughout the morning. I was not surprised when she told me that this change alone had helped her lose nearly 10 pounds in a couple of months. Even giving up a full serving of pineapples alone can make a difference. This can amount to around 16.3 g of sugar (slightly over 4 teaspoons) according to the nutritiondata.self.com website.

Pineapples are very high in vitamin C, which is good but sugar overload can overshadow the good nutrients. And if you are like me, having been accustomed to the message that eating multiple servings of fruits and vegetables is healthy, it's easy to take this message and run with it. And while rarely does anyone overconsume vegetables, it's much easier to overdo it on fruits.

 * Some fruits are low in sugar and can be consumed regularly in moderation: Whenever they are available, the best choices are green apples, raspberries, blackberries, blueberries, kiwi, and unripe bananas. Because apples are on the list of the Environmental Working Group's list of the dirty dozen, which includes fruits and vegetables with the highest amount of pesticide residues on them, I no longer eat them unless I can find organic choices. This is easier when I am based in the United States. Where I am currently based in Monrovia, Liberia, the only fruits I can safely eat are local bananas as well as papayas, choosing unripe ones because they are known as prebiotics that feed the good bacteria. Even with these, I am careful not to overdo it, paying attention to serving sizes. Sometimes I make a green papaya salad also a prebiotic. Otherwise, papayas contain digestive enzymes that help me with regular bowel movements. Success in making fruits work best for me required a higher level of learning and awareness as I made further attempts to keep sugar intake in check.

* No fruit is good when trying to conquer yeast overgrowth and lose weight: The quantum leap of my knowledge about nutrition, health, and balance came after I enrolled at the Institute for Integrative Nutrition (IIN) in the Fall 2012. Listening to one of the lectures by Donna Gates sometime in early 2013, I gained a much broader picture of how sugar works in the gut and throughout the body, creating imbalances that manifest themselves through various symptoms, some of which are not easily diagnosable through conventional approaches. Her lecture became life-changing for me. Not long after this lecture, I purchased

Body Ecology Diet, the book she co-authored with Linda Schatz and read it front to cover. My interaction with sugar is much more comprehensive because of it. She is therefore highly influential in my own views and understanding of food, and dietary choices needed to promote the growth of friendly bacteria in particular, as well as other lifestyle factors that help to restore gut balance and healing of body and mind. She not only helped me gain clarity on the reasons why my fungal infections and yeasts recurred, but I also learned a new way of eating and living.

Donna Gates helped me understand better what I had been missing. She helped me come to terms with the fact that getting rid of fungal infections and yeasts requires more than giving up the two teaspoons of sugar in my morning tea, bananas, sugary sodas, and all the other steps I had made to limit sugar intake. These were all good steps, but they were not enough. One of the missing links that I will get into when I introduce the health benefits of ferments, was that I was creating an environment for the bad bacteria to die down, but I was not recolonizing my gut with a diet that would be most appropriate for the friendly bacteria to thrive and take over with a stronger immune system. This diet that rebuilds the colony of good bacteria, also helps to counter the effects of sugar and antibiotics on the body. Without such a diet, the gains to my health and weight remained partial and unsatisfactory. The diet I needed had to maintain all the sugar control habits I had adopted as discussed above, but it required a few additional dietary modifications that I will discuss in the chapters on starches, fats, and ferments. That I favor green or unripe bananas is based on my understanding that prebiotics feed the friendly bacteria, a habit I never paid attention to before.

Do not be complacent

I slowly but surely discovered that there are other triggers I must pay attention to.

Hormonal changes in my body: Just as I thought I had sugar intake under control, I ignored a major change inside my body and that I knew very little about: hot flashes! I had entered perimenopause, and midlife was affecting my weight in ways I was not expecting. I had not paid attention to hormonal changes I had experienced before, not knowing how to make sense of these internal communication channels. I had to deepen my knowledge of how hormones work and communicate with one another. I knew I had to increase my understanding of insulin and any other fat-storage hormone, especially those linked to this phase, such as estrogen.

Changes in gut microflora that occur as women approach menopause create a fertile environment for yeasts to resurface. I did not want to slide back, especially resisting the urge to turn to antibiotics. I had come to realize that they are an incomplete solution at best. Instead, I registered for a class, *Cooking for Hormonal Balance*, offered by Magdalena Wszelaki, and continued narrowing down the root causes of yeasts and stubborn belly fat in midlife. This time, I started adding nutritional supplements where I knew I had gaps. I reintroduced probiotics and continue taking them, looking for better choices regularly. Good probiotics recolonize your gut with friendly bacteria, but as I will explain later, without a diet rich in prebiotics, their most important feed, they can be a waste of your money. Otherwise, probiotics are needed to help the body fight off yeast overgrowth. I introduced new supplements in the form of green powders, as well, to help keep my immune system stronger, which is necessary to prevent infections, including yeasts. I started taking spirulina and moringa *oleifera* powders for this reason. Both powders are high in anti-oxidants, as well. I continued to refine my diet and lifestyle to see if I could improve results around my weight and waistline. Although a focus on sugar control alone was not enough to allow me to reach a breakthrough around my belly fat, managing sugar intake better benefitted me in many other ways, including some I was not expecting such as stronger and healthier hair.

Environmental triggers: These include mold and high humidity, that became challenging when we moved to Liberia.

* Mold: When we moved to Monrovia, mold in our apartment and the humidity in the air, allowed the skin rash and yeasts to resurface in ways that did not make sense to me, given that I was still keeping a much-improved diet. Mold is indeed defined as yeasts' cousin. I have never seen so much mold around me as I saw in Monrovia. You cannot imagine how much mold can grow, not just on the walls of the enclosed bathroom where there is not enough natural air circulation, but also on clothes inside the closet, whether hanging or folded, and on the shoe rack, completely discoloring sensitive shoes. The two steps that help keep it in check are: painting walls when mold starts breaking through and showing discoloration, as well as keeping the air conditioning (AC) on. While my preference would not be to keep the AC on, I have become used to it. We have not been able to find any alternative, natural solution that would not require wasting so much energy.

* Humidity: Unfortunately, because of the heat and humidity in Monrovia, the skin rash and yeasts that thrive in damp and humid environments are hard to control completely. Several female friends here have similar complaints as well. Living in such an environment, requires that we remain on the alert. Keeping the AC on, minimizing sugar consumption, including giving up fruits off and on, taking a probiotic and high fiber foods as well as other healthy habits I adopt as my knowledge increases, continues to help.

Signs of improvement in controlling sugar and its effects on my health

With the above steps, along with a few others I outline in the next few chapters, I was actually able to see that my health was improving. Some of the signs of improvement include the following.

Yeast die-off: I could tell when urinating that some yeast-like strings were being pushed out of my body. They were being starved by my diet.

Sustained energy after a meal: Managing sugar better helped me keep a sustained level of energy over four, even five hours at a time before I felt the need to eat something. I used to feel sleepy after eating foods that raised my blood sugar fast. This was a sign that my insulin was not able to keep up with the amount of sugar I was ingesting at once. Eating in a way that allows hunger to come gradually, and not abruptly, is a big sign of improvement for someone like me, who is pre-disposed to diabetes. I no longer feel that I must find something to eat fast before I nearly faint or have a headache.

Healthier hair: My hair started to grow and look healthier again when I significantly controlled sugar intake. I used to have a thick Afro until my late 30s, and by African hair standard, it was quite long when I used a chemical relaxer to straighten it. When my hair started losing its natural thickness, straightening my hair only showed just how much thinner and unhealthy it had become. It also stopped growing. I tried going "natural" but it stayed short. I tried giving my hair a break by braiding it, but that worked only for a short while. I added extensions to look more professional when I had to attend a special event or had an important meeting to go to. I even tried wigs. These were only cover-up solutions for the real need I had to invest in: a culinary overhaul! I will discuss further what this overhaul meant in the next three chapters, looking at other carbs aside from sugar and sweet foods, as well as fats and ferments. These additional changes helped my hair grow thicker and look so much healthier than I have seen it in at least a decade. It became clear that my belly fat was consuming all life out of other parts of my health, including my hair. I am proud of myself when I get compliments on my big Afro, knowing the efforts I have made to get here.

A stronger immune system: Reducing sugar and improving my diet overall helps my immune system stay stronger, with only the occasional cold, once a year perhaps, but even then, it will get better quite fast. I am much more resilient, rarely feeling weak and sick.

Weight loss: Although the steps to manage sugar intake are combined with other dietary and lifestyle improvements, I could not succeed at losing the excess weight without controlling sugar intake. To date, keeping a low-sugar diet is one of the most beneficial steps of all the dietary steps I have taken. But it isn't the only step.

These improvements were what continued to motivate me to maintain the changes I had made thus far. Keeping sugar intake in check was part of a strategy to lose excess weight and the fat around my belly. I did not have to ask around for others to notice that belly fat had become the most obvious part of my physique. In fact, it was those around me who raised my awareness that my belly was visibly bigger than my overall structure. Breaking my sugar habits was an important step in the right direction of conquering yeast infections, but this step alone left me quite some distance away from my ideal weight and a waistline I would be comfortable with. Going deep involved applying other dietary and lifestyle practices that would help to keep yeasts and the skin rash in check and contribute better to shrinking belly fat.

CONCLUSION

I hope the breakdown of food choices and preferences offered in this chapter will help you create your own meal plan that will enable you to keep sugar in check. Dietary choices play a major role in how our body handles sugar. An inadequate diet can accelerate the emergence of symptoms such as a fungal skin rash or yeast infections, affecting both inside and outside our body. Yeast overgrowth, hormonal imbalances and excessive weight gain are all manifestations of an inadequate diet, unable to protect our immune system from assault. When this happens, yeasts start taking over the direction of our health. Losing weight is especially hard in midlife when yeasts still control our gut.

On the better side, a balanced diet can keep the friendly bacteria in control and our immune system strong enough to prevent an assault on our health. We will get more into ways to rebalance these gut bacteria with a regular consumption of fermented foods, particularly vegetables. As with all matters of our health, it was up to me, as it is up to each one of us, to know our individual threshold and to avoid foods such as those high in sugar that continue to exacerbate existing imbalances. Such imbalances contribute to building a wall around the middle, in the form of belly fat. In turn, belly fat increases our risks of diabetes, among other diseases associated with a dysfunctional metabolism.

In the next chapter, I will focus on the rest of the carbs and how making them work better for me was another key step in my efforts to keep blood sugar stable. This required significant shifts in my carb choices. As my thinking around them evolved, I continued to adjust my eating habits. While I may not always succeed at holding the gold standard in eating right, I know a whole lot more about diets aimed to keep blood sugar in balance than I knew before I started on this journey. I understand better that I have a threshold in terms of my tolerance of sugar. This is a place where I can eat without causing high spikes in blood sugar and without pushing my insulin levels overboard. I continue to rely on a low-sugar diet and I hope that this information will inspire you to find your own sweet spot when it comes to controlling your own sugar intake, your weight, and shrink your waistline as well.

Individually and together, we can hold each other accountable to make it to a place where self-monitoring is easy and adjusting meals that keep blood sugar stable is practical, affordable, and achievable. This is a place where our actions will enable us to keep our bodies free of debilitating yeasts, which in turn impacts positively our weight and belly fat as we continue to learn. So, stay tuned!

CHAPTER 3:

MAKE CARBS WORK FOR YOU

Let's be honest. What would the world of eating look like without bread, rice, potatoes, *chapati*, *ugali*, pasta, grits, corn, tortillas, or other starch we consider essential to our diet? What would your own eating habits be without starches, this most basic representation of food? What would you fill up on? In many cultures, including my own, bread in one form or another, is served for breakfast with tea or coffee, as toast with butter and/ or jam or other available spread or accompaniment. For many kids who grew up on the standard American diet (SAD), school lunches were often nothing more than two slices of bread spread with peanut butter and jelly. At home with my husband, we often relied on a bagel and egg or cream cheese for lunch for many years, starting before we got married. Although I would not say that this type of lunch ever became my favorite, I got used to it. I came to appreciate it because having bagels meant I did not have to cook lunch during a busy week filled with academic papers, professional work, taking care of kids, and/or tending to other chores.

However, a bagel for lunch was a new way of eating for me and others in my family of origin. I remember when one of my sisters, who had come to the U.S. to stay with me while finishing high school, asked if our usual lunch of bagels and cream cheese was a snack until the real lunch came. I could relate to her feelings. We were raised in a home where a complete meal with rice (or another starchy food such as potatoes or green bananas), beans and a vegetable were what we expected as a basic meal for lunch or dinner.

It did not take me long to realize that my boyfriend (later my husband) did not have many ideas for lunch. Since having bagels and cream cheese was a relatively cheap option, I adapted, and we maintained this habit of his, even after we got married and had kids. We introduced them to bagels at a young age and taking them to a nearby bagel place for lunch was a treat they appreciated. Our kids loved bagels, especially when they were served fresh and hot. It was a welcome break from the regular sandwiches they had for lunch at daycare or school. Naturally, going to a bagel place meant we would get something to drink. This, too, could add to our overall carb intake for the day, depending on the choice we made. For the kids, it was often a small bottle of orange juice. For the grownups, it was either herbal tea (unsweetened for me) or coffee (with cream and sugar) for my husband. Starchy foods dominated dinner, as well.

Bread was an important part of our diet, just as it is for millions of people around the globe. When my kids were younger, dinner rolls were often added to one or more sources of carbs such as rice, pasta, or mashed potatoes, that we considered critical parts of the evening meal. I could often find frozen dough balls that I only needed to reheat for just a few minutes and serve hot with the rest of dinner. Bread is such a valued commodity everywhere that its representation spans cultures and traditions, both literally and figuratively, and for centuries. In Christianity, for example, bread is a symbol of sacrifice, satisfaction and a source of life. It is broken to feed the hungry, as Jesus did during biblical times. Bread is also broadly earned as a reward, by those who value hard work, doing so to "put bread on the table," which applies both to those who live hand to mouth, as well as those whose hard work enables them to harvest the bounty in silos or bank accounts.

Until just a few years ago, I considered bread and all other starches to be of equal value. The only exception was that starches high in fiber are more beneficial, supporting regular bowel movements, something I never took for granted even as a kid. In my own very limited understanding of how we metabolize them, I considered starches as one food group that we must consume daily, representing the bulk of each of the three main meals of the day. Rice, pasta and potatoes occupied at least half of my plate, if not more, and the rest had to be added on the side or on top, for a full plate.

WHY DO WE EAT TOO MANY CARBS?

Since the advent of agriculture 12,000 years or so ago, carbs have become over-produced and hence over-consumed. Carbs are more readily available in all parts of the world. They are often cheaper than other food groups. For many, a meal without carbs is incomplete. With billions of people to feed on planet earth, few have been socialized to start their day with a low-carb breakfast. For this reason, I empathize with some of my clients who cannot imagine what they would eat if they gave up some of their favorite starches, even temporarily. This seems unrealistic, unfathomable and impractical. The response I often hear is: "If I stop eating bread or rice, what am I going to eat?"

This question is probably one that millions around the world would ask if the supply of starches was cut off suddenly.

Few can imagine what life would look like if we were forced to take a journey backwards and live according to the dietary habits of our hunter-gatherer ancestors. Contrary to what many would like to believe, our dietary needs are not that much different, and what worked for them would most likely work for us as well, provided we maintained, as they did, a more active and less sedentary lifestyle.

Their diet would work for us if we relied less on processed food choices and more on whole foods as nature provides. Our ancestors didn't rely on grains. Instead, fish and game, nuts and seeds, and seasonal fruits provided the bulk of their diet. Theirs was a low-carb diet as we understand it today.

Food production has made it possible for us to have access to different types of carbs all year round. Overproduction of grains and beans (another significant contributor to our intake of carbs, in addition to being a good source of fiber and protein) has made it possible for us to eat some of the same foods and in large quantities all year round. This is where we differ from even modern hunter-gatherers, whose diets and overall health shifts according to the seasons.

"The idea that we, 365 days a year, should be eating in the same pattern doesn't make evolutionary sense. I'm convinced, looking at our modern hunter-gatherers who still exist, that even their microbiome shifts on a seasonal basis as their food shifts" states Stephen Gundry, in an online interview with Joseph Mercola. Gundry is the author of *The Longevity Paradox: How to Die Young at a Ripe Old Age*.

Unlike our ancestors, we have become very dependent on excessive consumption of starchy foods, farmed in abundance for our indulgence. Access to carbs continues to increase on global markets, making it easier for people everywhere to find some of the same foods regardless of where they find themselves. Eating according to what's local and in season does not come as intuitively as it should. White rice from India or China is sold throughout sub-Saharan Africa as well as in the U.S. and Canada, making it possible for us to have access to it all year round, whether we grow our own or not. When eating out, rice is almost always on the menu. It is served at most restaurants, from the roadside makeshift kitchens of Liberia to the upscale restaurants of New York City and many other places in between, east and west, in the northern hemisphere and the south.

Quinoa from Peru is a highly prized "seed-like" grain in the United States and its market share continues to grow, reaching those who shop in higher-end food stores, even in Africa. While I hear that it is becoming more and more expensive in Peru, it is available for those who can afford it elsewhere. I have seen it even at the Harbel supermarket here in Monrovia, Liberia. Millet from India and Nigeria is sold in other parts of the world as well. And potatoes from Idaho are consumed not just throughout the United States, but also in Canada. French fries are available as an important part of the meal, not just in France, where supposedly they make the best you'll ever find, but also at many modest takeout places throughout the world.

Bread, porridge made of one or a mix of flours, *mandazi* (*beignets* or African donuts), bagels, cereal, pancakes, and other grain-based, high-carb foods feature prominently on the breakfast table. If this was the only time of the day when such foods were consumed, perhaps we would keep it to a safe intake level and maintain a stable and healthy metabolism, as well. But that is not the case. In most cultures, carbs are served in large portions at each of the three main meals of the day and often as a snack as well.

HOW DO CARBS IMPACT BELLY FAT?

"Carbohydrates is driving insulin is driving fat", George Cahill (former Professor of Medicine at Harvard Medical School) in Gary Taubes, *Why We Get Fat and What to Do About It* (10).

When it comes to body fat accumulation, the fundamental question addressed by many contemporary nutrition and health experts is: What regulates fat accumulation? Their findings point to the workings of the blood sugar hormone, insulin. Many experts agree that because of the way that carbs trigger the release of insulin, excess carb consumption, a bio-individual experience, is seen as the culprit when it comes to resistance to weight loss. When we eat carbs, the body's glucose levels rise and the pancreas releases insulin to bring this glucose to different cells in the body and to keep blood sugar levels in balance. Excess glucose is converted to glycogen, a carbohydrate with sugar molecules bonded together. According to Jeremy M Berg, John L Tymoczko, and Lubert Stryer, glycogen "is a *readily mobilized form of glucose* ... that can be broken down to yield glucose molecules when energy is needed." In this case, it "serves as a buffer to maintain blood glucose levels" between meals. A *UC Berkeley News* online article further explains that unused glucose is "with the help of insulin, converted into fatty acids, circulated to other parts of the body and stored as fat in adipose tissue. When there is an overabundance of fatty acids, fat also builds up in the liver," leading to fatty liver.

This is one of the reasons why a beer belly is not restricted to heavy alcohol drinkers. Overconsumption of carbs does the same thing, and anyone who struggles with the buildup of fat around the belly has an overabundance of fatty acids in the liver, as well. Belly fat in midlife is evidence of this strain on the liver and embracing a low-carb diet is one of the effective ways to shrink this fat around the waistline. The liver's glycogen stores are easily depleted when we are on a restricted carb diet. This requires that we only consume the amount of carbs needed for immediate energy and not more. This is the only way to prevent storing excess glucose that eventually converts to fat one meal after another. Mark Hyman in his book *The Blood Sugar Solution 10-Day Detox Diet* and other experts advise against eating carbs altogether, at least temporarily, if the goal is to lose weight fast and improve insulin function. In addition to weight loss, limiting consumption of carbs can curb cravings for breads, sweets, and other high-carb foods, as well as support blood sugar and heart health.

Gary Taubes explains how carbs affect blood sugar, insulin and weight in two distinct ways: "First, when insulin levels are elevated, we accumulate fat in our fat tissue; when these levels fall, we liberate fat from the fat tissue and burn it for fuel .... Second, our insulin levels are effectively determined by the carbohydrates we eat - not entirely, but for all intents and purposes. The more carbohydrates we eat, and the easier they are to digest and the sweeter they are, the more insulin we will ultimately secrete, meaning that the level of it in our bloodstream is greater and so is the fat we retain in our fat cells" (8-10).

In this chapter, I will take you on my personal journey, and share insights into some of the challenges I faced in the process of managing carb intake and how I overcame them. What took me at least five years to internalize and feel well-equipped to successfully apply, can take you much less time because the lessons I learned along the way are included here, so that you can follow along the shortcuts rather than having to reinvent the wheel for yourself. You will discover, like I did, that when you reach midlife there are many good carbs that still do not work when you want to shrink belly fat. There are many reasons why I reached the conclusion that carbs are not just another food group that I must always consume for a satisfying meal. I now know that they act as sugar's best "partner in crime."

Sugar is a carb in its simplest form, but even complex carbs are not always helpful when it comes to weight control.

Carbs are a food group that I must be vigilant about in my own meal planning and food intake, if my goal is to keep consistent energy throughout the day, maintain stable blood sugar levels, as well as restore or maintain a healthy weight.

While carbs have always been the biggest portions of my meals, how I metabolized them changed when I reached midlife. Adjusting carb consumption had to be a part of the change I needed to make if I wanted to lose some of the belly fat. To succeed at making carbs work better for me, I had to ask myself the following questions: Are all good carbs good for me? How often can I have these starchy foods without losing my battle to lose excess weight? And how much can I consume without losing the belly fat battle? The answers to these questions are not straightforward. Complex carbs are healthier than simple carbs, there is no doubt about this. However, not all complex carbs support weight loss. They must be managed carefully, and some are better at supporting this goal than others. The better ones include all leafy greens and select starchy vegetables, as well as some nuts and seeds. These contain starch and fiber and overall a limited amount of total carbs.

Other complex carbs include minimally processed foods that maintain a relatively high amount of the nutrients and most of the fiber contained in the whole food, such as whole wheat pasta, oat groats and steel cut oats. These can be healthy if you can digest gluten, but if you struggle with stubborn belly fat, they can keep you from losing it in spite of your efforts. If your weight is normal, these complex carbs and a few others such as whole grains, brown rice and quinoa, are considered by some to be important for an efficient metabolism. According to a study published in the *American Journal of Clinical Nutrition* and cited in a blog post by Leah Groth on boosting your metabolism, whole grains:

- Increase overall calorie loss by reducing the calories retained during digestion;
- Aid with fiber absorption;
- Enable the body to speed metabolism and burn calories;
- Lower risks of certain chronic diseases such as diabetes; and
- Benefit weight management.

Groth's blog post summarizes the findings of the above study looking at the practices of 81 men and women. Among them, "those who maintained a diet rich in whole grains while matching the recommended daily allowance for fiber based on age and sex lost an additional 100 calories per day due to a combination of increased resting metabolic rate and greater fecal loss." It is important to note that the USDA recommends a minimum of 3 ounces of whole grains per day for women. This is around one and a half to two cups of whole grains such as brown rice or oatmeal per day. It is the equivalent of 3 cups of dry cereal, 3 slices of whole wheat bread, or three small, six-inch tortillas, according to the University of Rhode Island website. While this amount is reasonable for anyone with a healthy weight, it can be excessive if you are trying to lose belly fat. In fact, until I started paying attention to the impact of grain-based carbs on my weight and blood sugar, as compared to other sources of carbs, sometimes I was consuming nearly this much per meal, rather than per day. It's no wonder efforts I made to lose weight failed, as well.

Taubes' work greatly informed my thinking about carbs. He highlights several important points related to the impact of carbs on weight, and summarizes the reasons why many health and nutrition professionals had been refuting, for decades, the idea that gaining weight and accumulating body fat is "a disorder of energy balance or eating too much." Taubes specifically highlights the key assumptions of past research that link the tendency to gain weight to the amount of carbs we consume (152-154).

Robert C. Atkins is one of the most recognized experts regarding the link between carb consumption and a resistance to weight loss. Rachael H. and Richard H. Heller, in their book *The Carbohydrate Addict's Diet*, also make the case for limiting carb consumption to promote weight loss. They observed that patients who seemed to be "addicted" to carbs needed targeted interventions, much like alcoholics and drug addicts. In this context, Heller and Heller define carb addiction as the inability to control hunger and a greater preference for processed carbs and sweets when struck with hunger (15). Mary Dan Eades and Michael R. Eades support the classic "slimming" regimes that many practitioners in the United States and the United Kingdom relied on to support patients with weight issues. They advise their patients to embrace a carb-restricted diet as a key step to managing what they call the "midlife middle."

What exactly do the above health and nutrition experts mean by carb restriction? They mean avoiding many foods that currently take up most shelves in conventional and even health food stores. They include "all forms of added sugar, all foods with added cornstarch or flour, all starchy foods including potatoes, pastas, beans and peas." Sugary soft drinks, bread, cereals, milk puddings, and white root vegetables were also included on this list of foods to restrict. However, in the 1960s and for a few decades to follow, diets were judged on the basis of how heart friendly they were. Carbs were considered as heart-healthy. In fact, even the U.S. Department of Agriculture issued a food pyramid in 1992, and on it, carbs were at the bottom of the pyramid, representing the largest proportion of recommended caloric intake. At the top of the pyramid were oils and sweets that we must "use sparingly."

Amidst this dietary confusion coming from high authorities in the field of nutritional policy and guidance particularly in the United States, people learned to adapt, relying more on carbs and less on other sources of macronutrients, and especially shunning dietary fats. Even the American Heart Association was comfortable recommending foods that did not contain fat. Many in the United States turned into heavy consumers of carbs, not questioning their nutritional value or effects on health and weight. After all, who in their right mind would question the importance of protecting the heart? Today, there is more evidence that a diet high in carbs contributes to weight gain, just as low-fat and no-fat diets do, while causing other negative side effects to our hormones and overall metabolism. As we will discuss later in the chapter on fats, this recommendation to lower fat intake while also giving carbs a thumbs-up, was based on shaky research and misinformed dietary conclusions.

HOW DID I END UP OVEREATING CARBS?

Did my move to the United States in 1991 result in overeating carbs? Perhaps. Pasta was cheap. A loaf of bread could last as long as a week or as little as a couple of days depending on what else I chose to eat with it. Potatoes and rice were abundant. A variety of morning cereals were easily accessible, for a quick breakfast. I developed the same eating habits as housemates, favoring like them, pasta and its pre-cooked and packaged sauce for a quick dinner, sometimes with or without a vegetable. Looking back, this reliance on a high-carb diet was not new to me. I grew up eating lots of starchy foods. We grew corn, potatoes, wheat, peas and beans on our family farm and these were our staples until I moved to boarding school at age 13. I never spent much time at home after that, and my diet, though slightly different each time, still placed carbs over and above all other food groups. Cassava was more prevalent at times and it was cheaper than rice, our preferred starch for lunch and dinner. Bread and tea were what we had for breakfast. While moving to America introduced me to culinary abundance, relying on a high carb diet was not a new habit I developed there. The move only made it possible for me to dive right in and enjoy the bountiful of starchy and processed foods that the country offers, often at affordable prices, even on a student stipend.

What I should have questioned then, if I had known better, was the quality of my food choices. It would take years to reach that point and even longer before I would question my carb choices. Generally, I thought that my carbs were good given that I was not very much into sweet foods. Once I had kids, my choices were similar to those of other parents around. We all relied mostly on what is known as the Standard American Diet (SAD). Through interaction with a few health-conscious friends and relatives, I was quickly convinced that switching to organic food choices was worth the extra cost. Questioning our dietary choices ended there, however, at least for a while. We continued to make many assumptions that turned out to be wrong. Clearly, just because a food is organic does not mean it is the right food for everyone all the time.

> *When it comes to carbs and their impact on blood sugar and body weight, it almost does not matter whether they are organic or not.*

The only difference may come from the micronutrients they contain, especially when they are whole and unprocessed. There seems to be no consensus among food scientists on this point, however. Two main schools of thought dominate the discourse on the differences between organic and conventional foods. One seeks to convince us that the nutritional value of organic foods is not much different from foods grown through conventional methods, whether as genetically modified organisms (GMOs) or not. The other pushes forward the evidence that organic foods are generally significantly more nutritious and advocates for organic food production methods.

In comparing the two approaches, I am inclined to believe that organic farming methods are safer for the environment, and for us, as well. They appeal to me, because I can often taste the difference, with a bolder flavor in 100% organic fruits and vegetables, for example, especially when they are also grown locally. Could it be only psychological? Even if it were, the peace of mind of knowing the foods I am consuming are pesticide-free would still be worth the extra cost. Ultimately, we all have our own reasons why we value food, but nothing will make it more valuable than the health benefits we gain from it. I believe that whole, unprocessed foods are better for us than highly refined ones, just as foods grown in naturally rich soils are healthier than those that rely on the application of chemical fertilizers and pesticides to keep the crops alive.

Relying on the physical appearance of produce, whether grown organically or in conventional ways, can be deceptive. Without the label that helps to distinguish the two at grocery stores, especially in the United States, consumers can barely distinguish one ear of corn or a grain of wheat from the next, based purely on physical appearance. While the two may look the same, they are not the same in their own natural integrity.

Our eating habits are also rooted in traditions passed down from one generation to the next, which leaves us trusting our food choices even when they lack some of the nutritional values that kept previous generations healthier.

This is a point many clients struggle with. They'll say, "We have been eating wheat bread [or rice] since we were kids. Our parents and their parents before them ate the same type of bread as. Why should it suddenly be a problem now?" I can understand and empathize with this point of view.

Carbs have undergone so much transformation through ultra-processing. This has left us with some of the least nutritious choices, which also are the most highly marketed by processed food producers. To keep up with demand for these foods, farmers apply chemical fertilizers to force the land to produce a yield that it would not be able to achieve without them. Plus, pesticides applied to crops are not all clean and cleared before harvest or before the foods are displayed on shelves in food stores or market stands. What we consume is no longer the same even if it comes from the same farms that generations before us used to grow their own foods. Then, they relied on less, if any, of the artificial inputs now required for a normal yield. When we consume these foods that our parents grew up with, without ever questioning their nutritional profiles, we may never know how they may be affecting our health and our waistline, and why previous generations did not have the same health problems we have today. Similarly, when we grow up without ever reflecting on what our caloric needs are, we will not be able to judge the value of a meal or adjust what we eat accordingly.

Being used to consuming multiple servings of carbs at each meal, means that replacing them in an informed manner is not as straightforward as we may like to think. Nonetheless, finding the sweet spot in terms of carb consumption, is an important component of what it means to eat right to support the changes we most certainly experience in midlife. This entails eating in such a way as not to exceed our body's needs for energy and nutritional balance. It entails eating in such a way as to prevent unhealthy weight gain and unstable blood sugar. The resources I have consulted, and the experts whose knowledge inform my practice both in terms of keeping my own carb intake in check and coaching others to do the same, agree that reducing carb consumption is a key step on this journey towards preventing weight gain, especially in midlife. Failing to do so only sets the stage for further fat accumulation around the waistline, a sign of and often a precursor to insulin resistance. Preventing excess fat accumulation is critical because once stored, it is not easily accessed by the body as a source of energy.

We were not meant to have access to, nor to consume carbs in large amounts without taking a break from them in between seasons of bounty and seasons of shortage. Even when consumed with other foods, the energy that carbs provide must be depleted before the body triggers the use of any fat that is already stored. Unfortunately, whenever our consumption of carbs exceeds our immediate needs for energy, the remainder of the carbs eventually converts to fat. Overconsuming carbs with each meal creates an over-accumulation of fat that settles especially around the belly.

In their book *Good Carbs, Bad Carbs*, Johanna Burani and Linda Rao write that "when it comes to getting quick sources of energy from food, your system almost ignores dietary fats, although they do make an important contribution, by providing you with the form of energy you can easily store to use later ... fats contain the most calories. And because of the chemical structure of these calories, your body chooses them as its favorite nutrients for body-fat storage. Because many people ... don't have a chance to dip into this stored fat for energy ... it goes on your thighs, middle, and butt! Your system just loves to store fat and has an almost unlimited ability to do so" (9).

Now you understand why your middle suffers when you continue relying on excess carb consumption for energy. You realize also, I hope, that relying on medical treatments and surgical procedures to help us recover from preventable ailments, especially when dietary changes can bring the results we want, is not just an unfortunate choice. It gives our power of choice, healthy choices, away to the promise of quick but much more costly and unsustainable fixes. The less we take care of ourselves, the more we are leaving our wellness into the hands of others. There are always companies in search of newer technologies to sell to vulnerable and at-risk clients. For those who prefer such an approach to health and wellness, the potential for new treatments of diseases often associated with high abdominal fat as Sarah Yang explains, can sound promising. Yang summarizes some new research conducted at the University of California, Berkeley as follows, " A gene that helps the body convert that big plate of holiday cookies you just polished off into fat, could provide a new target for potential treatments for fatty liver disease, diabetes, and obesity."

It's helpful to know that as science evolves, newer and more effective treatments for any of these diseases may become easy to reach by targeted patients. Until these treatments hit the market and are affordable enough to reach the millions of people who struggle with excess weight, belly fat, insulin resistance and the cluster of diseases known as the metabolic syndrome, we can limit carb intake and make other effective dietary and lifestyle changes that can bring us to similar results. Other forms of therapy and treatment not only cost more, but they often have unwanted side effects as well.

Being an informed consumer or patient helps us to achieve results in a sustainable way as well. There is nothing to lose but a lot to gain. Among the millions of women who, like me, have found themselves wondering why in the world midlife came with so much build-up of fat around the belly, managing carb intake carefully and wisely can serve as one of a number of strategies that can help revitalize our changing body. When fat accumulates around the waistline, it triggers the onset of ailments that we most often associate with the natural process of aging. Here comes midlife, we think! But does it have to be that way? No, it does not.

MANAGING MY CARB INTAKE

Testimonials from different sources shared by practitioners who recommended carb restrictions motivated me to try it myself. I went through many steps before I was able to identify the carbs I could consume without losing the battle to lose weight and belly fat. I knew that continuing to put insulin in overdrive, a sign of sugar overload was a warm welcome to more fat storage as well as an invitation to diabetes. What I share is a synthesis of lessons learned over the last five years I spent carefully learning and adjusting my carb intake. As I put carbs to test, I wanted to know exactly which carbs would help me shrink my belly. I hope that what I share in the remainder of this chapter will serve as a useful guide for you to create a simple and manageable plan that will yield intended results for you and help you lose inches around your waistline as you get closer and closer to your ideal weight.

I will explain how my consumption of carbs has evolved over time, and how this has impacted my short- and long-term weight, waistline, and blood sugar management goals, keeping in mind my genetic predisposition to diabetes. You may be ready to act now but are still wondering, what would be the simplest and most effective way to manage carb intake? Is there a straightforward path, an easy to follow formula or a quick way to reach the results you most want? I am sharing my evolving understanding of, and approach to, restricting carb intake. First, I will provide general considerations to keep in mind in order to prepare for success. I will then share the steps I took to achieve this success.

General considerations

Knowing your overall caloric needs: At any given time, our level of activity, age, body size and our metabolism, will dictate the most effective diet and the amount of carbs (or other food groups) we must consume to maintain a healthy balance. Reducing our intake of starchy foods, even slightly, may be sufficient sometimes. However, giving them up, even temporarily, may be required to help us achieve intended results more efficiently and effectively. This is not a new concept. It is in our genetic makeup, as Eades and Eades remind us: "Our metabolic machinery was designed to cope with an unpredictable food supply. We had to store food away [unused calories] for the lean times ahead. The hormone insulin did this for us. Unfortunately, a diet heavy in carbohydrate also sends our insulin levels soaring, and our body interprets this as a need to store calories, to make cholesterol, and to conserve water - all important to our survival way back then" (21). Fortunately for many, we do not have to worry about food shortage. In fact, what we need to understand and apply is how much and how often we can consume certain foods such as carbs, without pushing ourselves into a metabolic overload. Skipping carbs requires knowing individual caloric needs, so that we can intelligently replace them with other foods that provide similar caloric content and nutritional value, as needed. If you are in the habit of overconsuming carbs, it is challenging at first to know how to eat a carb-restricted diet.

How are you going to consume the calories you need without carbs? You will be surprised when you start adjusting your carb intake and realize, as I did, that you can survive and even thrive on much less starchy foods. Nutrition researcher Kris Gunnars writes that "If you eat a 2000-calorie diet, you should aim for about 225 to 325 grams of carbs per day. But if you need to lose weight, you will get much faster results eating around 50 to 150 grams of carbs." Eating is as much about physiology as it is psychology. It's important to reach a point where you can go for three, four and even five hours, without feeling hungry, while also eating less overall, and especially less starchy foods. It requires knowing how much food you need to fuel you and avoiding excess. It requires combining foods appropriately, as well, so what you give up in carbs, you can gain in other food sources for adequate calorie intake. This varies from one person to the next. This general rule requires getting into the specifics of your individual needs, what you can access, and your preferences among healthy substitutes.

"With Diets, most of us forget common sense. We pick a diet at random, giving little thought to our needs, our preferences, our strengths, our weaknesses, or specific metabolic levels. We take what may (or may not) be appropriate for someone else, and assume that it should be correct for us .... Then we blame ourselves when, in the long run, it doesn't work .... Maybe, just maybe, that's because it wasn't an appropriate plan in the first place", Rachel F. Heller and Richard F. Heller, *The Carbohydrate Addict's Diet* (33).

Location and Access: To succeed at adjusting carb intake in terms of quantity and quality requires having access to the different types of carbs and other food groups to choose from in your location. Different carbs do not affect blood sugar, weight, and belly fat the same way. To make carbs work better for me, I had to know which of them affected weight and blood sugar the least and focus on those. To do this successfully depends on food availability in real time and place. In the United States, for example, I had many types of carbs to choose from. Once I knew which worked better for me to control weight gain, I could rely on them more in my diet, while giving up or significantly reducing those that are least helpful in supporting my goal. The US also offers a wide range of other food groups so that one can easily skip carbs and still feel satisfied with the meal you can put together.

Eating in season has helped me maintain a healthy weight even here in Liberia, where rice is dominant in most kitchens, whether at affordable local eateries or at expensive ones where expatriates tend to congregate. I will share more about my choices that help to keep my weight in check, while based here in Liberia. The concept of meal replacement should not be reduced to the concentrated powder sold in a pouch or as liquid in a can. Owning the process of choosing what we eat, focusing on local foods that are in season, is an important step. This will help us to know which of our foods bring the health benefits we are looking for. Either way, regardless of our dietary preferences and choices, an adjustment in carb intake is required in order to stop fat accumulation around the waistline.

My specific steps to manage carb intake

Similar to my approach to managing my sugar intake, I started out with the wrong assumptions. By the time weight became an issue, our carb choices were mostly organic, so I thought the changes I would need to make would be simple and straightforward. It turned out to be a bit more complicated as I started going deeper, making changes in carb consumption and adjusting one layer at a time.

Restricting processed carbs: Before I started restricting certain types of carb, I could not imagine that the pancake flour, as plain as it was before we had added anything to it to create the batter, could be a problem.

We consumed two to three relatively large pancakes whenever we made them, using eggs, sugar, milk and flour and sometimes butter. When the kids allowed it, we substituted white flour with whole wheat or mixed the two for increased fiber. I felt that by making them from scratch rather than using quick mixes such as the Aunt Jemima's brand would make a difference. And I believe it did, even though I now know it was not the best option in healthy eating, especially when I used white flour to make them. The quick mixes are convenient. They only require an addition of an egg or two, some milk, and a little bit of oil (or not) beaten together to make the batter. By making pancakes from scratch, I was sure to control the amount of sugar I added, usually less than what the recipe called for. Either way, between the sugar added to the batter and the syrup, bananas or strawberries on top, we definitely had our share of carb consumption at the start of our day. Thankfully, we had pancakes primarily on the weekend, when we had a more relaxed morning to prepare them. Cold cereal filled the gap the other days.

When I started restricting processed carbs, I continued limiting the amount of sugar we consumed, as well. My baseline initially was a can of coca cola, which contains as many as six teaspoons or 24 grams of sugar, in the form of high fructose corn syrup. I learned gradually to limit the amount of added sugar to no more than what I would add to a cup of tea, when I used to drink black tea. Two teaspoons or eight grams was my threshold. This worked when I chose processed foods, with a list of ingredients that included sugar in them. I learned to avoid processed foods with a long list of ingredients, even when my awareness level of what it meant to eat right for one's body was very low.

What I did then helped me to avoid those foods that Mark Hyman calls the "hyperprocessed, highly palatable, intensely addictive foods" supplied by "the industrial food complex" (17). Avoiding such foods with a long list of ingredients was a fact that even my kids had internalized and became a non-negotiable when selecting their own snacks or treats. When I look at the ingredients in some of them, including graham crackers and other brands of kids' snacks these days, I shake my head in disbelief that I actually used to buy them, eat them, and feed them to my kids! What type of artificial flavor is added to the popular Nabisco brand? And why not make the choice clear to consumers so that they know which oil was used to make the crackers instead of leaving up to us to make the call based on the list of ingredients that include "soybean and/or canola oil"? What if I can handle one and not the other? The devil is often in the details. Graham crackers were one of the first foods I gave to my kids when they were teething. A carrot would have been a better option, but what did I know? There certainly are other healthier choices as well.

Once a processed food passed the test, in terms of having a shorter list of ingredients, regardless of what these were, then I checked the amount of added sugar. Often, I failed to check the amount of sugar when buying organic snacks, especially when they were advertised as high in fiber or protein. I focused on these two and less on what the rest of the nutrition facts meant. I did not know enough to pay attention to the total amount of carbs then and remained focused on avoiding sugar to the best of my knowledge and ability. Though my full awareness of the real benefits of protein came much later, I knew that fiber on the other hand was good and the higher the amount, the better. This remains true, for the most part. Too much of a good thing can also backfire. Sugar and fiber were therefore the two initial factors I took into consideration when deciding whether or not I should buy a processed carb or whether I should look for a better alternative with less sugar and more fiber. The problem is that many carbs, including rice or pasta or even Irish potatoes, do not necessarily have added sugar. I ate these regularly and could not imagine that there could be anything I should have been concerned with, in any dietary plan.

Could I and the rest of the world be getting it wrong? I did not want to believe it. Either way, these carb choices counted among those "sabotaging [my] brain chemistry, [my] waistlines" (Hyman 17). To succeed, I needed to gain a better understanding of how carbs convert to sugar. Glucose is the body tissues' preferred source of energy. Of the two main types of carbohydrates, simple and complex, simple carbs trigger the highest and fastest increase in blood sugar and consequently the highest release of insulin. As noted in the previous chapter, sugar is a simple carbohydrate. It has one or two sugar molecules that are broken down easily by the body for use as a quick source of energy. Table sugar is the ultimate example of this. Complex carbohydrates on the other hand contain three or more sugar molecules making it harder to break down. Cooking and chewing them allow us to digest them better. Still, they release sugar into the bloodstream as well, but they do so slowly and steadily and as they do, they allow the body to absorb the nutrients they supply.

In normal amounts, sugar in the blood is beneficial as a quick source of energy. Many food sources of sugar are also healthy. Mother's breastmilk, the best first food, is a sweet but healthful source of nutrients for the delicate digestive system of a newborn and infant. It is one of the healthiest sweet foods ever available to human beings, and it contains healthy amounts of fat as well. In moderation, many food sources of sugar are also healthy, including the sugar that is released from complex carbohydrates such as fruits, starchy vegetables, grains, nuts, and legumes. The vitamins, minerals, enzymes and proteins in them assist the body in metabolizing sugar, causing it to be less harmful.

Ultimately, we were not meant to consume any food, including complex carbs, all year round, but instead we were supposed to enjoy them when they were in season and available in abundance, with some months of break from them when they were out of season.

Therefore, even with their health benefits, complex carbs can increase the overall amount of sugar absorbed with each meal, depending on individual sensitivity to insulin. Excess sugar, regardless of the source, whether from simple or complex carbs is not stored as an easily accessible source of energy to be used as needed. It is stored in fat cells and contributes to expanding our overall structure, and especially our waistline consistently when no effort is made to stop it. Carb restriction in our diet is one way to put a break on this expansion.

A targeted focus on fiber: One of the ways I distinguished one source of complex carb from another was to pay attention to their fiber content. As a rule of thumb, a minimum of 12 percent fiber was what I looked for on the nutrition facts label, to help me decide whether or not to buy a food. Twelve percent fiber content in a processed and packaged food source of carbs served as the baseline upon which I determined its worth and value. Once I was comfortable with this level of awareness, I shifted my attention to recognizing fiber content in terms of the number of grams in the food, based on a serving size. I had to do this because sometimes the percent was not included on the nutrition facts label. So, a food that had less than 3 grams of fiber did not meet my basic fiber standards. This is the same as 12 percent of fiber per serving of a specific food. In a general sense, the higher the fiber, the healthier the food was at this stage of my awareness.

Replacing most simple carbs with complex ones was meant to increase the amount of fiber in the foods I prepared. So, at home, we gradually shifted from white rice, white bread and white pasta for our go-to starch, to brown rice, whole wheat bread and whole wheat pasta mostly. Anyone raising kids knows, however, that they are not going to buy into this idea that we must eat whole wheat pasta mostly and that white pasta must be avoided or limited. So, with the kids, we negotiated that we would alternate between the two types of pasta, letting them have white pasta off and on, as they desired. The taste is not the same. I knew that, and I wanted to be flexible with them as I continued to pay attention to all the other adjustments that I needed to make so that my carb choices and intake would work best for me. Was eating whole wheat pasta, or brown rice or other carbs that I considered to have higher fiber contents, what I needed to lose weight and shrink my waistline? Not exactly. Nonetheless, understanding fiber better helped me justify the importance of eating complex carbs rather than simple ones, even to my kids.

Complex carbs are either unprocessed or minimally processed and they are the main suppliers of fiber. This makes carbs an important component of a healthy diet. Fiber has no nutritional value of its own, but it is beneficial in many other ways. It makes us feel fuller for longer, which can prevent overeating and snacking between meals. Depending on which we choose, snacks can significantly promote weight gain, adding to our overall calorie intake and a less efficient metabolism. On its website, WebMD summarizes the benefits of fiber: "Fiber helps you manage your weight, lowers cholesterol, keeps your bowel movements regular, and reduces your odds of getting diabetes and heart disease." Therefore, the idea is not to give up complex carbs altogether, but rather to focus on those that work best in supporting a healthy metabolism and a healthy weight.

A focus on net carbs: My next level of awareness came when I started comparing the total amount of carbs with the total amount of fiber to understand what impacted blood sugar and weight. By subtracting the total carb content from total fiber content, I was able to get the actual picture of the net carb. So, a food with a relatively high total-carb content but a low-net carb content because of its high fiber would create a low impact on insulin, a fat storage hormone. I came to value this simple equation: Total Carb - Fiber = Net Carb. This net carb is what matters when it comes to eating right for blood sugar control and preventing weight gain.

Placing my carbs on the glycemic index: I reached another level of awareness of the impact of carbs on blood sugar, when I was introduced to a tool known as the glycemic index. I started working with this index to make wiser carb choices. The glycemic index ranks foods based on a scale that goes from 0 to around 100. The closer to 100 a food is on this scale, the higher the GI of a food. I took a systematic approach that involved checking the glycemic index of the starchy foods I ate often and ranking them based on their status on this index. I focused on the foods I was eating at least two to three times per week. I relied on the online resource found at SELFNutritionData on the nutritiondata.self.com website to identify the glycemic index of the foods listed below with their GI. Another useful resource that identifies the GI of common foods is a Harvard Health Publications online article which includes a "[g]lycemic index of 60+ foods".

Flour-based foods and grains on the glycemic index
- Breads: whole wheat or whole grain bread: 74
- Brown rice: 50-68 (depending on source)
- Whole wheat pasta: mid-50s (depending on how you cook it. Al dente is best, releasing sugar more slowly)
- Quinoa: 53
- Gluten-free bread: 90

Legumes
- Black beans: 30
- Navy beans: 54
- Lentils: 32
- Garbanzo beans: 28-33

Starchy vegetables
- Potatoes (boiled): 78- 85
- Sweet potatoes (boiled): 61-63
- Butternut squash: 50
- Pumpkin: 64-75
- Plantain/Green bananas: 65
- Green peas: 68
- Carrots (boiled): 39

Snacks

- Hummus: 6
- Baby carrots: 71
- Green apple: 36

Regardless of how I sliced and diced it, my overall carb intake ranked high on the glycemic index. Simply put, I consumed unhealthy amounts of carbs. Had I stopped there in my quest for foods that are blood-sugar friendly, I would have dropped a few of the foods with a high or medium GI and, at the same time, I would have sacrificed their health benefits.

Foods with a GI below 55 are considered low GI. Those between 56-69 are moderate GI and those 70 and higher are high GI foods. Like peeling an onion, with each layer I removed came another layer that required further research and understanding. Just as I had never counted many of these foods as my carb sources when planning meals, there are several I assumed to be healthy low-carb choices but still added to my overall carb intake at each meal. Legumes such as beans, lentils and chickpeas are a case in point. There also are some moderate and even high GI carbs that turned out to be not as bad as they looked on the surface of this GI scale. I came to this conclusion after I was introduced to another tool known as the glycemic load.

Comparing the glycemic index and the glycemic load: Searching for the best carbs in my quest to shrink belly fat led me to another tool that most accurately assesses the actual effect of a food on blood sugar. This tool is the glycemic load. While the glycemic index assumes a serving of 50 grams of carbohydrates, which may apply to only a few of the foods on my list, the glycemic load takes into account the actual serving size and the carb content based on that serving. Let's use baby carrots as an example. With a glycemic index of 71, I would be tempted to give them up assuming they are going to raise my blood sugar too high and too fast. However, even if I ate a full cup of baby carrots, which I would rarely do, the amount of carbs in these would be about 16 grams. The glycemic load of these carrots would equal 16 x .71. This gives us a value of a little less than 12, which is moderate GL. Note that a GL of 10 or less is low, between 11-19 is moderate and 20 or more is high GL. Based on my actual consumption of baby carrots, I would most certainly keep my consumption of them to a low GL value. Having them with hummus, a naturally low GI food, does not substantially change their impact on my blood sugar. The same principle applies to other foods on my list of starchy vegetables and particularly pumpkins, a fruit that is eaten as a vegetable by many. I never consume as much as a full cup, which is the measure used for determining its glycemic load.

Removing gluten and dairy: As my diet continued to evolve (and it still does!), I took two additional steps after hearing a lecture by Donna Gates and then reading her co-authored *Body Ecology Diet* book. She introduced me to the world of food sensitivities and how they manifest themselves inside and even outside our bodies. I always had been intrigued by the symptoms I saw in my husband, in particular. Conventional prescriptions were not effective, so I decided to try a gluten-free and dairy-free diet on him in 2013. The results were amazing! For the first time since we met in 1991, his chronic runny nose cleared. Within a few weeks, he no longer needed to keep a handkerchief in his pocket. His cough, triggered by any subtle change in the environment, stopped. His eczema that came and went even after treatment with steroids and antibiotics, improved gradually, leaving him with healthy-looking fingernails. He had suffered from eczema since his college years, about 30 years earlier, he said. Today, there are occasional symptoms on one thumb and one big toenail.

There are always possibilities of food cross-contamination when we eat out, and there might be other dietary and environmental triggers that we might not be aware of yet to explain the occasional flare-ups on the thumb and toenail. All the other improvements we have seen in him continue to date. Even his receding hair line has stopped, slowing down the balding head that came as a surprise in his late 20s, when a young boy, the son of a friend from Zanzibar looked at him and exclaimed, "Uncle Paul, *hii ni nini* [what is this]?" The new hair growth, fueled most likely by the dietary changes we made, is long enough now to cover some of the bald spot on the back of his head.

He also lost nearly 20 pounds and has been able to keep this weight off. His snoring also got better. We did not need a medical diagnosis to confirm these results. He felt better. He looked better. We were all pleased, and we knew we needed no more incentives to maintain these changes. Given that I was the one preparing most of our meals, I ended up supporting him by going on a gluten-free and dairy-free diet, as well, although I reintroduced dairy, off and on, especially milk kefir and raw cheese when I could find it, which now is limited to just a few times a year.

Did these changes help me lose weight? Possibly. At this point, I was implementing several new habits at the same time. With my husband, we had eliminated all foods that were not labelled gluten-free from our diet. We removed white and whole wheat pasta and all breads made with wheat flour from the foods that we ate. For a change, we found brown-rice pasta, a gluten-free choice, to be "acceptable" on the culinary scale. Gluten-free bread was also becoming easier to find, and we used these for sandwiches at lunch sometimes. We stopped eating regular oatmeal and other cereals for breakfast. We gave up bagels and cream cheese.

We also snacked less as gluten-free options we enjoyed were not as plentiful as wheat-based ones. We replaced regular milk with almond or rice milk to go with our gluten-free cereal. In addition to brown rice, we started eating quinoa, millet, and amaranth, three gluten-free seed-like grains that I learned from the co-authored *Body Ecology Diet* book. We minimized sugar intake, giving up ice cream and many wheat-based desserts. We were going for regular walks, as well. I did lose some weight but I could not tell how much of it was triggered by removing dairy and gluten and how much came from a combination of factors that blended diet and lifestyle in the mix. Still, none of these efforts brought me to the waistline I wanted. So, the search continued.

Managing servings: A more accurate understanding of how many carbs I was consuming required a grasp of what an actual serving was. Up until I reached this new level of awareness, I counted a full plate as a serving, with carbs covering one half and vegetables the other. I never was a heavy meat eater; even when I had the opportunity to indulge, meat was never something that I ate in excess. Perhaps meat was the only food group I was eating in moderation, skipping it when I was not in the mood for it or adding it to flavor the rest of the food rather than having a real serving. So, there you have it, a regular size plate, as a baseline for a meal. My full plate gave me more than enough carbs, especially when the vegetables I had were also starchy, and my protein of choice was beans or lentils. Going for seconds did not just give me a second serving, as you may realize. In many cases, it was giving me a third serving of carbs in one meal, especially at dinner time.

This pattern of eating was not unique to me. There still are many who define a meal by how full a plate is. It is paradoxical because even at my level of awareness, I still feel sometimes tempted to tell people to get more when they take what I consider small servings. What looks like small servings are more accurate representations of how we should all be eating when we have not outstretched our stomachs. Easy access to carbs everywhere in the world makes it possible for us to overeat. Counting servings based on how much one can fit on a dinner plate is a dangerous way of eating, especially when what's on the plate is mostly carbs, even unprocessed ones. Nonetheless, a plate full of leafy green vegetables is not the same as one full of starchy carbs when it comes to their effects on weight and blood sugar. And an excessive consumption of red meat, chicken, or even fish is simply not sustainable. So, here is what my typical first serving at dinner looked like:

- 1 cup (estimate) of rice or pasta, or several small potatoes (2-3 servings), often covering at least half of the plate (about 90 grams of total carbs);
- 1/2 cup of beans or lentils (about 20 grams of total carbs). I ate less when added to meat or fish;
- 1 cup of cooked vegetables, non-starchy choices such broccoli, cabbage, cauliflower, or sauteed string beans and/or starchy varieties such as peas and carrots (or a large serving of salad when available). Amount of carbs varied depending on choice; and
- 1 cup of mixed fruits with breakfast and/or for desert after dinner.

Note that except for the animal proteins (meat, chicken and fish) and the non-starchy vegetables, the other food choices were starches with direct effect on blood sugar. Depending on our fruit choices and what we ate with them, we easily pushed our carb consumption over healthy limits. The nutrition facts label helped me again on this journey. I checked for the number of servings in a packaged food before estimating how much I should be eating at any given meal. So, if a package contained six servings, I knew that having it all over only three equal meals meant that I was having two servings each time. If each serving for example, provided 47 grams of total carbs, with two servings, I would have to count 47g x 2 = 94 grams of carbs. Given our habit of eating legumes as our main source of protein or as a side dish, they could easily add another 20 grams of carbs to my meal, as well. Adding fruits for desert after dinner meant that I could easily have nearly half of my carb requirement in my largest meal of the day, dinner. Evenings are the time when we need the least amounts of calories to sustain us, but that is not how I ate.

My intake of carbs was simply excessive, even before I had weight issues. Estimates based on the number of servings in a package are good enough if you rely on it to guide you before you serve yourself. Sometimes a serving is the equivalent of a cup, sometimes it is half or even a quarter. I started making it my goal to stay as close to the recommended serving size as possible, or to have less than a serving of carbs, in order to reach my weight goals faster. It helped. Another useful tool I found on MyPlate.gov website has come in handy in this regard as well, as it divides the plate in 4 portions. On one half, it has vegetables and fruits. The other half is divided in two, with 1/4 or less for protein and the other 1/4 for grains. Because I often skip fruits to limit my sugar intake, I generally double the vegetables in the half that holds fruits and vegetables according to MyPlate.gov guide. This generally helps me keep my carb consumption under control. The weight gain of mid-life called for additional adjustments to my carb choices as my knowledge continued to increase.

Switching to whole unprocessed carbs: Gradually, I shifted away from almost all processed foods to focus more on whole foods, not the name of the upscale chain food store in the United States, but the types of foods that we eat as nature produces them. These foods have not gone through any level of transformation that turns them into a different food product, often with added ingredients to add bulk, enhance flavor, and/or to increase profit margins for an otherwise denatured food. As an example, we can think of the difference between an apple and an apple pie, a carrot and a carrot cake, a banana and a banana nut bread. We can think of brown rice as opposed to rice milk as well. And whole almond nuts are not the same as blanched almonds or almond flour, nor are soybeans the same as soy milk or soy protein isolates.

Such processed foods may still contain the natural whole food ingredient in significant amounts, but what's added or removed is what will determine how wholesome the pie, cake, bread, milk, flour or isolate is in the end, as compared to the unprocessed food in its natural form. Even whole wheat bread is not the same as whole wheat grains. With the bread, there is often something else added. Also, whole wheat bread is often better than wheat bread that often looks like white bread, even if it might be made from wheat flour. With white bread or even wheat bread that is not whole wheat-based, something has been removed from the whole grain of wheat to produce the final bread product, with a few other ingredients added often to enhance flavor, add bulk or to prevent mold.

Thousands of processed food choices are sold as containing natural ingredients, but without knowing what these ingredients are, it is easy to be fooled by marketing gimmicks. Once a food is processed, it loses many health benefits of the whole food and what's added rarely makes up for what's removed. The other issue with processed foods, and especially highly processed foods, is that they lose the fiber and its many benefits as mentioned above. Lack of fiber in a food makes it quickly raise blood sugar, cause hunger faster, and also feeds yeast.

When I switched to whole unprocessed carb sources, quinoa became a regular grain in our diet. It is a good source of fiber, with 3 grams in each serving. I prefer quinoa to brown rice also because it is a good source of proteins as well. Millet and amaranth are also our other sources of gluten-free seed-like grains that we rely on when we can find them. I even started mixing these gluten-free grains and cooking a pot of hot cereal that we would then have for up to a week at a time. We eat these in the place of processed cereals in boxes that we ate prior to this increased awareness of the higher value of whole unprocessed foods. Were these beneficial in terms of supporting weight loss and shrinking belly fat? Not really, at least not in my case initially. More adjustments were needed. What were they? Skipping all carbs altogether, even for a few days at a time, as some experts recommend, left me lacking sufficient energy to make it through the day without taking a nap. I also had muscle cramps at night when I skipped starches completely for several continuous days. This was therefore not practical for me, but I still had a few other options. Keep reading!

Replacing whole grains with root and starchy vegetables: Informed by Mark Hyman's book *The Blood Sugar Solution 10-Day Detox Diet*, I decided to try his recommendations to remove all grain-based foods from my diet to see if I would notice any change in my weight and blood sugar control. I slowed down on quinoa, brown rice and other gluten-free grains, having them once instead of three times a day, sometimes skipping them completely and opting for other starchy foods. In the place of grains, I would eat one of the following: winter squash, pumpkin, red skin potatoes, sweet potatoes or yams, green or unripe bananas, or cassava root. I gave up Irish potatoes, a high glycemic index food that makes it easy to eat more than a serving at once. This step worked the best out of all the other attempts I had made to control carb intake and its impact on my weight. I did this because as Hyman notes, "all grains ... even gluten-free ones - can spike blood sugar and insulin." My goal was to follow his advice to "shut down insulin production as much as possible" (78). Remember insulin is good at storing fat.

Removing grains brought me another step closer to a breakthrough. What I noticed was that whenever I ate grain-based starches, even "healthy" choices such as quinoa or brown rice, within a couple of weeks the few pounds I lost started creeping back. When I got off grain-based carbs for a few days, my weight started normalizing again. I have tried this way of eating many times, off and on, and I see the same results each time. I now know that to stop myself from this carb-induced weight gain, I have to limit my intake of carbs and especially remove grain-based carbs until I return to the weight I want. From there, I am careful not to get carried away again and keep controlling grain-based carbs in my diet by limiting them to one serving per day. This has enabled me to better control my overall weight. Reducing my frequency of consumption of grain-based carbs helps me to consistently maintain a low GL diet, to continue supporting my weight loss goals. I get my sources of energy, primarily from eating fish or chicken, and occasionally red meat for protein. Moderate amounts of nuts and seeds are my other sources of energy as well as healthy sources of fat that are low in carbs. I continue to eat a limited amount of fruits, though not every day, and I eat large servings of non-starchy vegetables, for the vitamins and minerals they provide, while also supporting my caloric and micronutrient needs.

Adding winter squash, pumpkins, and even green bananas and cassava root to my list of preferred starches has improved my ability to keep my blood sugar in check, partly because I never need to consume more than a serving of these in one meal. Although pumpkins rank high on the glycemic index at 75, their glycemic load is low because what counts as a full serving is more than I can consume in one meal. Registered Nurse and nutrition expert Anne Tourney discusses the impact of pumpkins on blood sugar based on the following consumption estimates: "About four-fifths of a cup of pumpkin contains only 4 g of carbohydrates - and has a glycemic load of 3. A total of 4 g of carbohydrates represents 5 percent of the total content of a serving of pumpkin, which means you would have to consume a large amount of boiled pumpkin to increase your blood sugar significantly." This is the best way to understand their metabolic effect because the glycemic load, as noted earlier, accounts for the carb content, the serving size, and the glycemic index of the food. Pumpkin is now one of the few starchy vegetables I rely on to keep myself on a low-carb diet, and to limit regular consumption of grain-based carbs as well as their impact on my weight and my blood sugar. Knowing my specific carb tolerance and diversifying my choices have made such a big difference in my ability to keep a healthy weight.

The additional benefit of this step is that it no longer requires the extra effort of double-checking each food's GI and calories. I rarely need to eat as much of the non-grain based starches, such as pumpkins, sweet potatoes, or green bananas, as I needed to feel satisfied when I focused on grains such as rice, pasta, potatoes, or even quinoa. I no longer need to worry about raising my blood sugar and insulin caused by high carb foods, especially grains. When I plan a meal, I ensure that my total carb intake stays within the limits of a serving. If I have prepared more than one source of carb, such as winter squash or pumpkins (as my starch) with lentils (as a vegetarian protein), I make sure that the vegetable of choice to go with the meal is a non-starchy one, such as spinach, broccoli, cauliflower or cabbage. Lentils and pumpkins are both significant carb sources, but by having less than a serving of each, I know I will be able to stay within the carb consumption limits that my body can tolerate without spiking my blood sugar levels. Sometimes I have a small cup of lentil soup as my source of carb, with an egg or chicken leg and lots of non-starchy vegetables for a very low-carb meal, especially at lunch. Midday seems to be a time when I tend to react to carbs more than I do in the morning, for example. I must always pay attention to how I combine foods and to serving sizes to create meals that are satisfying without affecting my blood sugar almost instantly or causing other medium- to long-term effects on my weight and my health.

Increasing animal protein: Following Mary Dan Eades and Michael R. Eades' recommendations in *The 6 Week Cure for the Middle-Aged Middle*, I learned the importance of including animal protein consistently while taking necessary efforts to shrink belly fat. The Eades informed my choices and contributed further to the knowledge I needed to support my success. The book focuses specifically on what it takes to shrink belly fat in midlife, for both men and women. The timeframe is shorter than what I experienced, partly because dietary changes happen in the context of other aspects of our lives. When you are the one who prepares meals for your family, which is my case, it will most likely take longer than six weeks to reach your goals because you have to also keep the dietary needs of other family members into consideration. When you add food sensitivities in the mix, you have to be even more flexible with your choices.

An important lesson I gained from *The 6 Week Cure for the Middle-Aged Middle* was related to the importance of adding animal protein to meals (while also limiting carb intake) as a strategy for better management of insulin and its fat storage effects. The Eades define insulin's role as "designed to drive nutrients (glucose, amino acids, and fats) into the tissues ... play[ing] a minute-by-minute job [of keeping] glucose from accumulating in the blood after meals in part by accelerating its entry into the cells to either be burned for energy or stored for later use, but chiefly by suppressing the liver's ability to make glucose." Knowing this helped me to internalize the importance of protein in countering the effects of insulin. Proteins, according to the Eades, in fact "cause an anti-balancing release of insulin's opposing hormone, glucagon, and thus the net hormonal consequence is quite different from consuming carbohydrates" (29).

Eating a meal that contains protein, fat and fiber is one of the best ways to start your day, Magdalena Wszelaki counsels in her *Cooking for Hormonal Balance* course and book. Her farmer's wife breakfast is a combination of lamb sausage cooked in ghee (a good fat if dairy is your thing), fresh green mix and fermented vegetables for fiber (with olive oil and apple cider vinegar for dressing). Add a few slices of avocado (a good fat as well) and *voilà*. Wszelaki is a strong proponent of a diet based on protein, fiber and fat, and this is a type of diet that continues to inform my food choices as well. Such low-cab meals prevent insulin from being released, a key step in blood sugar and weight management.

Nonetheless, animal proteins and fats are both higher calorie foods than carbs per gram of serving, and they take longer to digest. So, it is important not to assume that one needs the same amount of proteins and fats as one needed of carbs, especially when using a dinner plate as a measure for how much one should consume. With proteins and fats, less of these will still go a long way. Paying attention to serving sizes will help in this regard. On average, we only need about 50 grams of protein per day. As for fat, we need anywhere between 44-78 grams total fats and of these, only 22 grams should be from saturated fat sources, according to Registered Dietician Katherine Zeratsky in an article on the Mayo Clinic website.

Protein Power, also by Eades and Eades, highlights further the benefits of protein in a balanced diet, which helps to:

- Modulate the body's metabolic hormones, including insulin;
- Control the storage of fat;
- Direct the flow of amino acids, fatty acids, and carbohydrates to the tissues;

- Regulate the liver's synthesis of cholesterol;
- Function as a growth hormone;
- Control appetite; and
- Drive the kidneys to retain fluid.

By modulating insulin, protein plays a role in the prevention of a cluster of diseases known as metabolic syndrome, which is associated with the development of cardiovascular disease and type 2 diabetes, as noted earlier. As diabetes runs in my family, I do not take it lightly, knowing how devastating it was for my parents. Eades and Eades consider elevated insulin as "a primary cause of or a significant risk factor for high blood pressure, heart disease, obesity, elevated cholesterol, and other blood fats, and diabetes"(6). Since legumes are significant sources of carbs, they are not the best choices when it comes to protecting the body from a surge of insulin and its long-term effects, especially when combined in a meal with rice or another starchy food, the way of eating in many cultures, including the one in which I was raised. I now know that I cannot rely on plant proteins such as legumes to control blood sugar. While they are also a good source of fiber, their carb content can make them less desirable on a low-carb diet.

Therefore, the only sources of proteins that will not directly increase carb intake are animal proteins. However, increasing animal protein can cause the body to become acidic. Heartburn is one of the ways I know that my meal was acidifying. If you are a vegan and you need to lower carb consumption, it may be challenging for you to do so without adding some source of animal protein. Even adding eggs can make a difference. Replacing carbs with some animal protein, and some good fats from almonds, ground flax seeds or an avocado, continue to help me maintain healthy caloric requirements while staying on a diet that minimize carbs' impact on my blood sugar and my weight. Without animal proteins, it is easy to overconsume carbs with each meal to feel satisfied for at least a few hours at a time. Any excess of carbs, beyond what the body needs as an immediate source of energy, will be stored as fat. Belly fat, here I come!

Adding good fats: Adding good fats as another important source of calories and energy also has contributed to balancing meals without the need to overconsume carbs. Nevertheless, replacing carbs with an increased intake of some good sources of fat may not be feasible for everyone, either. Coconut oil, for example, is a good fat for some, not others. Some highly respected health professionals including Mark Hyman swear by it. However, I am still careful not to overdo it in my diet because I notice that its high saturated fat content does not work for me. I prefer avocadoes and almonds that also contain fiber. When I use it for cooking, I take a probiotic with lipase and other digestive enzymes, and this helps me enjoy it and a few other sources of beneficial fat that would be harder to digest otherwise. In my case, fats sometimes cause constipation. I will discuss the benefits of fats further in Chapter 5. For now, let's keep in mind that the three macronutrients, protein, fat, and carbohydrates each brings its own health benefits, but in the context of weight management, excess carbs contribute most directly to weight gain. Their intake must be managed carefully when weight is an issue. Many of the most popular diets and ways of eating in many cultures are high in carbs, and such diets remain among the biggest health challenges of our time, making it particularly challenging for women in midlife to maintain a healthy weight. This is because all other changes that take place during this life stage make it also easier to accumulate fat around the waistline, as we will discuss further throughout the rest of the book.

Increasing non-starchy vegetables: Being able to load up on non-starchy vegetables has become an easy solution in my attempt to balance meals without affecting insulin. Non-starchy vegetables help to lower acidity that meat can cause. These vegetables also supply various micronutrients. Consuming enough fresh foods that contain their own natural enzymes helps to alkalize the body. Vegetables contain very limited amounts of carbs, and unlike all other carb choices and even other macronutrients, the risk of overeating vegetables is rare for most people, including those of us who are veggie-lovers. It would be quite an exception for anyone to eat enough to trigger insulin. While these vegetables add little to our caloric needs, they provide vitamins and minerals, the micronutrients that are essential for health, perform many cellular functions, and are involved in the regulation of metabolism. Although we need them only in tiny amounts, micronutrients are, according to the World Health Organization (WHO) website, "the 'magic wands' that enable the body to produce enzymes, hormones and other substances essential for proper growth and development." Eades and Eades add that micronutrients' functions, include "the efficient use and disposal of the macronutrients" (3-4). Joel Fuhrman concurs that a diet rich in green vegetables has health-promoting benefits, including the ability to help the body to reach a healthy weight: "To achieve superior health and a permanently thin physique, you should eat large portions of green foods.... Eating large portions of these super-healthy foods is the key to your success" (75).

Surprise! Reintroducing resistant starch: You may recall in the previous chapter on sugar that an important lesson I learned from Donna Gates' lecture (and book) was to remove from our diet foods that feed yeast. Sugar was the main target but it was not alone. Other foods, especially processed carbs or even unprocessed ones when overconsumed or not combined properly in a meal, have the ability to cause digestive discomforts. This, in turn, creates an environment for the bad bacteria to proliferate and multiply, while depriving the good bacteria of the nutrients they need to support proper digestion, a strong immune system, and good overall health. One of the foods included on the list of foods to remove from our shopping list was white Irish potatoes. While I did not consider myself as an excessive potato consumer, especially since I moved to the United States in 1991, I ate potatoes frequently before then, either boiled or sautéed. What's the problem with potatoes, you may ask? They are a high glycemic index food, with one medium potato containing 26 grams of carbs and only 2 grams of fiber, according to the livescience.com website. Consuming more than this, is more of the norm than the exception. Therefore, depending on the level of tolerance of carbs, potatoes can quickly elevate blood sugar in the body, hence feeding yeast. As we'll learn later, yeast overgrowth is linked to resistance to weight loss.

However, cooked and cooled potatoes become a source of resistant starch that feed the good bacteria. Joseph Mercola writes that "digestive-resistant starches - found in chilled, cooked potatoes, seeds, tapioca starch and unripe tropical fruits such as banana, papaya, and mango - can be considered a ... type of starch, differentiated from insoluble fiber by the fact that many of their benefits result from the fermentation process that occurs as they move through your large intestine." He adds that "like insoluble fiber, digestive-resistant starch is not broken down as it travels through your digestive tract and therefore adds bulk to your stool. They're also powerful prebiotics. By slowly fermenting in your large intestine, they feed gut bacteria that support optimal health." I learned how to make a cold salad with red potatoes in cubes that I spice and roast, and then set them aside. Once cooled, I store them in the fridge, and then I eat a few cubes with other foods as part of a meal or on their own, with a tablespoon or two of sauerkraut, a little olive oil and salt as a snack and to feed the good bacteria. For the same reason, I also now make a green papaya salad, especially when in Liberia, where papayas can be easily found all year round. I have come to favor foods that feed good bacteria and consistently include them in my diet.

My other go-to snack these days is cold green banana that I cook with the skin on. Then, before I eat it, I remove the skin and bake it to dry up all the liquid for a crispier snack. I will discuss further the benefits of probiotics and prebiotics in the next chapter. For now, it is important to keep in mind that many sources of carbs are beneficial beyond supplying a good and easily accessible source of energy. Digestive-resistant starches are still starches, but when prepared and consumed appropriately, they are less impactful on blood sugar. What a nice surprise!

CONCLUSION

Making carbs work for me includes the important step of maintaining a balanced diet that replaces certain carbs with others that are less impactful on weight and blood sugar. Low carb diets require getting the needed calories from the two other sources of macronutrients, namely fats and proteins. Both are required for a balanced diet. However, as noted above, not everyone digests fats easily. Therefore, it's up to each of us to support our body to function at its best. Taking digestive enzymes has helped me tolerate fats without causing constipation, something that in the past had forced me to give up even some of my favorite sources of good fats such as avocadoes and almond nuts. By reducing carb consumption and focusing more on these two other macronutrients, along with a balanced supply of micronutrients from lots of non-starchy vegetables and small servings of fruits, is an important step in helping to stop unnecessary weight gain. For me, reducing carb intake was an important step in this process. Choosing carbs that least impact weight was another. Giving up certain carbs even temporarily is yet another way that we must be willing to take when the other steps do not seem to bring the results we are seeking. I did try this as well and I know it works but it can leave unwanted side effects such as low energy or leg cramps.

Not doing anything is not an option. It only makes matters worse because the body seems to have such an amazing ability to continue over-expanding if we do nothing to stop it. For women in midlife, the body does so by adding a layer of fat around the belly in particular (and/or the butt for some). On top of not liking ourselves in our favorite dresses when the waistline is expanded, belly fat is a health risk. Managing carb intake is critical to the success of shrinking belly fat.

When I eventually succeeded at understanding the different sources of carbs and choosing the ones that worked more effectively to shrink my waistline, I knew I had a story, a tool, and a resource to share. I want you to have access to this knowledge and information that can help you prevent some of the health risks associated with an over-expanding waistline. What I want to highlight, however, by taking you along my journey of managing carb intake, is that you can do yourself a favor by putting what I recommend into practice sooner, rather than later. Dietary changes, such as those rooted in restricting carb intake, can slow down or prevent the accumulation of fat around the waist in midlife, an important step in the prevention of type 2 diabetes and the diseases in the metabolic syndrome category.

I do not pretend to have created a resource that other women in midlife can use as a "copy and paste" guide, as we tend to assume. Instead, I want to provide a tool that must be adapted by those for whom the information shared resonates, first and foremost. Then, adapting to your situation becomes easier, as the foundational knowledge is what I share here. You can refer to the shopping list included at the end of the book, instead of having to create your own from scratch. This will save you time as you choose from the list of carbs, a few of which you may not have considered as carb choices before. My plan cannot be copied verbatim because my journey has required continuous adjustments in food choices based on a number of factors, including knowledge base, location and food availability, as well as trial and error. To make it work requires adaptability and flexibility. For example, since we moved to Liberia, I have given up on the attempt to find organic food choices. In fact, except for a small selection of imported frozen vegetables, I cannot find other organic foods here, and local food production and supply is, in my opinion, overall underdeveloped.

Ultimately, what I want you to walk away with is this simple message: *We must listen to our body, and help by giving it what it calls for to feel grounded and in balance.* Ever-expanding belly fat is a sure sign of imbalance and a body crying out for help.

Because there is no one-size-fits-all when it comes to our individual needs for food, supplying our body with the amount of carbs it needs for energy is an important step in embracing a responsive approach to eating right and maintaining a healthy weight.

Because of the changes that occur as women enter midlife and that many of us know so well, our dietary and other lifestyle choices must be geared towards recognizing that our specific needs are not the same as those we needed as younger adults. Specifically, the amounts of carbs we consumed in our younger years must be adjusted in midlife to prevent any excess calories from accumulating as fat around the middle. This is an important step I have taken to help me reach better results when many of the other changes I had undertaken weren't working. I remain committed to these dietary changes because I realize that shrinking my belly fat is no longer an aesthetic goal but a health goal, tied to my predisposition to type 2 diabetes. Adjusting carb intake was a key step to my success, and it is an important step in yours if you consume carbs daily and you want to shrink belly fat. Do what you can. Any step in the right direction is a good step!

CHAPTER 4:

NOURISH YOUR GUT WITH HEALING FOODS AND HABITS

In the *Body Ecology Diet*, Donna Gates and Linda Schatz describe fermented foods as the "missing link in all other systems of health" (13). My kids used to call them the stinky foods. And I can understand why, judging from the smell in our hotel room when they first made the comment. I had been sold on the importance of eating fermented foods regularly. So, I packed a jar of sauerkraut in the cooler we travelled with to keep supplements and a few snacks. The kids were not amused by the smell when they returned to our room after breakfast. I had just opened the jar to take my daily dose. *What is that smell? Did someone just fart?* I laughed and showed them what it was. They looked at me and asked: *And you eat that?* Needless to say, they left the room and waited outside for my husband and I to join them and proceed with our trip. And the questions they were asking were somewhat rhetorical because they knew my husband and I had been eating sauerkraut, religiously, daily, ever since I discovered it weeks earlier. But opening the jar of ferments from inside our kitchen at home with more room to absorb the smell did not create the same intense assault of their senses as it did in our hotel room, without a window to let in fresh air.

I was not raised to appreciate the benefits of fermented foods, and therefore, I did not raise my own kids to appreciate the taste and flavors of cultured foods. I learned at a much younger age however, about tending to a garden. I did not do much work on the farm during my youth, and I did not necessarily enjoy the little bit of work I did. I did, however, learn a lot by observing and helping when needed. I paid attention to the details of getting the soil ready for a new crop, planting, mulching, weeding, harvesting, and storage. Years later, I did start my own vegetable garden. I learned what it needed to thrive. I developed the skills I needed to do it right.

In a similar way, I have come to think of our gastrointestinal system as an inner garden that requires the same level of care and attention to bear the "fruits" of a strong immune system.

Reflecting on what I had to do to keep my garden healthy, when I was introduced to the importance of the gut and why we need to take care of it, the analogy of a well-tended garden came to mind. Taking care of the gut requires a similar level of diligence as tending to the garden that supplies the foods we eat.

The gut is a long tube that starts inside the mouth and extends all the way to the rectum. It plays many essential roles for us, including the intake and absorption of nutrients into our body. What we eat matters as it must pass through our entire gastrointestinal system - and help us either stay healthy and strong or make us struggle to maintain a healthy balance. It is this digestive process "that provides the building blocks the body needs to live, to function, and to stay healthy," notes Dr. Lisa Ganjhu from the New York University Langone School of Medicine. The health of the gut is dependent on a well-functioning digestive system. In fact, as a general rule of thumb, you must work on improving digestion of your food if you want to heal your gut and lose belly fat.

GENERAL STEPS TO IMPROVE DIGESTION

There are many habits that support a healthy digestive system, which is required for the health of the gut and overall health of the body. I will highlight six of them below as these are the ones that I apply consistently and that help me prevent constipation and acid reflux, two of the main symptoms of indigestion even when I was much younger.

Eat whole, unprocessed foods

Taking care of the gut requires choosing whole, unprocessed, fresh and local foods as much as possible. Whole foods are generally good sources of fiber, which feeds the good gut bacteria and not their opponents. Whole foods provide natural nutrients including vitamins and minerals that can get lost during processing and refining. Nutrient deficiencies are often linked with poor gut health and a weak immune system, which makes it easier for pathogens to proliferate. Eating a lot of fresh vegetables is beneficial as they contain their own enzymes, which make it easier to digest the vegetables and other foods that require the enzymes they provide. However, subjecting fresh vegetables to high heat during cooking can destroy some, if not most, of the enzymes they contain. Therefore, proper food preparation is key to preserving the nutrients in foods, while at the same time improving their digestibility. Soaking legumes prior to cooking for example, helps me digest them better than I used to before I learned about the phytic acid they contain that can make them hard to digest.

Add digestive helpers

Fermented foods and drinks, prebiotics, and digestive enzymes all offer gut-healing benefits and act as digestive helpers. As whole and raw foods, fermented vegetables are an excellent source of good bacteria that build a strong immune system, which in turn help to defeat pathogens including bacteria, fungi and worms, and protect us from getting sick when the pathogens invade. When vegetables are fermented, the process of fermentation increases their bio-availability as raw, nourishing and easy to digest foods. Undigested foods become breeding ground for yeasts, and other harmful pathogens in our gut, making us more susceptible to other infections. Undigested foods weaken our immune system as well. In fact, both good and bad bacteria are always present in and on our body. "Both good and bad bacteria scope out the territory and settle on the best spot for themselves and their families. And when you notice certain smells coming from your body, that's bad bacteria letting you know they've chosen to live under your arm, between your toes, or in your mouth" (Pescatore and Gazella 34).

- helping to digest foods;
- processing and manufacturing important vitamins;
- managing and eliminating toxic substances; and
- killing harmful bacteria" (Pesatore and Gazella 34).

The good bacteria are "some of the hardest working molecules in the human body ... perform[ing] a wide range of important tasks that include:

As "live" foods, fermented foods are increasingly recognized as important "super foods". Joseph Mercola writes that "eating fermented foods can help improve your gut health by 'reseeding' your gut with beneficial bacteria. In turn, the bacteria convert sugars and starch into lactic acid, a process called lacto-fermentation, boosting the nutritional content of the food and producing essential amino acids, short-chain fatty acids and beneficial enzymes, and increasing the bioavailability of minerals." Fermented vegetables are on top of my list of gut-friendly foods that I consume regularly whenever I can access them. The combination of eating fermented vegetables and taking probiotics enable me to harvest the many health dividends described above – and more.

I don't remember exactly when and who had recommended probiotics to me previously, but I do remember that I discontinued using them because I was not convinced that they worked without leaving behind any future side effects. I did not want to become dependent on them, either. And there was a part of me that considered them - and all supplements - as disguised pharmaceuticals. While I thought that probiotics may be better versions of the pharmaceutical products we take as medicines, I was not sure how effective they really were. This is why I did not trust probiotics enough to take them on a regular basis. I often ended up holding onto them beyond their expiration dates and throwing them away. Cash in trash! What did I know?

Understanding the importance of fermentation and recognizing that quality probiotics may supply some of the benefits we get from fermented vegetables, I decided to give them a try again. I now choose them carefully, paying attention particularly to the diversity of strains, with more being better. Obviously, I follow the instructions on the box of these supplements. The higher the strains of bacteria in a probiotic supplement, the more likely it will supply some of strains that match with individual gut health needs. As a rule of thumb and based on many expert recommendations, I look for those with at least ten different strains of beneficial bacteria. I have tried one with as many as 85 strains as well and it contains enzymes that help me digest fat better.

Fermented vegetables enhance digestion of fats and overall nutrient absorption inside the intestines. "The microflora in fermented foods produce B vitamins. B-3, B-6, and B 12 play a critical role in the assimilation of fats. Once your inner ecosystem is established with lots of vitamin B-producing friendly bacteria, you'll find it easier to digest fats .... Digestion of fats is greatly enhanced when they are eaten with cultured vegetables, daikon, leafy green salads, apple cider vinegar, and lemon juice" (Gates with Schatz 105, 106). I started adding ferments to our shopping list and eating a heaping tablespoon or two at once in the morning and often also in the evening. You can take them with each meal if you can afford it.

I also prefer probiotic supplements that are considered safe without the need for refrigeration even though I keep them refrigerated whenever I can. This enables me to travel with them and not worry about losing their potency. I have no way of knowing whether this practice works or not. The probiotics I use generally work to prevent constipation which I have learned to expect whenever I cannot control what I eat on the road. By promoting regular bowel movements, these probiotics help to remove toxic waste out of the body. The probiotics I buy no longer expire on me, although I will skip them whenever I have fermented vegetables around. This is because I take probiotics for what they are, supplements to complement all other efforts I make to give real foods, fermented foods in this case, their true place and a real chance to support the health of my gut, build immunity and bring digestive balance and healing.

By diversifying the brands, my goal is to take probiotics that carry different strains of bacteria so that taken over time, and with repeat use, they supply the types of beneficial bacteria that my body needs. In the additional resources at the end of the book, I will share where I source my probiotic brands I have been using. However, there is nothing better than naturally-fermented vegetables that come straight from your healthy garden, if you can grow your own. Fermenting these local vegetables enhances the beneficial elements that they already have in their natural, fresh form. How balanced or out of balance the gut is, determines for each of us the degree to which we benefit from taking a probiotic supplement, in addition to fermented foods. Working with a health professional who is equipped to assess your needs and recommend the best supplement for you is therefore a good practice.

However, unless there is a known sensitivity to crucifers (all vegetables in the cabbage family including broccoli, cauliflower, brussels sprouts) or dairy (which many with a challenged immune-system do not tolerate), consuming sauerkraut and probiotic-rich fermented foods can only benefit us. As pre-digested natural sources of probiotics and enzymes, they are easy for the digestive system to absorb and gather the nutrients in them while enhancing access to nutrients from other foods we eat. Fermented foods also supply a much higher dose of these good bacteria with guaranteed improvements in digestion and an almost instant relief from heartburn. That is my experience. You can appreciate the fact that fermented vegetables prevent constipation as well and with no harmful side effects. I have experienced this too.

In fact, one of the side effects I hear repeatedly and that I have experienced is that you may have two or three bowel movements a day, something that many find unusual but need not worry about. In fact, this can help with your weight loss efforts as your body releases the excess it never needed to hold onto in the first place. You can therefore understand why fermented vegetables are considered superfoods. They indeed help cleanse the colon naturally. And if you are wondering if acidic foods such as fermented vegetables may increase the acidity of your body, rest assured. Naturally fermented raw vegetables are acidic in taste but they are not acidifying. In other words, they do not increase the body's acidity. On the contrary, fermented foods are one of the best allies and helpers for strong digestive and immune systems, which are both needed to keep yeast under control and to alkalize the body.

Unlike digestive killers that I discuss further below, digestive helpers, including enzymes and probiotic-rich foods and supplements, build a strong and healthy gut which translates into a healthy and strong immune system. If as much as 80% of our immune cells are located in the gut, you can understand why taking care of the gut should be everyone's priority. While we expect our digestive system to do its job and break down the foods and extract nutrients from them, how it works depends on how well we support it to continue functioning well, if it ever did. I know people who can eat almost anything and they claim to digest it well. I have a brother who, unlike me, almost never complained of indigestion. For those whose digestive system runs smoothly, the health of the gut, and the dominance of friendly bacteria, can claim a good part of the credit. For those whose system runs poorly, extra help can always be enlisted. Naturally fermented vegetables are one of the most potent helpers I have found to enhance digestion. Fermented vegetables and drinks as well as quality probiotics create an alkaline body, enhance the acid/alkaline balance, and build a strong immune system.

Let's note here that probiotics are not a new health trend. In the grand scheme of things, the mass introduction of artificial preservatives and sugars into the modern diet are what is relatively new. Fermentation helped us long before we knew much about how it helped us. It was one of very few ways to preserve food before refrigeration and artificial preservatives. Nonetheless, science is not fully caught up yet in figuring out what these microorganisms do and how to best enlist their full potential in supporting our health based on individual needs. What we do know is that they convert food into useful nutrients for the body. In addition, they help to remove and kill impurities and prevent diseases. Each new research reveals that they do much more, including influencing weight as discussed in Chapter 2 on sugar. A healthy gut is central to mental health as well.

> *Therefore, losing weight and body fat is not just about how much we eat and how long we exercise. Improving the genetic makeup of our gut microbiome can have profound weight management implications as well.*

This is what fermented vegetables and quality probiotics provide. We need probiotics just as we need fertilizers for our crops. Besides promoting the general health of our plants, fertilizers create viable land for agriculture. The viability of our intestinal population of microbes also varies based on whether they are receiving a regular supply of fertilizers in the form of probiotic-rich foods and supplements as well as prebiotics and the additional support to the lining of the intestines that bone broth supplies, for example.

Gut microbiome can vary substantially from one individual to another. There are cases where two people's microflora may be only 10% identical, for example. Either way, the greater the diversity of gut microflora, the healthier the individual is. Gut-healing foods and practices that increase the diversity of our gut microflora increase our likelihood of success in losing excess weight as well.

Other digestive helpers I have introduced to my diet are bone broth, coconut milk kefir, and coconut water kefir. When I can find marrow bones from local grass-fed cows, I make bone broth and drink one cup a day. Bone broth is known to seal the lining of the intestines, which otherwise leaches particles back into the bloodstream when the gut has been damaged. Finally, I have added prebiotics to my diet as well. These are the foods that the good bacteria like and a diet that lacks prebiotics does not allow the beneficial bacteria to crowd out the bad bacteria. Prebiotics are less talked about than probiotics. However, they are just as important in your diet as probiotic-rich foods are. The prebiotics I rely on include green bananas, cold red potato salads, green papayas, and when I can find them, tiger nuts, a high fiber and nutritious food I was introduced to on my first visit to Ghana in 2018. Coconut oil pulling, as well as brushing and flossing regularly, help to take care of my mouth and remove yeast that may be spreading out on the surface of my tongue. Coconut oil pulling is "an oral health routine that involves swishing oil in the mouth ... for 15-20 minutes to reduce harmful bacteria in the mouth and on the teeth," writes Kat Gál in an article on the Medical News Today website.

Limit use of or avoid antibiotics and other known digestive killers

"When you take antibiotics, especially if you take them repeatedly, many of the friendly germs in your body (especially those in your digestive tract) are 'wiped out.' Since yeasts aren't harmed by these antibiotics, they spread out and raise large families (the medical term is 'colonization'). When yeasts multiply, they put out toxins which circulate through your body, weaken your defenders and make you sick" (Crook 11). You may recall that in Chapter 2, I shared that I took repeat doses of antibiotics to address a recurrent skin rash. Then, I knew nothing, about the harmful side effects they cause. While probiotics mean "for life," antibiotics mean the opposite, "against life." Yet they were considered "magic bullets" or "miracle drugs" when they were first introduced.

Today, antibiotics are recognized for having two faces. They kill "not only disease-causing bacteria; they also kill beneficial bacteria, upset the body's inner ecology, and allow unfriendly organisms to take over" (Gates and Schatz 4). As my knowledge and understanding of antibiotics has expanded, I now compare the antibiotics to chemical pesticides. While antibiotics destroy the good and bad bacteria in our gut, chemical pesticides kill the good and bad in plants and soils. Some pesticides are known for causing further damage to our health when we eat foods that contain their residues.

It is for this reason also that I am careful and try to avoid consuming meat and poultry that have been treated with antibiotics. I consider antibiotics as digestive "killers." They affect the natural balance of microbes in the body. We must be mindful of how often we take them and equip ourselves with their antidote, fermented foods, prebiotics and probiotics, as these are gut/digestive helpers. We must be ready to take probiotics as soon as we have finished taking a dose of antibiotics. Whenever we can avoid antibiotics, we should. Whenever what we are diagnosed with is a virus, we have no reason to take antibiotics because they are not meant for viruses.

Chew your food properly

The third aspect of caring for the gut involves chewing food properly. Recognizing that the stomach and the rest of our digestive system have no teeth, we must be mindful that we have teeth not just to smile when we are happy, but also and especially, to chew our foods. When we mix food with saliva in the process of chewing, we generate digestive enzymes in the saliva. In fact, saliva is released even before we put the first bite inside the mouth and digestion begins here. Chewing foods releases the digestive enzymes that help to break down the cell walls of the food and begin the process of gathering the nutrients that the foods contain. Author and physician Alejandra Carrasco concurs that "as you chew ... saliva coats your food with the enzymes amylase and lipase. These enzymes begin to digest fats and starches right in your mouth." Chewing is like an alert system for the rest of the digestive tract signaling to the stomach and the pancreas to prepare to release their own enzymes that will facilitate digestion.

Ignoring this key step can indeed hamper digestion, keep undigested foods in the stomach longer, affect digestion of fats and carbs, and negatively impact the gut. When food is not properly digested in the stomach, and it stays there longer than is considered healthy, food starts fermenting in there. An article on the WebMD website explains that foods that stay in the stomach too long often lead to a growth of bad bacteria." This contributes to the body's acidity, creating yet another breeding ground for yeasts and other unfriendly bacteria to proliferate. Chewing food properly helps to prevent food from overstaying their welcome inside your stomach. Proper digestion is key to healthy weight.

Avoid overeating

It is important to avoid overeating as it causes a strain on the digestive system, and as noted above, food that stays in the stomach longer than it should will start fermenting in there, and feed yeast. Conventional wisdom is to apply the 80/20 rule, which means that you should stop eating when you are about 80% full to leave room for digestion as this process makes you feel fuller, and it takes about 20 minutes after you stop eating to have the sensation of fullness. When you feel full by the time you stop eating, you will have overeaten because when food settles and starts to break down in the stomach, you will feel bloated and overfed! Chewing properly also helps to avoid overeating as the brain will process the feeling of fullness better when you give it time to recognize that you have been eating for a while.

Practice food elimination

In the United States, food packages indicate the main food allergens and make it easier for consumers to avoid those foods they tend to react to. For example, "Free of gluten, soy, nuts, dairy, and corn" is an important piece of information in marketing a processed and packaged food product to consumers who may have a known food sensitivity or allergy to any of these. The list continues to get longer as vegans avoid anything that is made of animal products, including eggs, butter, and anything derived from cows, pigs, chicken, fish or other animals. "Vegan-friendly" is a marketing tip for those in this category. Therefore, food elimination means removing from our diet any food that causes any form of digestive discomfort or distress. It is our job to pay attention and know which foods do not agree with us. Eliminating these foods, either temporarily depending on individual level of sensitivity, or permanently in the case of food intolerance, is a step each of us must take to maintain the right balance in our gut and overall health.

We must also know when it's time to replace certain foods with others that we digest better. For example, I used to have a difficult time digesting beans. I would always have heartburn within an hour or so after eating them. This went on for years until I decided to give up beans. I later on learned that beans contain phytic acid, and other enzyme inhibitors. With my predisposition to serious heartburn, eating beans only made matters worse. When I learned that soaking them overnight can remove these enzyme inhibitors or significantly reduce them, I started soaking them before cooking them, and it made all the difference. An article in the *Journal of Food Science and Technology* confirms that "soaking markedly decreased the activity of enzyme inhibitors. Cooking of presoaked seeds was even more effective as greater reductions (78.7-100%) were observed for all pulses."

Gates and Schatz also emphasize the importance of soaking beans, writing that "[w]hen the digestive tract is weak and lacking an inner ecosystem, it will not be able to break down the phytic acid found in all grains, beans, nuts, and seeds. Soaking removes this enzyme inhibitor" (89). Because I now soak legumes before cooking them, I am able to eat them regularly, managing serving sizes to maintain the right balance in the amount of carbs I consume as mentioned in Chapter 3. I suffer from heartburn only occasionally now and I know how to get rid of it with the right foods and food combinations.

It is not unusual for people to continue eating foods that make them feel miserable, when they have not been trained to slow down and establish the connections between what they eat and how they feel afterwards.

I can relate because I too used to accept the fact that heartburn and constipation were normal and that I could not do anything to change how I was created. Books now have been written on this very topic, aiming to challenge this way of thinking. One that comes to mind is *Junk Foods Junk Moods* by Lindsey Smith. In this book, Smith seeks to establish the connection between what we eat and how we feel, recognizing through her own lived experience that if you rely on a junk foods diet, you can expect your moods to reflect that as well.

Not everyone agrees that soaking legumes is required for proper digestion. Naturopathic medical doctor Alan Glen Christianson does not consider soaking beans prior to cooking a requirement for healthy digestion. He highlights some health benefits that come with eating foods that contain phytic acid when he notes that "those who consume more phytic acid have lower risks for diabetes. It is also a good detoxifier against heavy metals, in particular, lead and cadmium." This is a reminder that not everyone needs to remove a food simply because someone else does not digest it. Also, applying the principle of moderation is key always. It is important to understand individual level of tolerance of phytic acid. In my case, soaking has helped me digest beans better. Now that digestion has improved, I have made another modification by boiling water first and then leaving the beans to soak in that water for about 1-2 hours instead of overnight. Then I rinse them and cook them afterwards. This continues to work for me, and I no longer have any problems digesting beans.

There are other foods that are known to be harmful to the gut, and that I have removed from my diet when I embarked on my food elimination journey.

Added sugar: I almost always avoid foods that contain high amounts of sugar. As discussed in Chapter 2, sugar feeds yeast. Allowing for yeast overgrowth is a sure way to weaken your immune system, just as a weak immune system cannot fight off yeast infections effectively. I eat fewer fruits than I used to. I used to eat all fruits liberally without realizing that the sugar in fruits - fructose combined with glucose - is just as bad for keeping weight and yeast in check. Fruits therefore contribute to weight gain when consumed carelessly. Other types of sugar including the artificial sweeteners listed in Chapter 2, are just as harmful.

Gluten: Food sources of gluten - a protein that many react to especially when they suffer from yeast infections - include wheat, couscous, semolina, spelt, barley, bulgur, and rye. Breads made from these grains are high in gluten, and therefore, sandwiches are no longer my "grab and go" lunch. When I eat bread, I limit myself to a slice because most breads are high in carbs and because they raise blood sugar, they too feed yeast. Limiting bread and other starchy foods go a long way in starving harmful bacteria and yeasts.

Red meat and alcohol: I limit consumption of meat, especially red meat, and have given up on alcohol because these two are more acid-forming foods. Yeast love to hang around an acidic environment.

Peanuts: I rarely eat peanuts because they tend to attract mold. Eating raw peanuts for a few consecutive days once caused such digestive distress that took a long time to heal. Later I was able to link the distress to this change in my diet. I have developed a repulsive feeling about peanuts ever since.

Dairy products: They are hard to digest for me. I can have a slice of cheese here and there, usually at parties and other social gatherings. I prefer raw cheese when I can find it. Otherwise, I have a hard time digesting other types of dairy products. Undigested foods, including dairy, feed yeast and weaken the immune system.

Soy: I went through a phase early on in midlife when I drank soymilk instead of dairy milk. I stopped drinking soymilk when I learned that soy has plant-based estrogens, which may increase our risks of breast cancer.

Not enough evidence exists to make such claims conclusive and in fact, there are others who claim that soy may even be more beneficial and offer preventive benefits against cancer and osteoporosis for menopausal women. I tend to err of the side of caution. So, I gave up soymilk and other soy products except for organic fermented tempeh or tofu, and organic edamame beans. I digest these better. In addition to these health concerns, other soy products cause too much gas for me.

Eggplant: Even when I was much younger, eggplant caused heartburn for me. I continue to avoid them whenever I can, because of this association. In addition, eggplants are included on the list of nightshades, which include tomatoes, potatoes, and green bell peppers, that tend to negatively impact the lining of our gut and overall digestion.

I consider all of the above potential digestive "killers" (Gates with Schatz 107) and believe that they must be managed carefully to support proper digestion, which is required for a healthy gut and a healthy weight. Below is another habit that took me, almost by surprise, on a gut-healing journey!

GARDENING: A HOBBY THAT TOOK ME ON A GUT-HEALING JOURNEY

When my family moved to Malawi, I experimented with edible and inedible plants by starting a nursery with more than 20 varieties of plants and hundreds of seedlings. I grew lettuce, green peppers, tomatoes, Swiss Chard, and amaranth, as well as herbs such as basil and parsley. I stayed on the look-out for pests every day and applied natural pest control methods, including manually removing any bug before it multiplied and spread to other plants. I monitored the health of the plants to see which among them were most vulnerable and I either moved them away from the rest or removed them from the stock. I added mulch regularly, moved plants around to ensure their placement would enable them to gain the necessary light and shade they required for good health. I added flowering plants that would attract bees and butterflies and not harmful pests. I dedicated a few minutes each day, to checking it out and ensuring all was well before I worked on other projects on my schedule for the day. It was not always easy but diligence always pays off.

My goal then was to destress while also decorating our yard with different colored plants and shrubs that would delight my family as well as our guests. As it turned out, I did succeed at delighting at least one young mind - my older son - who was in the fifth grade then. He gave me one of the best compliments a gardener could ever want. He told me that other than the United States Ambassador's residence (the only ambassador's residence we had the privilege to visit), ours was the best-looking garden he had ever seen in Lilongwe. This was enough to make me feel like I had succeeded at testing my skills as an amateur gardener!

Before we left Malawi for good, I received another gratifying compliment from someone I least expected - our landlord - an older gentleman of Indian ancestry! He came to see us the night before we vacated the house. We did not have a long conversation but as he was looking out into the garden and observing what we were leaving behind, he turned to me and said: "Too bad you have to leave before you have fully enjoyed all the hard work you put into this garden!" He knew how it looked when we moved in. Not to blame him or anyone else, what we saw was typical of many compounds in early September, which is during the second half of the dry season.

When we walked in, the compound looked dry and dusty and not well-cared for at all. The scattered perennials around looked dead. With the exception of an old tree in the back, which served as home for baboons raised by the previous tenant, as well as a small shrub off to the side of the house that smelled like perfume when it started blooming, the large yard was quite unappealing to anyone who cares about being surrounded by green and flowering plants. That is what we inherited. The house and the yard around it were spacious, and I saw the potential. This was the first time I took gardening seriously and I tested my gardening skills there as well. It worked! What I did then, I continue to do whenever I have my own garden.

I appreciate gardens that are pleasing to the eye, productive, and disease-free, with flowering plants, fruits and vegetables that are tasty and health-promoting. This is what I imagine happening when I take care of my gut by eating such healthy and gut-healing foods. These are the foods that starve or "weed" out bad bacteria, and instead help to maintain the right balance between the good and the bad ones. "Mulching" with gut-healing foods, particularly fermented foods and prebiotics - the foods that feed the good bacteria like resistant starches - build a healthy gut, which is the foundation of a strong immune system. Just as I never spray any chemicals on my vegetables in the garden and use only organic mulch and compost as fertilizers, I favor organic choices when I am shopping for vegetables to ferment or for immediate consumption. Just as I fear that herbicides and pesticides would destroy the good and the bad in the plants and vegetables, I limit my consumption of foods that are laden with pesticide residues.

When I am based in the United States, my main resource for knowing how to shop wisely to avoid these harmful pesticides in my diet is the Environmental Working Group's (EWG) Guide for Healthy Eating, which includes a link to what is commonly known as the "Dirty Dozen and Clean Fifteen." This resource ranks produce based on the amounts of pesticides residues on them that end up in our bodies as consumers. The "Dirty Dozen" have the highest amounts of pesticide residues. I try to avoid these as much as possible. I lose the battle when I'm based in other countries as many do not have such a resource. I have not seen anything similar in the countries where I have lived on the African continent.

"Unless you have been eating organic foods, the chances are good that you have been ingesting foods exposed to pesticides, insecticides, antibiotics, herbicides, fungicides and estrogen", Eric Berg, *The 7 Principles of Fat Burning: Get Healthy, Lose Weight and Keep It Off* (107).

It is for this reason that I have stopped eating strawberries if I cannot confirm that they were grown organically. Since I started referring to the EWG tool, strawberries almost always rank on top of this "dirty dozen" list, showing the highest amount of pesticide residues. Is there any reason why you and I shouldn't question these chemicals in the environment and in our food supply? Shouldn't we be concerned that such chemicals may end up in our gut as well and that over time, they will weaken our immune system and get us sick? The liver is one of the organs that takes the hit from pesticide-laden foods and drinks.

Toxins in the environment, including DDT, an insecticide that has been banned in the United States but is still in use in many other countries, is a known liver toxin. A toxic liver cannot do a good job of detoxifying the body. It is sluggish. These toxins also compete with the beneficial bacteria in the gut and over time, without the help of these bacteria, constipation will knock on our door. With it, the liver gets further congested and losing weight is even harder to achieve. As mentioned earlier, use of antibiotics only worsen *candida* symptoms, yet another liver toxin.

"A liver problem can originate from any different sources. One is constipation. If the bowels cannot eliminate, the liver will become backed up. The toxicity in the body will prevent weight loss," notes Eric Berg (103).

A liver problem can also originate from consumption of refined foods such as white rice, bread, pasta, cereal, pancakes, juice and sodas. These are quickly converted to sugar in the blood which rises insulin levels fast as well. As discussed in the two previous chapters, high insulin levels are a sure way to accumulate fat around the body, and particularly around the belly. Such refined foods that quickly raise blood sugar are generally stripped of their nutrition and force the liver to handle them, which it does with greater difficulty, each time they are consumed. Particularly, "... mixture of sugars with fats - in the form of ice cream, barbecue ribs and breaded meats - adds stress to the liver .... The liver produces substances to break down fats, but when it is deficient, an overload of fatty foods aggravates the liver .... Cravings for fatty foods come from the body telling you it needs something. What? It needs fat-soluble vitamins - A, D, E, K and certain B vitamins..." B vitamins and potassium are some of these nutrients whose deficiencies are also a known cause and a symptom of liver problems (Berg 104, 105).

Therefore, whenever I have the opportunity to grow my own vegetables, I focus on growing those that do not require the application of chemicals at any stage of the growing process. I have also learned to become friends with the earth worms instead of being disgusted by them or trying to scoop them out of the ground and taking them somewhere far from the plants. This is what I used to do when I did not know how beneficial they were to our gardens. And I have come to appreciate the fact that naturally rich soil without chemical fertilizers and weed killers produce healthy crops that nourish us without leaving behind harmful sediments that eventually harm our gut and our bodies. In *Body Ecology Diet*, Donna Gates and Linda Schatz concur with Rachel Carson, who expressed the concern that "the pesticides that seep into our food and water supplies, [are] affecting our health and the health of future generations" (Gates and Schatz 3).

Neglecting our food choices or tampering with our food supply and our environment is the same as tampering with our bodies that must ingest and digest such foods. And it is not a given that we will be able to digest properly those foods that rely on added chemicals to survive.

These chemicals ultimately alter the plants' DNA whether added during production, processing, or in storage. We cannot truly appreciate the beauty of wholesome foods until we have fully experienced the difference in taste, and the peace of mind that comes from enjoying local, in season, and as much as possible, 100% organic produce. The National Organic Standards Board passed the following definition of organic agriculture as "an ecological production management system that promotes and enhances biodiversity, biological cycles, and soil biological activity. It is based on minimal use of off-farm inputs and on management practices that restore, maintain, and enhance ecological harmony ... methods are used to minimize pollution from air, soil, and water .... The primary goal of organic agriculture is to optimize the health and productivity of interdependent communities of soil life, plants, animals, and people" (Mullin and Swift, 73). Once you have acquired the taste and are able to distinguish between fresh produce that was bought from the supermarket and shipped from thousands of miles away, to that which is freshly picked from your garden just a short while before it is prepared and served, you will also be able to value local farmers who grow and supply you with nutrient-dense, gut-healing foods.

Having enjoyed the taste of fresh, local, and organic produce, I can understand why more and more people are becoming pickier and are prioritizing health over taste or cost when food shopping. The numbers of farmers markets continue to increase because more and more consumers are looking for local and in season produce. The market share of fermented foods and supplements continues to increase as well. Fermentation is no longer a skill of ancient cultures; instead, new and trendy health food stores are diversifying their supply of fermented foods as well. These foods help build our gut, supporting the center of our being and the nucleus of our wellness. Many experts bring to our attention the benefits of ferments, prebiotics and probiotic supplements on gut health. Gates and Schatz highlight the following benefits of probiotics, especially those that we find in fermented vegetables and other suitable fermented foods:

- Help white blood cells fight disease;
- Control putrefactive bacteria in the intestines [These are disease-causing bacteria that are linked to the foul-smell due to decomposition of organic matter in the intestines];

- Provide important nutrients for building the blood;
- Assist digestion;
- Protect intestinal mucosa;
- Prevent diarrhea and constipation and contribute to bowel elimination; and
- Manufacture important B vitamins and are the most abundant source of vitamin B-12 (6).

Without seeking the expertise of a microbial ecologist, I have found that simply thinking about our gut microbiome as an inner ecosystem, as Gates and Schatz suggest, is helpful in appreciating the scope of its complexity. I have also started to imagine the gut, not as a filthy sewage system but as an extraordinary garden. I hope that as you read on, you too can imagine the gut and a healthy microflora as a nourishing garden for our cells, helping us to digest and assimilate foods better, getting nutrients from them. They help us build a stronger immune system that resists diseases. I now think of it in the same way that I think about the role of the soil for plants. Like the gut, healthy soil is home to microorganisms which convert, recycle, remove, and otherwise engineer materials that enter the ecosystem, to produce useable food.

Plants can only grow successfully in a well-developed community of microbes that extract vital nutrients from the soil. In fact, some micro-biologists hypothesize that a key "evolutionary innovation of animals was to scoop up the microbial communities [that were] necessary for survival and to take them along for the ride, achieving mobility," states Moises Velasquez-Manoff in a 2015 online article in *Nature*. Our internal microflora is like little parcels of soil that we carry around within us. Research shows that as many as 500 strains of bacteria live inside the human gut. A healthy human is host to as many as 100 trillion microorganisms. For comparative perspectives, the entire human body has anywhere between 20-30 trillion cells. A healthy gut has beneficial microorganisms that dominate those that are harmful, keeping us healthy when we would otherwise feel weak and sick. What we feed them determines which of the them will run our health.

Just as the organisms and bacteria in a naturally fertile garden break down the nutrients from the soil, a healthy gut has a wide variety of bacteria that support digestion by helping to break down foods, transforming them into beneficial nutrients for our cells.

To enhance soil performance - to make it more fertile - we apply nutrient-providing fertilizers. Similarly, we need to think of probiotic supplements and naturally fermented foods as fertilizers for our gut. Just as healthy soil requires care and maintenance by a farmer or gardener, a healthy gut requires consistent work and nourishment as well. Feeding the gut with fermented foods and drinks is one of the best ways to tend to our inner garden. Just as healthy soil has trillions of living bacteria, the health of our gut is also determined by the amount and quality of beneficial bacteria that it holds.

There are various strains of these friendly bacteria including *lactobacillus*, *plantarum*, and *bifidus*, all living inside a healthy digestive tract, as beneficial bacteria. Probiotics can be obtained from consuming fermented vegetables and drinks such as sauerkraut, kimchi, kombucha, pickles, kefir, yogurt, miso, tempeh and natto. These ferments are probiotic-rich foods that help the healthy bacteria in the gut thrive. Probiotic supplements are also available at many health food stores and other regular food stores. Knowing which of the supplements support your individual gut balance is key to success in restoring the integrity of the intestinal lining and rebuilding the colony of friendly bacteria as needed.

The quality and amounts of beneficial bacteria and worms in the soil distinguish a well-tended garden from one where pests and weeds dominate. In the latter, the plants are deprived of the nutrients they need to grow, thrive, and bear safe and nourishing foods. Those who recommend that we eat dirt, including Josh Axe in his book, *Eat Dirt*, and Brett Finlay and Marie-Claire Arrieta, authors of *Let Them Eat Dirt*, know that fresh produce grown in rich and preferably organic soil, have live bacteria hidden inside crevices of leaves or skin and roots of vegetables, that are not necessarily harmful to us.

This is what led me to become "friends" with the dirt and soil in my garden as I learned to appreciate how well-preserved mulch nourishes my vegetables. If I do not mind investing the time and effort required to keep my garden looking attractive by weeding regularly and adding compost and natural fertilizers, why would I mind putting in the necessary time and resources to create a healthy and immune-enhancing gut? If I have the reputation of being the "green hands" lady based on my success growing healthy-looking plants and vegetables, why would I not invest in keeping my gut healthy as well? I wouldn't mind having the same reputation of truly being the master of my gut, knowing what to do to keep my inner garden healthy so that I can share with others what they too can do to achieve similar results.

Fermented foods are becoming more and more popular because of their known anti-inflammatory and gut-healing benefits. This is why fermented foods and probiotic supplements are now a priority on my shopping list. "Fermented Foods Top the Superfoods List" writes Joseph Mercola, in a 2019 blog that references a survey of 1,000 registered dieticians. This annual survey, which began in 2014, looks at health trends in nutrition. The most recent one focused on such trends for 2018 and 2019 and ranked fermented foods on top of the list, with avocadoes coming in second position. The rest of the top ten foods on this list are seeds, grains, exotic fruits such as açai and golden berries, blueberries, beets, nuts, coconut products, and lastly non-dairy milks.

Interestingly, even though my interest and involvement in gardening started around the time when my health had started falling apart, I still considered myself to be one of the more nutrition-conscious among many around me. Some of my friends and relatives looked to me as a model. I was the one paying attention to and who recognized the close link between foods and health and had taken measures to improve my diet as a key step to taking care of my general health. Nonetheless, I still lacked a clear picture of what I needed to do to stop weight gain as a woman in midlife. Looking back, there are many things I was doing wrong. For example, although I knew that stress was taking a toll on me, I did not understand enough about how it affected my weight.

When I realized that certain activities, such as gardening, allow me to lose track of time as I become fully immersed in what I am doing, I learned to trust in the capacity I have, deep inside of me to enjoy the moment without worrying about how I was going to handle what's next. I did not think I had access to this inner power. But whenever I stepped out into the garden, particularly on Saturday mornings, I knew I could reconnect with my source of inner peace that I had neglected during a busy work week filled with meetings, report-writing, and project deadlines.

Gardening provided a healthy outlet for me to manage my busy life and stress better.

My interests and skills in gardening grew as I took advantage of the large compound we lived on when we moved to Malawi and later to Rwanda. Understanding all the efforts I put into those two gardens, hopefully gives you an idea of how diligent I became. Connecting with the outer garden and seeking to nourish and "heal the land" motivated me to do my best when it was time for me to start taking care of my inner garden. This is why I took on the art of fermenting vegetables and other foods. I consider fermentation an important skill to have and apply as through it, we increase the health benefits of produce and other fermentable food products that in turn nourish our gut with beneficial gut bacteria. A healthy gut is a key component of a healthy weight.

PRACTICING THE ART OF FERMENTATION

You may be asking yourself, why ferment? What happens when you ferment vegetables (or any other suitable food for that matter)? Through fermentation, we transform the usual taste of raw, fresh produce, and move their health benefits up a notch. To achieve the health benefits of probiotics described above, Kirsten and Christopher Shockey highlight the following perks of fermenting vegetables in their book, *Fermented Vegetables*.

Fermentation:

- Preserves vegetables raw and without heat, so it retains their vitamins, minerals, and enzymes;
- Enhances B and C vitamins;
- Does not require any chemical preservatives; and
- Supports the immune system.

Shockey and Shockey point out also that organisms that enable fermentation are also beneficial (21). Fermenting vegetables changes their physical/ cell structure and nutrient composition, while at the same time enhancing their flavors, and rendering them more beneficial to our gut and overall health. With experience and a little creativity, it is even possible to create a batch that comes out less "smelly" and more boldly flavorful and beautiful.

While eating probiotic-rich foods may seem to some as if it were a new dietary trend, fermentation has been practiced in many cultures for thousands of years when people knew of and enjoyed the many benefits of consuming fermented foods. In fact, pottery shards from the Chinese village Jiahu, dating back more than 9,000 years, were found to have residue of fermented fruit, rice, and honey, according to research conducted by University of Pennsylvania Museum archaeo-chemist Patrick McGovern. Wine, a product of fermentation, has also been found in Iran from 7,000 years ago. Ancient Egyptians, pre-Hispanic Mexicans, and indigenous Sudanese also fermented alcoholic drinks thousands of years ago. These ancient cultures must have known the many gains of fermentation.

The first scientific study of fermentation was led by Louis Pasteur, and initial results were published in 1857 and in 1860. Pasteur noticed "ferments" within yeast cells while peering into his microscope, hence becoming the first to "demonstrate experimentally that fermented beverages result from the action of living yeast transforming glucose into ethanol" write Luisa Alba-Lois and Claudia Segal-Kischinevzky in a 2010 article in *Nature Education*. Through Pasteur's work, we know that fermentation occurs in yeast cells during the process of beer or wine-making. Fermentation also occurs in microorganisms inside the human digestive tract as well. It also occurs in jars and vats when we fill them with our favorite vegetables, whose health benefits we enhance through shredding and pounding prior to starting the fermentation process or through brining in salty, filtered water.

Learning to appreciate the role of gut-friendly bacteria increased my awareness of the importance of our food choices in supporting them to live and support our health as well. The good bacteria are in a constant war with harmful bacteria that thrive on a high sugar diet, refined carbohydrates, chronic stress, repeated use of antibiotics, and hormonal imbalance including a decrease in estrogen production, which is expected as women reach midlife. Fortunately, many of the dietary changes discussed in the different chapters of this book are the same that you need to embrace to support the health of your gut. While some of the changes in hormone production are irreversible for women in midlife, there are dietary and lifestyle choices that help to ease the symptoms associated with the aging process and its manifestation during this stage. The appropriate diet limits sugar and refined carbohydrate intake, as discussed in detail in the second and third chapters. It includes probiotic-rich foods and supplements as well as other general eating habits that support a healthy gut and that I discuss in detail in this chapter. It includes healthy fats and the lifestyle habits that I will discuss in detail in the next four chapters. They all have a bearing on the gut.

Many clients have asked if the sauerkraut on shelves in regular food stores are fermented. Unfortunately, the answer is no. These products are most likely sour cabbage and other vegetables that are pasteurized (i.e. heated) and then soaked in vinegar and salt, which creates the sour taste that an unexperienced consumer can mistake for the real thing. If that were the case, I could have made a quick trip drive to the nearest grocery store for a large jar instead of driving across town to a health food store for a jar of fermented vegetables that is much more expensive than those that are simply pasteurized with vinegar and salt. Naturally fermented cabbage has no added vinegar.

With this increased level of awareness and appreciation for sauerkraut, I was convinced that I should test myself again, like I did with the vegetable garden, and learn how to make my own fermented vegetables. Whenever I can find fresh organic produce, I make it a habit to ferment vegetables regularly and I did so for three years while based in the United States, until we moved to Liberia towards the end of 2017. I take a probiotic supplement on a regular basis while I am here but take a break from the supplements when I travel to a place where I can access fermented sauerkraut.

To ferment, we rely on the freshness of vegetables (or other produce or drinks) to enhance their nutritional value. Vegetables are naturally covered with micro-organisms, some are beneficial (the lactic acid bacteria) and others are not (including pathogens such as yeasts and molds). What we want to achieve with fermentation is to create an environment that encourages the multiplication of the lactic acid bacteria and discourages the growth of the pathogens. This happens with the process of cutting or shredding, which allows the natural sugars inside vegetables to become more readily available as the cell structure of the vegetables are broken down to feed the gut-friendly bacteria through lactic-acid fermentation. The natural sugars in the vegetables are, in fact, what turn into lactic acid through the fermentation process. With the addition of salt, which pulls the juices out of the vegetable cells, a salty brine is available, creating a new environment that enables the lactic acid bacteria to survive and thrive while the molds and yeasts that require oxygen are unable to live when submerged. These foods are in fact, considered "live" because they have active bacteria (live cultures) inside them commonly known as "probiotics."

These days, cabbage is the first vegetable that many people tend to use when they learn the art of fermentation. Green cabbage is what I initially experimented on as well. However, many other vegetables and drinks can be fermented and over time, I too tried fermenting red cabbage and also combining red and green varieties as I started feeling more confident with my fermentation skills. I sometimes added chopped leeks, as well as shredded root vegetables such as carrots and beetroots. Adding caraway and/or dill seeds and these other vegetables also changed the smell of the ferments in the end. These combinations added a flavor and color density that green cabbage alone could not offer.

Fermented cabbage straight out of a newly opened jar has a smell that can be embarrassing for those who are not familiar with the actual smell of this superfood. I have found that even adding leeks alone creates a "more manageable" smell by those who are repulsed by plain sauerkraut. Adding spices and creating different flavors also helped produce a final product that even my kids were willing to try and eventually, they were more open to taking this superfood with dinner on occasion. They eventually stopped complaining about my diligent reminders to have a spoon full when they too started experiencing the benefits. They began to realize that with ferments, constipation could be avoided and their bowl movements improved. Sometimes they would even request some without being prompted!

Fermenting vegetables is a time-consuming and carefully crafted process that requires tender care and extra cleanliness, from planning through preparation, until mason jars are filled, closed and ready for fermentation. Even when fermentation has begun, taking care of the fermenting vegetables prevents spoilage and ensures a final product that is worth all the effort that goes into its preparation. Fermenting reminds me that all good things come at a cost and I can see why those who have made fermentation their trade, do not sell these foods cheaply. Learning how to make your own ferments not only helps to control quality and taste, but it also saves money. To cut my costs down significantly is what led me initially to start experimenting with making my own. Then I enjoyed the taste of homemade ferments better and that convinced me to keep fermenting. In the additional resources at the end of the book, I will share my basic fermentation tips and hope you too will start fermenting your vegetables and start enjoying the benefits that your own ferments will bring to your health.

I have also made milk kefir using regular low-fat milk, and I have used canned coconut milk to make coconut kefir as well. When we moved to Liberia, where I could not access a regular supply of good quality fresh vegetables, I stopped fermenting vegetables. However, I often make coconut water kefir and this helps us to keep consuming ferments, this time in the form of a drink. In the additional resources, I will share my recipe for making coconut milk and coconut water kefirs. These are much easier to make and much less time-consuming, so long you have access to good quality raw materials.

When fermenting vegetables, the color changes over time and eventually, it settles for its true nature as the vegetables reach their fermentation potential.

When consuming these, I do it because I have come to understand that I cannot expect to reach my health potential without taking care of my gut. I have come to understand that I cannot reach my genetic potential without a healthy gut. I have come to think of a healthy gut as a reliable nucleus and center of my being, from which I receive clear messages regarding who I was created to be and what I was created to do. After all, don't we all have a purpose for which we were created, whether we know it or not?

GARDENING AND GUT HEALING: A SPIRITUAL JOURNEY

Did you know that our "gut feelings" are not just about the digestive tract, but that they also involve the physical and emotional components of our lives? The interconnection of these two is what causes us to feel the urge to use the bathroom when we are nervous. Together, a healthy body and a healthy mind bring balance that enable us to manifest the best versions of ourselves as spiritual beings as well. A healthy gut enables us to reach deeper into the spiritual part of who we are. This level of understanding and awareness caused me to stop thinking of my gut as if it were a refuse for everything that must eventually be expulsed from my system - where eventually everything left in it smells, like the sauerkraut in the jar inside our hotel room or worse. Instead, I started reflecting further on why I should make taking care of my gut a priority.

My gardening experience and learning how to make fermented vegetables, became a spiritual journey towards the center of my being. This is the place where "the divine in [us] abides," as Oprah Winfrey shares in one of her inspirational podcasts. Gardening gave me the gratifying feeling that came from watching a little seed transform itself into a beautiful and sometimes majestic plant. I never thought that the work of my hands, combined with some mental creativity, could nurture a plant in a garden and bring its beauty to full life. I never imagined that watching the beauty inside healthy and colorful plants could be a source of serenity and inspiration for me. I also never imagined that this journey inside the garden, watching, tending, smelling and nurturing, would become part of a divine messenger of who I was to become, seeking to feel equipped to serve and help others to reclaim their own power to take better care of themselves, physically, mentally and spiritually.

That peaceful reconnection with the center of who I am that took place initially through my work in the garden subsequently fed into my work as a wellness coach and a new hobby as a *fermentista*. It opened the possibility that I could, If I chose to and when the time was right, re-focus my career towards doing what I felt was part of my identity, my DNA, my calling. I wondered whether I could find work that would give me the same level of satisfaction and bring a sense of peace and fulfillment as that which I was able to experience while working on my vegetable garden or watching my raw and fresh vegetables turn into healthier and much more healing superfoods once fermented.

The work I do now teaches me how to support my body and prevent self-inflicted abuse that included eating foods that were not nourishing to my cells and that allowed yeast overgrowth. Stress overload, poor sleep habits, and lack of exercise all contributed to this self-abuse. This is what eventually broke me at the core, as I became overweight, tired, and with intense lower back pain that at one point kept me home from work for a couple of days, unable to move on my own or even sit up. All these were signs of a poorly running, dysfunctional system. While I already appreciated organic foods, and had tried to invest in buying organic foods whenever I could, I came to another level of recognizing that in foods, especially gut-healing foods, there is a message that we must equip ourselves to decode.

I came to believe that by eating wholesome foods that are fresh, local, and preferably organic, and including fermented vegetables, we are able to connect with the center of our being and receive messages that we may miss when we do not pay attention to what we eat and where our foods come from.

Remembering that nearly 80% of our immune cells are located in the gut, and with a better understanding of the gut-brain axis, with pathways sending messages from the gut to the brain than the other way around, could I really believe in all honesty, that what I feed my gut is inconsequential?

When I entered midlife, I retraced my steps to understand when I lost myself and from there, I started learning what I could do to recover the lost self again. Supporting my gut with fermented vegetables, combined with other healthy eating and lifestyle habits, have given me a level of self-awareness, at the physical and mental levels, that enable me to better understand the keys to my health and no longer allow myself to get lost again. Working on these areas have built the foundation for spiritual maturity as well. I know myself better. I recognize my strengths and try to make the best use of them. I know that each strength and skill and ability I have, and all the resources I make use of, were given to me by the grace of God. I did not do anything to deserve any of them.

I know my limits as well, and I accept them with much less self-judgement than I used to in the past. I manage stress better and do not fear to fall. I know that the power to rise again is within reach and is up to me to use every time I need it. Therefore, while the initial experience and the thoughts and actions that followed came to me while getting my hands dirty, working my plants and vegetable garden, what followed eventually led to the gut. It is from this long inner tube I now tend to, as I would my healthy garden, that helped me to appreciate my place in this world as a spiritual being.

With a healthy gut, I have come to believe that we are better equipped to manifest the best versions of ourselves. When I give my very best to the work I do, and I am fully present while doing it, bringing head and heart, mind and soul to what is aligned with this nucleus of who I am, I can co-create with the Ultimate Creator – God – and cause the things that I deeply desire and work hard to achieve, to manifest themselves into my life. I have seen this happen more than once in my life, and it happens in ways that I cannot fully understand. This has caused me to pause and reflect on my life's journey and purpose. I no longer doubt that there is a supernatural force working in my favor when I allow it to. What confirmed to me about our power to co-create with a greater universal force in us and around us, is what came about when we entered our compound in Rwanda after we moved from Malawi.

There was clearly a message that the universe sent me unambiguously then. Recalling all the efforts I made to create a beautiful garden in Malawi, when it was time for us to leave, my regret was not that I was leaving it all behind. I was happy that the next tenant will enjoy the yard because of the hard work of my hands, my head and my heart. I was happy that my efforts guiding and training the person who helped regularly keep it in good shape, did not lose his job but instead was hired to continue the same work with a neighbor who bought many of my plants in big pots when we left. I was happy because the perennials I planted on the compound around the house were there to stay and contribute to creating a greener Area 3 as our neighborhood was called, around the corner from Bishop McKenzie International School. I was happy that I had discovered a passion I did not know I had, and that I could pursue it as much as I could, and for as long as I wanted to.

However, there was a part of me that was weary and uncertain. I wondered whether I had the stamina in me to start over again knowing that we may be in Rwanda also for about the same time, two years, as we did in Malawi, or perhaps a little longer if we had the opportunity to. I wondered whether two years was long enough to want to start over again and again as our lives as a family were on a trajectory that might require moving from country to country in pursuit of the next work opportunity. I wondered where I would find a nursery and a potter, and the variety of plants that I had really enjoyed in Malawi. I wondered how long it would take for me to create equal beauty around our new home in Rwanda.

What truly convinced me that we can manifest what we feel in our gut when we put our thoughts into action, was that when we arrived in Rwanda, an even more bountiful garden was awaiting us. Most of the plants that I first discovered in Malawi were scattered around the layered compound in Rwanda, the country of a thousand hills. An untrained eye would have missed many. Not I. I started multiplying them. Moving them around. Finding better spots for some. Placing several in the few pots I found around the house and buying more pots and plants to create a truly impressive nursery around our home. I even had many potted plants inside the house. No one complained, so I was happy. And on the outside, lots of old trees and shrubs reminded us that this was indeed one of the oldest neighborhoods in Kigali. Bananas were bearing fruits, soon ready to be picked when we arrived. My brother who came from neighboring Burundi to welcome us when we arrived said, "God truly is bringing you to the land of plenty." I told him about the garden we left behind in Malawi and the mixed feelings I had. He said, *God had it all planned and you have an even better one here.*

As I recall again a podcast by Oprah Winfrey that inspires me again and again, I wonder whether what we call luck is a misrepresentation of a universe at work in our favor, when we are working in alignment with the center of who we are or who we are meant to be. Oprah does not believe in luck. She believes that "[t]here is no luck without you being prepared for that moment of opportunity." I did not know I was being prepared for an even better garden when I left the fruits of my labor behind in Malawi. But there I was, in awe of what the universe, God in my world, had already prepared for me in Rwanda.

> *This seemingly mundane experience taught me to focus more and more on doing the best I can and to trust that what I am pursuing that is meant for me will manifest itself in due time.*

I began to see that in the realm of the spiritual, I am connected to a power, a source and a force that is greater than my own and that I need to stop worrying and start believing that God will take care of me and fulfill the desires of my heart. I need to stop thinking that it's all up to me to make things happen to become successful at what I do. I stopped believing that I can rely only on my own energy, independently of the divine force in and around me, to help me reach my full potential.

Indeed, if you can relate to my story and are still reading, I do believe and hope you too will consider taking care of yourself, and not neglect your gut as an entry point for improving your physical and mental health, as well as reaching a higher level of spiritual awareness and transformation. Maintaining a healthy gut is, in my opinion, required to live a spirit-driven life, which is your door to a fulfilling life. Such a life combines better self-care and service to others. "By rebuilding our health and immunity, we can restore our inner ecology, and we will have a much better chance to achieve all our goals, including restoring the ecology of our outer world," note Gates and Schatz (4).

You do not have to take gardening lessons nor do you need to enjoy playing in the dirt like I do, to heal your gut and bring balance to your physical, mental, and spiritual health. However, the gut is a messenger of how well our body functions. Taking care of it ensures we receive the intended message that drives us to action to do the good that benefits us and inspires or brings needed change to others. Focusing on healing my gut and my health have helped me embrace a new career as a wellness coach, teaching and supporting others in search of what I had already found. Writing this book is one of my ways of contributing to the knowledge that many others may be seeking as they approach or enter midlife. This phase of life is a prime time to reflect on the urgency of living a life of purpose.

Being able to inspire others and model what I "preach" has allowed me to reach a higher level of self-awareness and wellness, and it has brought me to a place of greater relevance in this world. I do believe that practicing self-care, and healing the gut, with regular consumption of fermented vegetables, probiotics and prebiotics, is key to unlocking your physical, mental and spiritual potential. This level of health and healing equips you to better manifest the best version of yourself. It also frees you to embrace your true nature and your genetic potential.

With such a level of self-awareness and healing, there is little that holds you back.

Taking care of our inner garden, our gut, the nucleus of our immune system, therefore helps to clear body and mind of the clutter that tends to keep us focused on individual, self-centered needs. With a healthy body and mind, which require a healthy gut, we can feel "full" and are better positioned to share the excess with the world in a selfless way knowing that there is enough to go around. By understanding the importance of a healthy gut, and knowing what I needed to do to restore my own balance, I was able to focus my work better, recognizing what I should prioritize. I was able to bring a unique perspective to my community, starting with my family and on to my readers, clients and friends, to be of meaningful service to them. Keeping my gut healthy remains a priority. It always will. And I hope I have convinced you to make yours a priority as well.

WHAT ARE THE SIGNS THAT PROBIOTICS AND FERMENTS WORK?

There are several measures of improvement that I observed in myself that resulted in a healthier body and gut.

* Seeing string-like threads of yeast die-off that showed inside the toilet bowl often when I urinated was a sign that the bad bacteria were slowly being defeated and the good bacteria were being supported to thrive. The yeast die-off did not cause any pain or any other symptoms, but I could tell that it was not just urine coming out. Yeast overgrowth does not die easily, however, but consistently eating fermented foods and maintaining a diet that minimized sugar consumption along with other dietary and lifestyle habits aimed to strengthen the gut, helped to restore my health to a level of balance I had never experienced before.

* A stronger immune system, rarely getting sick.

* Improved digestion, rarely suffering from acid reflux or constipation, two health issues that haunted me for years when I relied on various antacids for relief of acid reflux. I can promise that if your system works like mine, you can experience almost instant relief from the occasional acid reflux with a heaping tablespoon or two of naturally fermented vegetables. This does the trick and works better than any pharmaceutical antacid that I have ever tried and believe me, I have tried many, including Maalox, Tums, Zantac, and Tagamet that my doctors recommended. They provided short-term relief. None prevented constipation. Fermented vegetables and a quality

probiotic helps prevent both acid reflux and constipation. They even help relieve the discomfort of indigestion that happens sometimes when I eat out, or when I combine foods poorly even at home. I am convinced that fermented foods are a superfood that can prevent digestive distress when taken as part of a balanced diet and lifestyle.

* I am able to keep vaginal yeast infections and the skin rash under control.

* My hair is thicker and healthier.

* My waistline is normal. I am no longer self-conscious about it even though I do not have the super slim waistline of my 20's.

Please note that keeping a normal weight and building a stronger immune system and healthier hair have come as a result of a combination of all the strategies outlined in this book, with each strategy compounding the effectiveness of the others. All are important. None must be left out!

CONCLUSION

Learning that regular consumption of naturally fermented foods can reverse a number of diseases linked to a weak digestive system, including recurring acid reflux and constipation, as well as get rid of yeast infections, it seemed like a no-brainer to try these foods and keep them in my diet. With my own creativity and inspiration from experts to create flavors that differed from those I was getting at the health food store, ferments became a known and appreciated commodity in my home. And it was out of frustration over not getting better, in spite of years of trying to eat healthy, combined with a determination to get to the root cause of recurring yeast, skin rash, and an unresponsive middle, that I left no stone unturned.

I kept searching until I found the answer. I did not know where it would come from, and when it would come. But perseverance most often pays off. I discovered ferments, and ever since, I have become an advocate of fermented foods and probiotics with anyone who will listen. Therefore, instead of spending valuable time thinking that there is nothing you can do to change the way your body works, keep searching for where the imbalance comes from. Provide your body with the support it needs and experience the amazing power and energy your body will put into its own healing and restoring lost balance for you.

Nowadays, eating fermented vegetables and taking probiotics have become a way of life, important practices I rely on to keep "mulching" my inner garden and support my inner tube, the home of my immune system, the digestive tract. While I have come to trust that raw sauerkraut and other fermented vegetables consistently help with digestion, not all probiotic supplements work as well. So, I pay attention to where I source mine and urge you to do the same. I try to buy from trusted vendors, or those recommended by health experts I trust, and from there, I find two or three that work for me, and that hopefully "reseed" the gut with friendly bacteria and provide the health benefits I am searching for. With prebiotics, I am able to give the beneficial bacteria what they require to thrive. Adding ferments in my case was an important key to my success. This habit became the missing link to all else I had tried.

You will, I hope, realize that if your body seems to suffer frequently from acid reflux, constipation, recurring yeast infections, and/or stubborn weight, these are signs that your gut needs help to rebuild the colony of friendly bacteria. And there is no better food to do so than ferments. I had believed in the lie in my head that my body was dysfunctional. I had believed for years that I was born with a weak digestive system and that sooner or later, digestive distress would kill me. Never did I think that my food choices had anything to do with it and that solutions existed within reach. I did not even have the necessary awareness to be able to make the connection that whenever I took probiotics, they helped relieve symptoms of yeasts or prevent constipation. This is why I took probiotics off and on, almost as if I had to try them out, test them, and see if they worked each time.

It was not until my level of awareness increased that things would change. I was ready to listen and develop habits that helped. I was ready to internalize the information and trust it, once and for all. I was ready to practice what I was hearing, this time intently so that I could get to the root cause of what was eating me. I was able to trace vaginal yeast and the rash that discolored the skin on my back to yeast, in the same family of a fungus that becomes systemic when gut bacteria are out of a healthy balance. Fermented foods truly are a superfood, and they came to my rescue. I now consider spending time teaching others about the benefits of such foods and equipping them with knowledge and the skills they need to start practicing healthy habits such as the art of fermentation, as key to helping them reach their own balance. This is what will help us all embrace or continue to live a life of purpose.

CHAPTER 5.

EAT GOOD FATS

"…[T]he body adapts to fat deprivation by *conserving fat*, not burning it …. Your body needs fat on board and responds to fat-deprivation diets by hoarding fat. It thinks you're starving", Will Clower, *The Fat Fallacy* (25).

It was not in my family traditions to avoid fat. Dietary fat was part of our natural way of eating. When I was a kid in Burundi, we drank all the fat from raw and fresh milk. For cooking, we used raw butter that we collected from milk after we cultured it, a type of fermentation whose value I ignored then, focusing instead on the fact that the sweet fresh raw milk turned sour once cultured. It was also a low-fat milk as I understand it now because to get it ready for drinking involved adding some sort of fermentation starter to fresh milk, keeping it in a covered gourd for several days, and then shaking it for about an hour or so. This process enabled the butter to rise to the top, and it was then separated from the milk underneath it and used for cooking. The sour milk was not my favorite, but I did enjoy food cooked with the butter, another source of fat for us. Even later on as I grew up, many of the foods we ate at home included good fats: plain yogurt (flavored options did not exist then - thank God!); cassava leaves cooked for several hours with meat bones and with large amounts of cold-pressed palm nut oil that was required for a full flavor that we enjoyed; avocado slices spread on bread or served with other meals; as well as small fish that we cooked, from head to tail, with green bananas.

These are the sources of healthy fats as I understand them now. No one questioned the wisdom in these eating habits. In fact, I had no awareness of low-fat and fat-free options. I did not throw away the extra fat from cooked beef or chicken. It was part of the gravy. My family did not throw away the liver either. Eating organ meats was the norm. And being overweight was a rare exception in our village and other surrounding villages and towns. Then, and even later in my 20s and early 30s, I had no reason to worry about my weight. If anything, I needed to put on a few more pounds. I remember that those who saw me prior to leaving for the airport when I first left home for the United States thought that I was "skinny". In our context, this meant that I was underweight and unhealthy, even though I was not sick. Questioning my diet was only limited to my own concerns with acid reflux, which got worse especially when I went to college. There, I learned the term endoscopy for the first time, as it was required to diagnose persistent stomachache that turned out to be a stomach ulcer I had developed. My diet was not the best, but my weight was normal.

I could not imagine becoming overweight, not anytime sooner nor later. I do not come from a family of heavy people. Neither my parents nor any of my siblings or close relatives seemed overweight. Losing weight was what concerned people, not gaining it. When I was getting ready to leave for the United States, I lost a few pounds running around, missing meals sometimes, and working extra hard to pull together the resources I needed to buy the plane ticket, a requirement before I could access the scholarship I had from the American Association of University Women to cover the cost of one year of graduate training in Women's Studies in the United States.

Once I was admitted and made it to Indiana University, in Bloomington, this initial grant opened doors for other financial support, enabling me to walk away with much more than I thought was possible when I left for the States. Upon graduation, I felt prepared to join the workforce and to make a contribution in any of the areas of my multi-disciplinary training, which included classes in folklore and women's studies, my major and minor respectively, but also many courses that were cross-listed with anthropology, sociology, African studies, as well as a year-long course on the general topic of global change and world peace that I completed as a MacArthur Scholar. With such a training, the last thing on my mind was to worry about diets and foods. With any employment that I would land at my level then, I could afford any food that appealed to my palate. I had achieved the goal of getting a degree from a reputable higher education institution in the United States, a sure ticket to a life of comfort. Questioning foods in such a developed country was not a priority. I had better things to occupy my time, and in fact, I could not imagine why anyone would even want to study nutrition! I had enough to eat, sometimes more than I should have. Some of my food was good, but some not so. I kept an open mind, observing and applying the eating habits of friends, housemates and peers.

HOW I TURNED AWAY FROM DIETARY FAT

It was never my intention to shun dietary fat, but once I did, it took at least a couple of decades before I would make a turnaround to understand that I had no reason to make dietary fat a foe. As I reflect on how my awareness evolved, I realize that my habits around fat were determined by food availability and often, I had no control over what I ate on a regular basis. This was certainly the case when I was in boarding school and to a lesser extent, throughout college. Other times, I was influenced by friends and peers who informed my choices. This is what I did after I left college and became more independent in my food choices. Below I explain the trajectory I took as I shifted positions on dietary fat based on inadequate knowledge about its health benefits for most of my life.

In boarding school

I left home for boarding school at almost age 13. This is when my inadequate consumption of fat started. There, we ate meat more frequently than at home, usually as cooked beef or as canned corned beef. We almost never had any organ meats until we went home on holidays or during summer vacations. We never were served avocadoes either. We drank powdered milk that was added to our tea before it was served. I'll never know the fat content nor the source of that milk and how it was produced. For cooking in our campus kitchens, the cooks used liquid vegetable oil, and it was known as *amakoto* in Kirundi. In Burundi, *amakoto* (*Kirundi* for cottonseed oil, as "koto" stands for "cotton" in French), was most likely the first vegetable oil extracted from cotton seeds and that was introduced on the market. Other refined vegetable oils are sold on the market these days including soybean and corn oils but locally, they are referred to by the brand name rather than the actual seed, nut, or legume used to produce the oil. In the United States, cottonseed oil is also still used for cooking, and it's added to many processed foods including margarine, shortenings, whipped toppings, as well as French fries, mayonnaise and in animal feed, according to Joseph Mercola's 2019 blog post on "cottonseed oil." Cooking with oil was the norm. No one questioned the quality of the oil at the time. If sources of healthy fats such as avocadoes and raw butter had been served at the cafeteria, I certainly would have enjoyed them. I ate what I was served during that time.

In college

Our diet in college was similar to what I had in high school. In both cases, quality was nobody's business. This was "free" food. We were to eat it, enjoy it, and move on with our lives. You should never look a gift-horse in the mouth anyway. Should you? Were we not students, after all? Are students living in campus dorms supposed to eat well? Having enough food to eat was sufficient to keep us motivated to work hard until we graduated and became independent. Then we could choose our foods and how they would be prepared. Nonetheless, with a student stipend in college, we were able to supplement our diet, especially buying fruits such as mangoes and bananas as well as a variety of other tropical fruits that were in season. Avocadoes seemed to always be in season, and we bought them off and on, taking them for granted. Although I do not remember the exact time when margarine was introduced, I know I had it regularly throughout college. There, I was in good company. In our college dorms, we used margarine on bread that we had with tea, either when we were delayed and could not make it to the campus cafeteria for breakfast, lunch or dinner, or when we needed a snack any time between meals. Margarine (Blue Band was the brand) was a "must have" in the limited food pantry among our group of friends on the college campus. We took turns buying it and sharing it. Since none of us had access to a fridge, margarine came in handy. It was readily available in food stores and at open air markets. It resisted tropical heat and lasted a long time without attracting bugs or going bad. The bugs knew better!

We valued this commodity so much that it was also a gift that we would share among friends and relatives. In fact, when a cousin went to study in the Democratic Republic of the Congo (Zaire at the time) and she could not access it easily, Blue Band was the one gift she asked that I send her when we knew someone who was travelling there. As you can imagine, I sent her the largest can I could find and afford. It was not unusual to find margarine at the dining room table in many urban homes. For those with more resources in Burundi, margarine and jam were spread on bread and served with hot black tea with milk sometimes in pasteurized liquid form, other times powdered. "Nido" was everybody's favorite powdered milk brand. How was it made? What was in it that created such a distinct flavor we all enjoyed? It is still sold and enjoyed by many who remain oblivious to the fact that it may be as "fake" a milk product as margarine is to butter. It's always a good habit to check the list of ingredients, just to be sure all that's in a food meets our expectations. Margarine is creamy, salty and easy to spread, unlike regular butter that is harder to spread, especially when taken right out of the fridge. Butter requires refrigeration as well. Owning a fridge was not a choice for us in college. None of us could afford it and even if we could, access to electricity was unreliable. Not knowing any better, I assumed for years, that margarine was a more practical version of real butter.

In graduate school and afterwards: Observing and following peers' inadequate knowledge

From early 1991 when I arrived in the United States until as recently as 2012, my consumption of fat became carefully controlled. I followed the practice of friends and peers and stayed away from fatty foods. I used the cooking oils they used, but like many of them, I did not know enough to worry about liquid vegetable oils or other types of fats that may have contained unhealthy compounds. I limited all sources of fat as much as possible. I continued to avoid the fat in red meat and chicken and even preferred a vegetarian diet over other diets. In fact, during the time when one of my younger sisters came to study in the United States and stayed with me in a campus apartment, we relied mostly on beans, and occasionally fish and eggs as our sources of protein. She did not eat red meat and only started eating chicken years later when she became pregnant and was concerned about an inadequate diet that might affect the baby in her womb.

Otherwise, during that time, I ate like her, and we were both mostly vegetarian. Was ours a better way of eating? I doubt it. While I am still not convinced that a high meat diet is healthy for most people, I now wonder whether our diet that avoided meat during the time we stayed together and also limiting all sources of beneficial fat for at least twenty years in my case, may have established the right conditions for me to build a thick layer of fat around my waistline that expanded much more visibly as I entered midlife. I associated fat with fast foods, which were mostly unhealthy fried foods. I also associated meat with high amounts of fat that are artery clogging and that cause the body to put on excess weight. I believed that foods with fats must be consumed only occasionally in order to protect the heart and avoid other health risks. Like my peers, I did not know that fat was a key macronutrient that must be included in our diet for good health. I did not know that certain sources of fat were essential and that we must obtain them from food or else, we become deficient and out of balance.

Studying in the United States was an eye-opener in many other ways. I quickly realized that not everyone there was living a life of comfort, as I had assumed. It soon became clear also that not everyone had the resources to maintain healthy eating habits that included avoiding fattening fried foods served especially at fast food restaurants. And I heard stories of people getting depressed especially during winter months, when they were stuck inside and without the extended social networks that we relied on back home in Burundi. Winter months were also times when many turned to food for comfort and gained weight as a result.

You can imagine my disbelief when I first saw people who were so morbidly overweight during my first visit to Indianapolis, Indiana. The only thing I could attribute this to was over-eating, taking advantage of what I assumed to be the excessive access that the States, the land of plenty, had to offer. I contrasted these people's fate to that of the homeless I had seen when I visited Washington D.C. for the first time. There I saw people begging on the streets for something to eat. I could not believe my eyes. *Is this America?* I wondered quietly. Homelessness and begging for food were rare at home when I left. How can a country so rich and so developed not have enough food to go around? How could people live side by side in the same country, or even the same town or city, with some eating too much, while others did not have enough to eat? What kinds of foods were the obese ones eating that caused so much fat accumulation around the body? Was there something wrong in their bodies that made it easier for them to become so overweight to a point of reaching such a horrific metabolic overload? Although many of these questions crossed my mind, I did not have time to dwell on them. I had other learning to do that would keep me busy and help me stay away from too much fattening food, I hoped!

Nonetheless, these questions left me unsettled. They left me with many assumptions and misconceptions that would take years to resolve. First impressions do matter. These assumptions were my introduction to what is commonly known as the Standard American Diet (SAD). This was to become, in part, my diet too. I did not rely fully on this diet because I had registered in the back of my mind that if I was careful, I too could gain more weight than I wanted. I had seen clearly how bad things can get if one fails to tame one's eating habits. Remembering the saying I had learned in my English classes in high school that "prevention is better than the cure," I avoided fat to prevent obesity. I did not know yet about the link between excess body fat and high blood pressure, heart disease, or diabetes. I was still young and did not consider myself vulnerable. Turning to dietary fat for health seemed counter-intuitive.

Although I proceeded with misguided awareness, I still believe I made the right choice by avoiding fast food restaurants and their large servings of french fries. I ate at home initially, hoping to rely on the foods I was most familiar with. Bread and tea for breakfast had been my morning tradition, and I kept bread and butter in the fridge and replenished them when I ran out. Soon enough, I was introduced to cereal and milk, which replaced bread and tea. Because I could not find time to go back to our house on South Grant street in the middle of the day for a full meal with a starch, some vegetables and a protein, I figured that learning how to make sandwiches to bring along for lunch would not be a bad idea.

An avocado sandwich would have helped, but I was not impressed with the avocadoes I saw at the food stores. They were small and hard, clearly picked before they matured. They were also expensive and just simply unappealing. You would have to visit Burundi and taste them there to understand what I am talking about. So, I rarely bought them when I was a graduate student. Eating lunch out became more frequent than I was used to or had anticipated. I had pizza often, the cheaper option in the campus cafeteria on the ground floor of the main library, where I spent hours and hours reading for my classes, sometimes working on a part-time basis and writing research papers. For dinner, I tried to maintain some of the eating habits I had developed at home, though. I cooked beans and rice regularly. They were a staple and still are today. Gradually, I introduced new foods in my diet, including new types of cooking oil, mostly vegetable oil.

Choosing between butter and margarine: In the United States, I learned from my boyfriend then (now husband) that I should switch to butter completely and stop buying margarine, an artificial spread that many still use in the place of butter. He too had used it for at least a year while teaching in Kakamega, Kenya because he did not have a choice. Butter was not available in his village. He knew margarine was not the same as butter, but he did not realize yet how it was made and how bad it was for him. When he returned to the US, he switched back to butter. And he made sure I knew that butter was better and that I should give up margarine once and for all. So, I kept butter in the fridge, even though I used it only occasionally and sparingly whenever I did because it was full of fat and I had started to shun fat. Not my husband, nor my kids later on, though. They spread it generously on their toast, using more than I ever felt comfortable with. They seemed to enjoy it and I had no sound reason to not let them be. Then, my husband ignored his sensitivity to dairy and would suffer for years before making the turnaround, as I mentioned in Chapter 3.

We never introduced margarine to our kids because I had understood that it was not as real as butter. What that meant, I wasn't sure. That my husband did not recommend it was enough for me to trust his preferences. His habits around butter came from traditions passed down from his parents and grandparents who used real butter and did not even discard other animal fat when cooking. Instead, they enjoyed the full flavor it gave to other foods. He relied on this wisdom as he had taken time to observe, listen and then follow through in his own kitchen. Could many of the home-cooking and eating habits he grew up with be what kept his grandmother alive and strong without many health complaints till she died, in her late 90s? Neither she nor my own grandmother, continents apart, ever believed that fat from milk or meat should be avoided completely. But at times even our intuitive knowledge cannot stand against "expert" advice, especially when the aging process starts kicking in, taking its toll on parts of our body that seemed invincible when we were younger. Eventually, even his parents succumbed to the suggestion to switch to "I Can't Believe It's Not Butter" and "Smart Balance." Butter lost its place and was replaced by these hardened vegetable oil spreads in their fridge. What happened to the real butter my husband grew up eating? How could his parents and many others who knew so much about how to eat real foods and who understood the blessings that come with a long life, start doubting their dietary wisdom?

Could replacing butter with margarine be among the factors that often precipitate our declining health, bringing us sooner rather than later to the point where what keeps us alive are the boxes of well-marketed pharmaceuticals? What would happen if we relied more on quality fresh and local foods, and not how long a food will stay "safely" edible based on the expiration date which can be as long as two years into the future? With such foods, we are almost guaranteed artificial preservatives as well. As we age, our bodies lose some flexibility and strength; that is normal. However, people age differently, and dietary choices play a role. Dietary fat supports healthy aging, when consumed adequately. Margarine contains dangerous trans fats and speeds up the aging process instead. Could relying on it in my teen and young adult years, and avoiding good fats later on have contributed to laying the foundation for my excess weight gain and rather extreme imbalances I felt in midlife?

Don't get me wrong here. I am not worried about getting old or even looking old. Ultimately, I continue to disguise my age well. What worries me is losing my senses and becoming dependent on others with the basics of living my life. What worries me is losing my memory, or my limbs. Alzheimer's is not fun. Diabetes is not either. I empathize with those caring for an elderly parent or relative whose memory has failed. I empathize and can relate to those caring for a parent or relative who has lost a limb due to diabetes complications. If consuming healthy fats will help to delay or prevent Alzheimer's, or diabetes, I am open to it and will do what needs to be done in this regard. Removing margarine from my diet was an important step aimed in preventing both, as well as other health problems we tend to expect as we age.

Was cooking with vegetable oil a healthy choice? In the US, I started using canola oil for regular cooking, and occasionally for deep-frying the African donuts (*mandazis*) and making French fries. I had heard, almost as a warning, that regular consumption of hamburgers, hot dogs, and French fries served in fast food restaurants were to blame for people's excessive weight gain. I stayed away from MacDonald's and Burger King for this reason. Even when I cooked at home, I did not make hamburgers or hot dogs, and making French fries and other high fat and fried foods were an exception and not the rule. When I ate out and my meal of choice included what I now consider to be good sources of dietary fat, such as olive oil with bread served at Italian restaurants, I did this not as an informed consumer. I never targeted this important macronutrient in my diet. Instead, I was attracted by the appeal of the dish as advertised on a package, the restaurant menu, or as I imagined it once I had prepared it in my own kitchen.

My peers preferred canola oil and so did I because they were my role models then. Was canola oil a healthy choice? It was refined, and there was nothing in its taste that was repulsive. It looked like the familiar *amakoto*, or cottonseed oil, that had become quite popular by the time I left home in Burundi. The freshly harvested and cold-pressed palm oil that I grew up consuming was no longer as popular, as *amakoto* became the oil of choice for many.

Would I have used palm oil if I had if I had found it easily in the local grocery store? Perhaps. My housemates in the US introduced me to their way of shopping and eating, and I embraced their habits without asking many questions. To a certain degree, there is a level of comfort that comes with knowing that we fit in, when we behave like our peers. This is especially the case when we find ourselves in a new environment, a new country that also happens to be considered a model to be emulated by so many across the world. In such an environment, we do not want to be seen as "uncivilized," not understanding enough, or basically not belonging. This is one the reason why I went along with the choices of my friends in the US. None of them were overweight, at least not in the way I would have considered unhealthy. They were well-educated, mostly pursuing doctoral degrees at a well-respected university.

I was learning from the right crowd and since they were mostly Americans, didn't they learn from the world's experts? Didn't they know where to find the right answers, if necessary? Wasn't I among the lucky few Africans to have the opportunity to study alongside them in the States, gaining both academic knowledge and life skills to prepare me for success in whatever I chose to do afterwards? In graduate school, our attention was focused elsewhere. We were there to get an education that would position us well to pursue our professional and life dreams. Ideally, our food choices would have helped us maintain health and balance then and long into the future, but we all relied on many false assumptions.

Without diverting too much, there is some truth in this. Student loans aside, the United States educational system is still among the best, in my opinion. The US has a lot to offer and teach the world, especially in professional work ethics and business. In the context of healthy eating or balanced diets, however, I would turn to other cultures or be more discerning and selective. But this awareness would come much later as, at the moment, the habits and practices of peers seemed to suffice for me to make it through graduate school. I focused on avoiding foods high in fats as a strategy to prevent becoming overweight or obese, like the people I saw in shock in Indianapolis.

So, I turned to canola oil and other liquid vegetable oils for cooking and like my peers, I did not think I had any reason to question their nutritional values. I wanted to adapt as fast as I could. I could find a whole line of cooking vegetable oils at reasonable prices at the few stores where I did my weekly food shopping. Like my peers, I started also eating more meat than I was used to as well. It was cheaper and always plentiful. So were different types of pastas and new types of fruits that I was not familiar with, such as apricots, kiwis, watermelons, and even apples. I enjoyed these as much as they did.

Looking back, those who served as role models in the kitchen were probably misguided by the conventional wisdom regarding healthy eating at that time, which was the 1992 USDA Food Guide Pyramid. This came out when I had been in the United States for only one year, but most likely the Pyramid followed previous years of research and some evidence, perhaps not so conclusive, that saturated fat was dangerous for the heart and that high cholesterol foods raised blood cholesterol. Hence, the USDA Food Pyramid recommended that fats and oils be used "sparingly," in the same way as sweets had to be! Animal fats and tropical oils were singled out for being among the unhealthiest. Therefore, I assumed that those who put on excess weight were eating a lot of foods with a high fat content. Actually, even before the Food Pyramid came out and as far back as the 1950s, leading health authorities such as the American Heart Association urged consumers to focus on "the prudent diet" that limited animal fats and tropical oils. Specifically, the foods to avoid were meat, milk, butter, lard, cheese, and eggs, as well as tropical oils especially coconut and palm. Margarine, corn oil, chicken and cold cereal were considered safer and healthier (Perlmutter with Loberg 83).

Therefore, margarine and other hydrogenated vegetable oils became popular when consumers were advised to avoid foods high in saturated fat. Different types of fats, including butter and other animal fats, as well as tropical oils that are high in saturated fat, were believed to be harmful in two ways. First, they were artery-clogging and even though I was still young and not worried about developing heart disease, it is never too early for one to take care of one's heart. Second, these fats and oils caused the body to put on excess weight. Then, I was still comfortable with my weight as well. My peers most likely were influenced by this misguided understanding of what types of fats and oils were better for them. This is how margarine and liquid vegetable oils ended up replacing butter on toast for breakfast and in recipes for fried and baked goods in many households.

This is also how I became less comfortable with rich foods and used vegetable oil instead. Recommendations to avoid food considered to be high in cholesterol, such as eggs, influenced my behaviors as well and explain why for years, I did not make eggs regularly at home. As you may now be aware, the link between eating foods high in cholesterol, such as eggs, and having high blood cholesterol, is one of those myths that no longer stands. Eating them in moderation (1 egg per day for example) is considered safe and a good source of protein for most people. It took some time for me to reach a new level of awareness regarding fats and oils choices that are better for us. Until then, except margarine that I was convinced I should avoid, I based my food shopping choices on my friends' preferences. I developed a preference for foods that were advertised as low-fat.

And I assumed that when I bought "vegetable oils," I was buying oils extracted from vegetables. With such a level of ignorance, I proceeded to think that if the oils come from vegetables, they must be good. I simply broke "vegetable oils" down into its components: vegetables and oils! Aren't vegetables some of the healthiest foods that even the sceptics will agree that we can consume in abundance, if we like them? Can anything bad come from vegetables? In an article on "What are the most healthful oils, clinical pharmacist Jessica Caporuscio states that vegetable oils are made "from oilseeds, legumes, nuts, or the flesh of some fruits." While 100 percent cold-pressed vegetable oils may have many health benefits, their chemical structure changes making them unhealthful when heated at high temperature. This change applies to canola oil as well as other vegetable oils such as corn, safflower oil, sunflower, and soybean oils. Speaking of canola oil, Dr. Guy Crosby of the Harvard T. H. Chan School of Public Health explains that "[m]ost canola oil is chemically extracted using a solvent called hexane, and heat is often applied which can affect the stability of the oil's molecules, turn it rancid, destroy the omega-3s in it, and can even create trans fats." Crosby adds that "[c]old-pressed canola oil exists but is very expensive and hard to find."

When eventually I learned from reading various sources that I must avoid hydrogenated vegetable oils because they contain trans fats, the worst of artery-clogging saturated fats, I knew that I could not take these vegetable oils at face-value. Michael Noonan concurs with Caporuscio when he writes in his 2013 blog post: "Are there really vegetables in vegetable oil?" Noonan's answer is unambiguous: no. "The majority of these oils are better described as seed oils," Noonan states. The United Soybean Board contends that "all plant-based oils (corn, canola, olive etc.) were called vegetable oils to differentiate them from the lard-based shortenings," Noonan adds.

In Dr. Jason Fung's 2018 online article on vegetable oil, he describes how cooking oils and fats evolved in American kitchens and what led vegetable oils to become popular. One of the reasons was that, up until the late 1700's, cotton fiber was used for making garments whereas the seeds were useless. In the 1800's, increased population and rising demand for cooking oil and for lighting lanterns before electricity, paired with improved extractive technology, led to commercial production of cottonseed oil. It was used as such initially, and later on, it was added to animal fats and lards, and eventually even to olive oil sold in the US. Thanks to the Proctor & Gamble company and newer technologies, hydrogenation of cottonseed oil began, transforming the oil into a solid fat that looked like lard.

This is how Crisco was born. It stands for "Crystalized Cottonseed Oil" which became a commodity in most American households, Fung explains. Other oils, including soy, safflower, and corn, were also hydrogenated and marketed as being "heart-healthy." This is what misled friends and peers who also influenced my cooking oil preferences. This is perhaps what misled the authorities who developed the US Food Guide Pyramid and their recommendations to use fat "sparingly". And it would take me years, if not decades before I would come to realize that I was misinformed and misguided in my choices of cooking oils. Hydrogenated vegetable oils, including canola oil, were not devoid of trans fats. Joshua Rosenthal summarizes well why we should avoid trans fats, stating that "[c]onsuming hydrogenated oil can interfere with your body's natural processes, leading to many health problems including increased coronary death" (2011, 227).

Therefore, regardless of their sources, cotton seeds, soy or corn or other plants, vegetable oils are not extracted from vegetables, and they do not provide similar health benefits as vegetables do, either.

The health risks associated with consumption of trans fats are actually many and the manufacturing process of these oils makes them particularly unsafe.

Mary Dan Eades and Michael R. Eades write that "... exponential rise in fatty liver disease has occurred contemporaneously with the misguided public health campaign to increase the use of 'heart heathy' vegetable fats in the diet" (26). John Douillard in turn writes that "the result [of consuming trans fats], over time, is thick or sluggish bile in the digestive process. This is not inconsequential because bile is what regulates hydrochloric acid (HCl) in the stomach, the digestive enzymes of the pancreas and duodenum, and the ability to process fats" (12). In fact, Douillard uses the analogy of the grease on a stove that has not been cleaned for 20 years to explain what happens with the digestive process when our consumption of trans fat has created sluggish bile.

Hydrogenated oils are made by heating the oil at very high temperatures and "in the presence of hydrogen and finely ground particles of nickel metal .... which gives the fat new chemical and physical properties," states Walter Willet (63). Like other hydrogenated oils, margarine is high in trans fats, which has been linked to an increase in cholesterol (LDL-the bad kind), as well as the risks of developing heart disease, diabetes, and cancer. Other health experts confirm the negative effects of margarine and other hydrogenated vegetable oils, on our health. To summarize, hydrogenated oils:

- Make sluggish bile, which is what regulates our ability to process fat;
- Lack beneficial ingredients;
- Are damaged by heat, making them hard to digest; and
- Take on the worst characteristics of saturated fat.

Dr. Lawrence L. Rudel described the link between trans fats and weight gain based on animal research conducted by a team at Wake Forest University Baptist Medical Center: "Diets rich in trans fats cause a redistribution of fat tissue into the abdomen and lead to a higher body weight even when the total dietary calories are controlled." Though results from human studies are mixed, a 2019 blog post by Joe Leech refers to a 6-year study in monkeys that concluded that "a high trans fats diet (8% of calories) caused insulin resistance and elevated belly fat and fructosamine, a marker of high blood sugar." Nearly a decade earlier in 1997, medical doctors William P. Castelli and Glen C. Griffin warned against a liberal consumption of foods high in saturated fat, cholesterol, and trans fats in their book, *The New Good Fat Bad Fat*. This, of course, was written during a time when low-fat and fat-free diets were the craze. The FDA recommends that less than 10% of our daily calories come from saturated fat. The American Heart Association recommends that we should aim for 5 to 6% of calories to come from saturated fat.

Now that I have a better idea of how margarine is made, I consider it as one of the worst culinary commodities ever invented. Margarine is just as bad if not worse than natural sources of saturated fat. I have no doubt that it is killing consumers slowly but surely, especially in uneducated communities. Trans fats are no longer considered safe in any amount in the United States because of their many health risks. According to a Harvard Health Publishing online article, "[f]or every 2% of calories from trans fats consumed daily, the risk of heart diseases rises by 23%." The article summarizes the different types of fats: trans fats (the bad), saturated fats that should be consumed in moderation (the in between), and monounsaturated and polyunsaturated fat that should be consumed regularly (the good). In the United States, food manufacturers are now required to include the amount of trans fats added to any food that requires a nutrition facts label, which includes all processed and packaged foods.

"Thankfully, trans fats will be phased out of the U.S. food supply by 2018, joining European countries like Denmark, Austria, Switzerland, and Iceland, who have already banned them" (Rosenthal 2018, 237).

While fat (like sugar) is almost always included on the label, the devil is often in the details. Trans fat, for example, can be marked at 0 grams even when the list of ingredients includes partially hydrogenated vegetable oils.

This is because for a while, in the United States, the Food and Drug Administration did not require food manufacturers to count any amount of trans fats that was below .5 grams per serving. Given that no amount of trans fat is considered safe anymore, the more servings are consumed, the more trans fats are ingested, and the easier it is to reach harmful quantities, regardless of what we may have been led to believe in the past. Therefore, to be truly accurate, bringing the levels down to 0 grams per serving on the label requires also that no hydrogenated or partially hydrogenated vegetable oils are included on the list of ingredients. Trans fats are found in margarine, solid vegetable shortening, donuts, commercial baked goods, and even in french fries sold especially at fast-food restaurants. These fried foods appeal to our taste buds, which is why they continue to be so popular even as more consumers have an increased awareness that deeply fried foods are not heart healthy. While I never consumed any of these foods regularly, I used canola oil or other vegetable oils for cooking almost daily between 1991 and at least 2002. And I did most of the cooking on high heat. I had used margarine on bread for years before I left for the US in 1991, as mentioned earlier in this chapter.

Margarine and other sources of trans fat continue to be used in many restaurants especially where cooks and chefs perhaps ignore the nutritional value of the foods they serve their customers. I can often tell that it was margarine that was used, even when the waiter insists knowingly or not, that it was butter or some other type of oil. I remember the taste of margarine very well, and to be honest, I used to like its smooth and salty flavor over bread with tea for breakfast. What did I know? A few months ago, I was bold enough to request the package of the oil used for cooking at one of the local restaurants in Liberia. The chef refused to show it to us, based on internal policy, which left me feeling even more suspicious. I can understand his decision. They had no reason to trust me (or not), but they trust some of my clients whom they have served for years. They show them the cooking oils without asking questions. They even let them take pictures of the container. Therefore, I know that vegetable oil, corn oil, margarine, and canola oil are used in kitchens at restaurants around Monrovia, Liberia. This is why my husband and I don't eat out if we don't have to.

We must all be discerning when making food choices. Buying or eating a specific food just because it tastes good or looks good enough, is as misleading as trusting the food advertisers to only sell you what appear in larger print on the package or what chefs choose to highlight on their menu, something that fooled me many times. Also, some foods may seem harmless, as advertised on the package, but when the actual list of ingredients is long, then most likely there will be undesired ingredients, including hydrogenated vegetable oils that work against our health. The shorter the list, the greater the chances of having a better food choice, and the easier it can be to detect undesirable ingredients as well. Otherwise, you are fortunate when you take that packaged food home or eat out regularly and what you eat causes no side effects.

The absence of short-term side effects does not guarantee that long-term effects do not exist, however. Some of these side effects of consuming hydrogenated vegetable oils include weight gain, insulin resistance and belly fat.

The nutrition facts label, together with the list of ingredients, is the most common tool for us to detect fat content and other ingredients in packaged foods. Failing to read the list of ingredients either because we are in a rush, or because we left our reading glasses in a different pocketbook at home, as I often do, is almost a guarantee that we will end up with an ingredient we would otherwise avoid if it were clearly marked and legible to help us truly be informed consumers. This is how we miss the undesirable ingredients and take home a food product that does not meet our dietary preferences. To say that I always avoided trans fats when I brought home a box of frozen chicken nuggets, or even a loaf of bread, would be a lie. Now that I know better, margarine has become so repulsive that I cringe every time it shows up next to bread at the breakfast table of a friend's home. It continues to be sold and it has reached neighborhood stores far and wide. In Liberia, margarine is sold in larger than usual containers even in the few upper scale food stores I have visited. These large containers of margarine at these stores have really caught my attention. Is someone trying to get rid of it, by packaging it in monster loads? I'll let you guess.

Although my awareness of the link between trans fats and various diseases did not come until years later, for over a decade now, the devastating impact of type 2 diabetes on my parents remains a constant reminder that I must be careful to protect myself from known risk factors. Trans fats are one such risk factor. I avoid them because I have started to consider myself vulnerable. Nowadays, I read carefully the list of ingredients to avoid trans fats and other hydrogenated vegetable oils. I can succeed as long as I eat at home. I doubt that I am successful on the few occasions when I eat out. Many restaurants unfortunately seek profit over the health of customers. They use the cheapest cooking oils available, including those that contain harmful trans fats. Margarine is a common source of trans fats used in cooking. Other popular cooking oils include polyunsaturated fats such as cottonseed, corn, soy, canola, peanut, sunflower, and safflower oils that can be healthy when not overheated and depending on how they were extracted. These oils are "... more reactive and unstable, especially at high temperatures .... and can form free radicals when they are heated during extraction and processing or when used for cooking. These free radicals can initiate disease," writes Rosenthal (Rosenthal 2011, 227).

As a preventive measure, I have embraced the habit of cooking most of my meals at home. I continue to avoid fast food restaurants whether in the US or elsewhere. I was not even tempted when one of my colleagues invited me to join her for a meal at a McDonald's in Tokyo, Japan. I could not imagine any good reason why I would want to go to a US-inspired, fast food restaurant in Tokyo. I opted for a vendor selling noodles, chicken, and vegetables with soy sauce from a trailer kitchen on the side of the road. Is it possible that the oil used for cooking was one of the hydrogenated oils I should have known to avoid? I cannot be certain that he did not. But McDonald's even in Japan did not seem like the way to go. "When in Rome, do as the Romans do" was another saying I learned in high school.

There is wisdom in eating like the locals when you travel outside your comfort zone, especially when what is served is truly local, unprocessed and wholesome.

The noodles in Tokyo were local. I knew they were processed, but that was a different time in my awareness of the difference in nutritional value, between processed and whole unprocessed foods. That many locals were stopping by for their lunch was enough to convince me that it must be better than what they served at the nearby McDonald's. Could what they served at the McDonald's in Tokyo have been healthier than what is served at such fast food chains in the US? Who knows? This was in 2002, and my level of awareness of diets was still very limited. Then, I was more concerned about limiting most sources of fat.

In fact, I even failed to apply what I was doing for my kids, adding more olive oil and when available, letting them sprinkle as much parmesan cheese as they wanted on their pasta. Could what I did for them have been what I needed to do to keep myself in better balance when I reached midlife as well? I did not know enough to make an informed decision then. However, intuitively I thought that raising two boys who were into sports, required keeping a large supply of carbs, particularly throughout their teen years. This is the time when many signs of change associated with midlife started kicking in for me as well. For the boys, the excess carbs they consumed seemed to be used up for the energy they needed to keep going and growing. The added olive oil and extra cheese on their plate helped them stay full for longer. Limiting the oil and cheese on my pasta was meant to limit fat consumption. As I did not limit carb consumption, I now know that I was setting myself up for failure in managing my weight, as you can imagine. Live and learn!

Are all animal fats created equal?: Not quite. I had assumed that they were all bad and limited them as best as I could. Even though I liked whole milk on my cereal when I first arrived in the US, over time I started tasting the fat in it, and I no longer enjoyed it. I made every effort to find low-fat milk. I made every effort to find lean meat as well, especially when I bought ground beef. My preference was always white meat, because that is what housemates preferred as well, telling me that it was less fatty, and therefore healthier. I often bought ground turkey instead of ground beef, based on my assumption that because it was, like chicken white and not red meat, it would naturally always be better, regardless of the feed. And if I used butter on bread, I spread as thin a layer as possible. Then, I could not imagine that there was anything nutritional in fat, or that I could rely on it as a source of energy as I did carbs. I never imagined it being an even better source of energy, especially for anyone at risk of diabetes, struggling to manage her blood sugar, or trying to shrink the excess fat tucked inside the belly.

My views evolved also, particularly when I started paying attention to the ways that animals that serve as our meat sources were raised. Their feed matters. I cannot help but ask myself if animals rely on a high carb diet, such a diet would not make them fat just as it makes us fat. I cannot imagine that chickens fed GMO corn and growing up in enclosed and overcrowded factories provide the same nutritional value as the ones that have been roaming freely while feeding on a diversified diet that includes nuts, seeds, grains, and insects, a diet which, in chicken-land, makes for a balanced nutrition. This diet not only keeps the chickens resilient, but I believe that it protects our health as well. The spread of diseases in highly crowded environments require frequent use of antibiotics to keep the chickens alive and looking healthy.

Overuse of antibiotics is a known risk factor for developing resistance to treatment with antibiotics. According to the healthline.com website, "[e]xcessive antibiotic use can increase resistant bacteria, making the antibiotics less effective for both animals and humans," The article emphasizes that consuming meat from animals that have developed resistant bacteria has serious health consequences for human health, which include the following: "Infections that would not have happened otherwise. Increased severity of infections, often including vomiting and diarrhea. Difficulty in treating infections and higher chances that treatments will fail."

With such harmful side effects on us the consumers, could we be getting it wrong when we favor white meat, such as chicken or turkey, over red meat, even if the cows were grass-fed and have been grazing on green, pesticide-free pastures without the need for antibiotics? I am not suggesting that red meat is healthier always. All meat, red or white, were not meant to be consumed liberally. Even with regular consumption of meat, we would not have to worry so much, if our lifestyles hadn't changed from that of hunter-gatherer ancestors, for better or worse. "Everything in moderation" is a common saying in most cultures! The red meat I had once a week when I was growing up is not the same as the meat that I buy at supermarkets from cows that might have been raised in feedlots.

Factory farming was not meant to yield the healthiest of animals, slaughtered for our indulgence.

Therefore, without the ability to trace our meat products back to their sources, I can understand why many have opted for a vegetarian or even to a greater extreme, a vegan diet. Unfortunately, because not everyone knows how to maintain the necessary balance, strict veganism can backfire. I have never been a heavy meat-eater, nor am I a strict vegetarian. I do, however, prefer a more vegetarian diet. And I love my veggies over every other food choice! What we eat matters. What animals feed on matters as well. Our health is dependent on what we feed it. If we eat meat from animals that graze less and rely on a high carb diet, then I do my best to remove the fat from inside the piece of chicken or beef, if I must have it.

I fear red meat from cattle raised in conventional feed lots that are known to be injected with harmful hormones such estrogen and the recombinant bovine growth hormone (rBGH), in particular. Even without being conclusive, Hassan Malekinejad and Aysa Rezabakhsh, in a June 2015 article published in the *Iranian Journal of Public Health* and also available on the NIH.gov website, warn that "[t]o this end and with respect to the considerable progress in developing of analytical methods and bioassays, it is critically needed to clarify the possible and potential impact of the present hormones especially estrogens in dairy foods on consumers health situation because it is already pointed out that possible unwanted effects on human health by consumption of meat from oestrogen-treated animals cannot be excluded." The most probable effects, they add, are "in the initiation and provoking of breast and prostate cancers." Ain't nobody got time for that! Right? Fat in red meat is therefore what I have shunned the most but I still try to avoid fat from chicken as well, especially when they are fried, which adds to the fat found naturally in them.

I have grown to avoid other rich foods also. Even on the occasional times when I eat a piece of cake, I am still tempted to scrape off most of the buttery icing and eat the rest, which is often more sugar than I would ever want. Oh, how I wish I had learned earlier that butter is not always bad and that the butter in icing or on toast, would actually have helped to slow down the absorption of the glucose into my bloodstream and would have provided a better source of energy than pure sugar in a piece of cake. Live and learn! Cheesecake remains my least favorite of all. It's too rich, and too full of fat, and the sweetness and pungent flavors in cheesecake do not work well together for me. I developed a distaste for rich foods, plain and simple, even before weight became an issue. Perhaps this is because in the back of my mind, I was protecting myself from getting fat from the fat I would consume. Perhaps I was relying on my misguided assumption that I was protecting my heart by doing so as well. How wrong was I?

Tropical oils, healthy with a caveat: Palm oil and coconut oil are both high in saturated fat, which is why many have turned them into dietary foes. However, there is a part of me that was never convinced that palm oil was bad for me. What I am concerned with these days is that with renewed interest and increased popularity, palm oil has come with a new health risk. Sales of this oil are made easy by the proliferation of thin plastic pouches and recycled plastic water bottles, especially in various countries in Africa. These plastics will most likely melt into the oil when they are near heat in the kitchen or even under strong tropical sun. I observe this over and over again at many open-air markets and makeshift kitchens where I have travelled across Africa. The plastic pouch makes it easy for buyers to get their daily supply if that is all they can afford, instead of a weekly supply in a dark glass bottle as we did when I was growing up. Then palm oil was the oil of choice in most kitchen that I knew. Plastic bottles had not made it to the country yet.

Could the blend between melted plastic and the palm oil create an unhelpful cooking oil for hormonal balance? Could this blend create a harmful byproduct that, together with other unhealthy dietary and lifestyle choices, make it harder to lose belly fat in midlife? While I avoid buying the oil sold in these thin plastic pouches, I am almost certain that the palm oil used in foods at a restaurant or that are served at a friend's or colleague's home started out in a plastic bottle. In *The Hormone Cure*, Sarah Gottfried discusses factors that are linked to high estrogen, which acts as a fat-storage hormone just like insulin. Among these are xenoestrogens particularly phthalates and Bisphenol-A (BPA), found in plastic containers used for storing or serving foods. Gottfried writes that BPA "has been known to disrupt estrogen receptors since the 1930s" (160).

Excess weight is also known to produce estrogen from fat cells. Excess estrogen in turn can "lead to higher insulin and insulin resistance, which tends to make you gain weight, which leads to making more estrogen. This is a downward spiral with seemingly no end in sight," Gottfried adds

(163). Even without the addition of plastic melting inside the cooking oil, knowing which oils are healthy is important. Having choices is even better, allowing us to diversify our diet and get the benefits that each choice offers. This allows us to limit consumption of those known to be detrimental to our health as well. We must continue to educate ourselves and weigh the pros and cons of all our options. With regard to the different types of oils commonly used for cooking, quality depends on who you ask. For example, cottonseed oil is considered healthy by those who look at its fatty acid profile. The oil is low in saturated fat which, makes it heart healthy. Also, it is high in polyunsaturated fats, which has been shown to lower the LDL (bad) cholesterol.

In addition, cottonseed oil is high in vitamin E, an antioxidant, which may be the reason why it has a longer shelf life than other vegetable oils. Cottonseed oil also does not require as much hydrogenation as other vegetable oils because it is naturally stable. However, as Joseph Mercola notes in the online blog post mentioned earlier in this chapter, as much as 93 percent of the cotton grown in the United States has been genetically modified, and GMOs are associated with many health risk factors, including those that in one way or another eventually lead to weight gain or resistance to weight loss. Mercola writes: "Several studies have highlighted the adverse effects of GM crops, including reproductive problems, organ disruption, digestive problems, and allergic reactions .... There are also reports indicating that cottonseed oil has a high pesticide load and mold contamination, which may lead to allergies." All these bodily dysfunctions increase overall toxic load in the body. Without the ability to properly detoxify, the body puts on weight. Poor digestion in particular, is often a factor in weight gain.

However, some sources of fat are good and they are even needed for healthy weight management. Will Clower notes that fat triggers the "satiety signals" (168-69). This is what we need to stop ourselves from overeating, a sure way to gain weight. This is what I wish I had known when I feared adding enough olive oil to my plate of pasta, not realizing that the oil would have slowed down the release of sugar into my blood. It is with this same level of ignorance that kept me from adding loads of butter to mashed potatoes as a friend did, but neither her nor other members of her family seemed to be getting any heavier than the rest of us who avoided or limited fat to the best of our abilities.

Other influential factors impacting my aversion to fat

The change that comes with pregnancy: The stretch around the belly that follows pregnancy is often what motivates many women to diet. While some may succeed at losing some or even most of the baby bump, there are still many who continue to struggle, turning to yo-yo dieting as a way to restore themselves to a shape they would be more comfortable with. Whatever one chooses to do, I believe that feeling healthy and strong and keeping it that way for as long as possible is more important than a slim physique, which is not for everyone. Some women are naturally big, but healthy. What else would anyone want? Nonetheless, I cannot help but wonder what makes the baby bump a permanent stretch on some and not others. For those who lose most of the baby bump and the significant weight gain of pregnancy but then gradually regain it in midlife, like I did, can we still blame it on the experience of bearing children? What about women who have never had children and yet put a thick layer of fat around the belly in midlife?

Pregnancy brings changes that many women know to expect. What might have been a flat belly before pregnancy is slowly replaced by what looks like a thick layer of fat inside the belly immediately after the baby is born and sometimes, even months later. For some, it becomes a permanent change. It all happens for a good reason. We accept it even if we may complain about it at times. The baby who was there stretched us. Regardless of how small we were before the bundle of joy started doing the stretching and growing, we cannot help it but be amazed at our capacity to carry him/

her to full-term on the inside. Women in many cultures, including the one in which I was raised, do not even see the stretch around the belly that stays permanently after the baby is born, as something to worry about. I did not worry about it either after my two boys were born, not even a bit. Perhaps this is because I learned from many other women in my family and in my circle of friends that postpartum weight gain is the norm and not the exception. The expansion of my waistline then was not something I paid attention to also, because I continued to fit into most of my pre-pregnancy clothes.

In fact, in my culture postpartum weight gain was perceived as a sign of wellness while being overfed. It was an indication that the family had the resources and the right attitude to provide the support a woman needed to recover from the hard labor of delivering a child. How much food is required for her to feel nourished and recover is not a question that was usually asked of new mothers or those expected to feed them. It was however, commonly accepted that women need a lot more food after delivery than they did before, and most certainly more than they needed before conceiving. What types of foods would provide the necessary nourishment was not a question many paid much attention to. I did not either. Having had both of my kids in the United States without the extended family support to put on the expected cultural weight gain, my husband and I did the best we could. If I had my kids back home, one good source of beneficial fat, avocadoes, would have been included in most of my meals. In the US, I never put dietary fats on my list of priority foods to consume regularly prior to or during pregnancy, or even after delivery. I assumed then that dietary fat will make me fat and keep me from losing the baby bump. My diet then seemed to work, at least in terms of keeping me in good shape with a healthy weight. It wasn't until sometime in my 40s that the shift in my weight became most obvious around my belly.

This is when I had no choice but to change my wardrobe as I no longer fit into my favorite clothes of my 30s. By the time this shift became obvious to those around me, I had been living in the US for nearly fifteen years. I had also shunned dietary fats during this period. Everyone I considered role models in healthy eating demonized dietary fat over and above all other food groups. Those I believed had healthy diets limited fat consumption, especially fat in fried foods, meat and milk. Nonetheless, friends and peers did not consider canola oil as a source of fat to avoid. So, I too continued to use it for many years. I was not in a position yet to question my food and lifestyle choices that contributed to weight gain. The only dietary change I made in my 40s was the introduction of organic foods, a decision I made based on the promise that such foods are health-enhancing for people of all ages. I continued to favor low-fat or fat-free foods as well. I assumed that the same habits that worked for me before midlife were going to keep me healthy and my belly fat in check for life. How wrong I was!

My own individual experiences with fats and oils: At some point in my 40s and even earlier, my body started rejecting certain fats. Was it in the taste? Was it the message I had internalized, for better or worse, that if I swallow it, I might end up clogging up my arteries? Was it because I had some bad experiences after eating certain oily foods? There is truth in each of these questions to varying degrees. Oily foods have made me sick on more than one occasion. The fear that it may happen again sometimes keeps me from enjoying foods that seem to be high in fat, even when they are healthy sources. I recall this feeling very well on a business trip with colleagues in rural Burundi. We had been travelling for a couple of days already and wanted to make it back to our office and our homes before dark on that day. To be in shape for the long day ahead, and not knowing if we would be able to stop for lunch, we ordered our breakfast the night before so that we would avoid wasting time that morning waiting for breakfast. Along with a couple of my colleagues, I ordered a simple vegetable omelet with onions and tomatoes. As expected, our breakfast was served shortly after we sat down. With each bite of the omelet on my plate, I could tell there was more oil than I liked. Every additional bite confirmed that I was not going to enjoy what I was eating, and the excess oil was repulsive. I tried to lift the fork and let the oil drip back before each bite. It did not work. The oil started overwhelming me. I gave up trying and left the rest of the omelet behind.

As we got up to leave, the discomfort started getting worse. I was almost throwing up. We walked out of the restaurant. My colleagues got into the car and waited for me to get in. I told them I needed to wait for my stomach to settle. I was able to get back in the car after about 10 minutes of walking without stressing over how I felt and trying to focus my attention away from the oily taste in my mouth and the discomfort in my stomach, and instead breathing in the cool fresh air typical of the region where we were. Although I lost my appetite for the rest of the day, I managed to keep going and to do what we needed to get done on that day. Was my omelet different from the ones served to my colleagues? I will never know. It is possible that their bodies could handle the cooking oil better than I could. While I remember this incident vividly because the reaction was almost immediate, it was not the only time I felt uncomfortable after eating oily foods.

Years before, my husband had made a special side dish of broccoli stir fried with lots of olive oil and garlic. It was part of a family tradition he learned from his uncle, he said. I wanted to enjoy it. We were still dating. I did not want him to think that I did not like his food choices nor question his cooking skills, but I could not hide it. I got sick. Then, I could not tell if it was from the extra garlic or the extra oil or both, but I do associate the dish with too much oil, much more than I was used to consuming. The same thing happened at a Christmas dinner, where they served a dish of eggs with loads of butter, another one of his family traditions. This time, even my husband felt the same discomfort I felt afterwards. Perhaps he too had developed some repulsion to fats and oils because his body had become accustomed to my cooking. Perhaps he had lost touch with traditional dishes his family served on special occasions like Christmas. I do make omelets at home and when I prepare them with lots of green vegetables such as spinach or with broccoli, I do not experience any digestive discomfort. And because I do not get sick after eating boiled eggs, I have more than one reason to assume that the problem has to be with the cooking oil used. Therefore, I suspect that the type and the amount of oil used for making eggs will determine if I will digest them or reject them.

The discomfort for me almost always includes getting constipated when I eat high fat foods, unless the meal includes high fiber foods such as steamed, not fried, vegetables. Legumes, especially chickpeas, black beans and French lentils, usually help as well. Unfortunately, these are not always as common on restaurant menus as I used to think. I am careful whenever I eat out. Food poisoning is a common experience when I move out of my comfort zone, especially when I eat at restaurants while travelling.

Either way, whether we have an immediate or delayed reaction, when a food is not good, it does not change its long-term impact on our health, especially when consumed regularly. Repeated food poisoning depletes the gut of beneficial bacteria, another reason why we must be careful about what we eat, in or out.

One of my brothers used to joke that his stomach is made of steel. Mine is certainly is not made to withstand too much pressure!

Could the fact that I avoided fat for so many years be among the reasons why it is still harder for me to digest fat? I have had to re-learn how to stop shunning fat but instead embrace expert recommendations to use digestive enzymes as necessary to better digest good sources of fat that my body had needed all along. Fortunately, increased awareness of the health benefits of fats came when I was in better control of my food choices as well. My consumption of fat therefore evolved both in a negative and in a positive direction as I continued to apply what I learned each time. Let me explain how my understanding of the benefits of fat evolved gradually, bringing me to where I am today, as I now am more intentional about adding fat to my daily food intake. I know that fat is essential to a balanced diet and a healthy body. I know that dietary fat is required for restoring lost balance in midlife as well. Below, I summarized what convinced me that I needed fat in my diet to lose it in my body.

GOOD DIETARY FATS HELP TO LOSE BELLY FAT

"You have more than 100 trillion cells in your body and every single cell should be constructed of high-quality fat," Mark Hyman, *How Do I Know If I'm Eating Enough Fat?*

A fat-free diet is actually one of the worst eating plans one can ever embark on. Expert recommendations that highlight the health benefits of dietary fat have convinced me that avoiding fat might have precipitated the apparent signs of aging that I felt in midlife, along with the excess weight that was piling on, despite my restricted fat intake over nearly two decades. Many studies continue to link healthy fat consumption to an increased ability to burn fat. In their book *Healthy Fats for Life*, Lorna R. Vanderhaeghe and Karlene Karst reference different studies that confirm the role of healthy fats in fat burning. One such study was led by Dr. M. A. Mir from the Welsh National School of Medicine, who shows that "GLA from evening primrose and borage oils activates a metabolic process that can burn close to 50% of the body's total calories" (Vanderhaeghe and Karst 30). The healthy oils Vanderhaeghe and Karlene recommend for encouraging fat loss are flaxseed, hemp, evening primrose and borage (33). There are others who would even put it as simply as to say that we must "eat fat to lose fat." With an understanding that the body's fat storage is not necessarily related to the fat we consume, Will Clower, in his book *The Fat Fallacy*, writes that "[y]ou need fat in your diet so that you don't have to keep it in your body" (76).

Joseph Mercola considers conjugated linoleic acid (CLA) to be "a very powerful fatty acid ... that has been linked to long-term weight management and optimal health." Interestingly, "[s]ome of the best sources of CLA are grass-fed beef and raw dairy products," Mercola writes in a blog post on "The Secret Sauce in Grass-fed Beef." He also cites a study published in the *American Journal of Clinical Nutrition* that found "individuals who took 3.2 grams of CLA per day had a drop in fat mass of about 0.2 pound per week (that's about one pound per month) compared to those given a placebo." Vanderhaeghe and Karst also refer to a study published in the *Journal of International Medical Research* that showed "participants who ingested 1.8 g of CLA per day for 12 weeks experienced significant body fat reduction versus the control group." Given that both groups did not change other habits including their diet, but were exercising at the same time, those on CLA supplementation lost body fat but maintained their weight, which is ideal in otherwise healthy individuals (32, 33).

Annie Price highlights the health benefits of butyric acid (found in butter and ghee) in a 2017 blog post on Joshua Axe's popular website. She explains that these dairy fats can assist in fat-burning, noting specifically that "butyric acid, a short-chain fatty acid ... helps regulate the balance between fatty acid synthesis and the breakdown of fats." In addition, "[s]hort-chain fatty acids are believed to play a positive role along with probiotics in preventing metabolic syndrome, which almost always includes abdominal obesity," Price adds.

Most foods with natural fats in them contain varying amounts of saturated and unsaturated fats. While we need both in our diets, unsaturated fats are considered the healthiest and they are divided in two types: Mono-unsaturated and polyunsaturated fats. This does not mean that we must avoid all forms of saturated fat. In fact, Eades and Eades remind us that "avoiding saturated fat and eating vegetable oils instead ... is the very regimen that makes fatty livers worse in lab animals" (32). Could the same thing be happening in humans? I would not be surprised.

Returning to Mark Hyman's blog post cited earlier in this chapter, he makes the case that eating the right fats helps you to lose the wrong ones "[b]ecause healthy cell walls made from high quality fats lowers blood sugar and insulin levels, meaning you're more likely to burn than store fat". To balance my intake of dietary fats, therefore, I had to rely on this expert knowledge to help me become an informed consumer of this nutrient that I had shunned for years. Mark Hyman lists several warning signs of healthy fat deficiency and these include: dry, itchy, scaling or flaking skin; soft, cracked, or brittle nails; hard ear wax; tiny bumps on the back of your arms or on your torso; achy and stiff joints; memory problems; Attention Deficit Disorder (ADD); diabetes; weight gain; and even cancer.

Dry skin especially on my legs and elbows, brittle nails, weight gain and memory lapses were among those early warning signs that I needed to increase healthy fat consumption.

I was aging faster than I would have predicted. Along with the general weight gain around my whole body, my face became rounder, and the fat around my waistline was especially noticeable, as many around me communicated more than once.

For someone my height at 5 feet 4 inches, and weight at about 157 lbs when I finally decided to take action, there was no doubt that I needed to lose weight. Anything over 145 lbs for anyone my height is considered overweight, based on Body Mass Index (BMI) calculations. This index places individuals in four categories based on their current weight and height. People are underweight if they are below 18.5. They are of normal weight if their BMI is between 18.5-24.9; overweight if their BMI is between 25-29.9; and obese if their BMI is 30 and above. My current BMI is around 21.5. It is normal because I have taken steps to address several dietary shortcomings and no longer believe in the misconceptions that led me to shunning dietary fat. "Remember those countries and areas of China with extremely low rates of Western diseases did not achieve them merely because their diets were low in fat. It was because their diets were rich in unrefined plant products - they were not eating fat-free cheesecake and potato chips", notes Joel Fuhrman (87). And Vanderhaeghe and Karst list several benefits of healthy fats consumption. They include reducing the risk of heart disease and diabetes, helping to burn fat, manufacturing hormones, improving our skin and boosting our immune system. They add also that "[g]ood fats are essential in weight management, a key component of maintaining health" (33).

STEPS I TOOK TO IMPROVE MY INTAKE OF DIETARY FATS

First, I learned to distinguish the bad fats from the good ones that are beneficial to our health. I had to even return to some old dietary habits that had worked for me as a kid and continue to work for others in many cultures that recognize and rely on the value of good fats to maintain health and balance. From there, I had to do what I did with carbs, finding which among the good ones would work best for me. I did this through trial and error sometimes, to see if what worked for others, would also work for me. Trying to imitate my husband, who can tolerate large amounts of fat, including coconut oil that is very high in saturated fat, has failed me many times. But there are certain fats that work and that I continue to integrate in my diet on a regular basis. Below, I explain how I was able to bring myself to where I am today, consuming good fats regularly and intentionally. I had to do this because I could no longer ignore the fact that avoiding fat did not stop the weight gain and accumulation of fat around my waistline as I entered midlife. I had to admit to myself that avoiding fat did not protect me from the many other signs of imbalance that started showing one after the other in midlife. I needed fat all along. Therefore, I had to play catch up in midlife.

While I learned that without beneficial fats in my diet, there is a level of balance that I cannot achieve, I could not succeed without removing the sources of bad fats as well, and the knowledge that informed my decisions confirmed unequivocally that margarine and all known sources of trans fats had to go forever. Refined oils, including canola, are no longer my favorite cooking oils. My choices of fats nowadays include tropical oils such as palm oil, coconut oil and coconut butter, nuts and seeds such as almonds, walnuts, pumpkin and sunflower seeds, hemp seeds (whenever I can find them), pumpkin seed oil, fats from fruits such as avocadoes, olives and olive oil, tahini (made with sesame seeds), and hummus (chickpeas and olive oil). They include limited fats in grass-fed beef, some fat in chicken and fish as well. Below, I go deeper into the step-by-step approach I took to remove unhealthy fats and which healthy ones I added.

Changing my attitude toward Animal fat

From the time when I entered the US in 1991, up until 2015, I could not imagine that natural fat in meat or even dairy could be beneficial. It was an even greater stretch in my thinking to consider liver as one of the healthiest organ meats. Therefore, I have had to change my attitude toward animal fat. Joseph Mercola recommends liver from grass-fed cows as one of the highest suppliers of choline, as he notes in a 2018 blog post on the importance of choline to liver health. This nutrient is known to play an important role in preventing non-alcoholic fatty liver disease (NAFLD). In this blog post, Mercola cites nutrition expert Chris Masterjohn, who believes that "… dietary fat, whether saturated or unsaturated, and anything that the liver likes to turn into fat, like fructose and ethanol, will promote the accumulation of fat as long as we don't get enough choline." A 2016 article by Jill L. Sheriff and colleagues also consider the link between choline deficiency and the accumulation of fat in the liver. They note that this "link has been recognized for over 50 years, leading to the establishment of choline deficient-diets to induce models of nonalcoholic fatty liver disease in animals. In humans,

NAFLD is the most common liver condition worldwide, affecting up to 30% of Western and 17% of Eastern populations."

Furthermore, they also discuss the link between estrogen status, genetic and bacterial factors on one hand, and dietary choline and the risk of NAFLD on the other. The article highlights the multiple pathways through which choline impacts human metabolism. One of the well-documented health benefits of eggs comes in part from their high choline content. Among populations that tend to suffer from low choline, Mercola includes postmenopausal women. In his blog post that explains why "Choline is Essential for Your Brain, Heart, Liver, and Nervous System," Mercola writes that: "postmenopausal women have a higher demand for choline, since their low estrogen levels puts them at a higher risk of developing liver and muscle damage due to choline deficiency." Mercola adds in his blog post focusing on the link between chlorine and liver health cited above that "… their requirements are higher than those of premenopausal women." Awareness of this has helped me to open up to the habit of eating eggs for breakfast more regularly than I used to... According to a WebMD article by award-winning journalist and health expert Salynn Boyles, the consumption of eggs supports brain health and enhances memory, which tends to decline as we age.

I started appreciating some of the fats in animal protein when I understood better the health benefits they provide. I eat fish and chicken more frequently than beef. I prefer wild-caught salmon and sardines as they are high sources of Omega-3 fatty acids and low in mercury. They are also on the safer side of sources of animal fat that I can afford, especially when I cannot trust the sources of my red meat and chicken. Either way, food safety matters always, regardless of which diet one chooses to follow.

There are two dietary trends that include different types of animal fats (and proteins) as key components of a healthy diet: the paleo and ketogenic, or keto, diets. Although both continue to attract many followers, I will add my own little *caveat*. Paleo promotes more animal protein and fat than I am used to nor am comfortable with. Thinking that I could, if I wanted to, eat meat or fish every day is an acquired habit I developed once I moved to the United States. I am still not convinced that eating this way is the best way to eat. We also need to consider the importance of dietary balance and environmental sustainability. The keto diet also focuses on healthy fats as the main suppliers of necessary calories, with less protein and a very limited amount of carbs, mostly from vegetables, nuts, and seeds. I have occasionally tried modified keto and paleo diets that have required adding enzymes to better support my digestion of some fats, as necessary. There is no diet that works for everyone. This includes the keto and paleo diets. Keto is particularly not practical for anyone who does not digest fat well.

Reintroducing tropical fats and oils

Palm nut oil: Perhaps the fear of tropical oils is subsiding as I can now much more easily find both palm and coconut oils in glass jars, especially in health food stores in the states. This is a sign that I am not the only one recognizing their health benefits. I now keep palm oil in my pantry and like we did when I was still living at home with my parents, I almost always use it for making *isombe*, the cassava leaves vegetable that requires this oil to create the flavor we are most used to. Palm oil is added in higher than usual amounts in this vegetable dish, perhaps because earlier consumers led by traditional wisdom, had learned that it worked better this way, lowering risks of cyanide poisoning. A WebMD article on palm oil also points out that palm nut oil's many benefits include treatment for cyanide poisoning. Sometimes I use palm oil to lightly fry salmon or other fish, which I do first and then bake for just a few minutes more before serving. It's a great way to prepare it.

Unlike cotton seed oil, palm nut oil is also high in saturated fat, which needs to be limited but not fully avoided in our diet. However, because both types of oil are also high in unsaturated fat and vitamin E, their benefits outweigh the potential harm of saturated fat to susceptible individuals. In addition, palm nut oil is high in beta-carotene, a precursor to Vitamin A. Both vitamin A and E are powerful antioxidants that protect the body from free radicals. Health expert Bryce Wylde identifies several benefits associated with raw red palm fruit oils. They act as powerful antioxidants because of the high beta-carotene and lycopene contents; they can reduce plaque buildup in the arteries; they help maintain proper blood pressure; they quench free radicals and keep inflammation under control; and they improve blood flow to the brain. With so many benefits, why would anyone with easy access to tropical oils choose vegetable oils instead? Should we be surprised that cancer, diabetes, heart disease, and high cholesterol cases are on the rise in Africa, for example? More and more people have made the switch from beneficial coconut and palm oils to hydrogenated vegetable oils. Could such dietary changes have anything to do with some of these undesired health outcomes we are seeing these days?

Palm oil has been a preferred cooking oil for much longer than all other vegetable oils currently used throughout tropical Africa. The high saturated fat content in palm and coconut oil impact the heart differently than the saturated fat in red meat. Either way, I have never had a problem eating a meal that has a high amount of palm oil. There must be something in its fats that just works for me, especially in African dishes that typically require it, such as *isombe*. You too should try it before discrediting its health benefits or making assumptions about health risks associated with a regular consumption of this flavorful tropical oil.

Avocadoes: Among the healthy sources of fat that I continued to consume whenever I could find them were avocadoes. Initially, I enjoyed mostly the rich flavor they added to foods, knowing little else about their nutritional value. Back home, we ate avocadoes because they were plentiful. We enjoyed them and used them as a cheap spread on bread or even over rice and beans. They were a topping on most dishes. We enjoyed their creamy flavor without knowing how they were supporting our hormones and even improving our skin. In the United States, I enjoyed guacamole, but otherwise, I found avocadoes there to be of poor quality. This was before we moved to Liberia. Since then, I'll take the avocadoes in the states any time.

Avocadoes are a fruit that is mostly made of good fats with many health benefits. Meghan Ware's 2017 blog post discusses "12 Health Benefits of Avocadoes". She points out that avocadoes are a good source of energy-boosting B vitamins including B-6, riboflavin, niacin, and folate, which also show promise of protecting the body against various types of cancers. They are also a good source of magnesium needed for sleep and potassium that is needed to balance water in the body. Avocadoes support the heart as well as the absorption of beta-carotene needed for healthy eyes as we age and they are a healthy source of omega 3 fatty acids, which are also good for the brain and the heart. The healthy fats and high fiber in avocadoes can help you feel full and satiated, preventing overeating and the weight gain that follows. Eating fat also slows down the digestion of carbohydrates, which helps to keep blood sugar levels stable. Sometimes when I am travelling and have limited breakfast choices, two boiled eggs and half an avocado are enough to keep me satisfied through the morning. When I have a choice, adding sautéed spinach makes a full low-carb breakfast for sustained energy and alertness for up to four or five hours. And I do not experience a quick drop in blood sugar that happens when I eat a carb-filled breakfast.

Regarding the importance of consuming healthy fats, Will Clower notes that the beta-carotene molecules that are found in many vegetables "only work for you if your body absorbs them, and they're only absorbed in the presence of some form of oil or fat" (77). A, D, E, and K are all fat-soluble vitamins found in many fruits and vegetables and they require healthy fats to be absorbed. We often hear that "we are what we eat" but more accurately, "we are what we absorb." Without the ability to absorb the nutrients from the foods we eat, we are wasting foods and losing out on the benefits they would bring to us. We can therefore understand how palm oil, a good source of vitamin E and carotenoids, which the body converts to vitamin A, can be part of a healthy addition to any vegetable dish, as its fats also support the absorption of its beta-carotene! Palm oil is definitely a source of good fat that I enjoy, and I digest it well.

Introducing new sources of healthy fats

Coconut butter and oil: Coconut oil has some powerful nutrients that make them an exceptional food for those who can digest it well. In Jillian Levy's 2018 online article, she explains that coconut oil contains lauric acid, a medium chain fatty acid that is associated with improved digestion, heart and brain health, along with fat burning and weight reduction.

I use coconut oil occasionally. It withstands heat better than olive oil and is high in monounsaturated fat, a healthy source of fat. Coconut oil has a very high saturated fat content. I learned from adding coconut oil to my diet that high amounts of saturated fat do not work for me. Generally, I limit such foods, consuming them in small amounts, so that I can have them more regularly. Digestive enzymes support the absorption of these healthy fats. A probiotic with lipase enzyme in it for example, helps. Similarly, having fats with non-starchy vegetables, ferments (cultured vegetables), apple cider vinegar, and fresh lemon juice support fat digestion as well. This is a tip I learned from Gates and Schatz in *Body Ecology Diet* (106). I digest coconut butter better than I do coconut oil. Coconut butter has some fiber in it, which is perhaps why I digest it better. However, coconut oil works well for my husband, even though he too prefers coconut butter. So, you would have to try them and see for yourself if one or both work for you or not.

Nuts and seeds: Almonds, walnuts, pumpkin seeds, sunflower seeds, and flax seeds are all sources of beneficial dietary fat and many other nutrients that I choose from and add to my diet. I make an effort to always have almonds and flax seeds, in whole or ground form, in my pantry or fridge. Since nuts and seeds are high-calorie foods, I pay careful attention to serving sizes, in particular. Often, a handful of these is enough to eat as a snack or to add to my cereal, smoothie or a salad. I sometimes use butters from almonds or pumpkin seeds and add them to a dish that calls for peanut butter. Almond butter is now my favorite nut-based butter. I add it to *isombe* as well. Instead of ground peanuts that the dish usually calls for, almond butter and sometimes almond flour add a similar rich and creamy flavor we would otherwise get from ground peanuts. My husband and I have eliminated peanuts from our diet just as we did gluten and dairy. Peanuts are actually legumes rather than nuts and they attract mold easily, which is why they are a known allergen for sensitive people.

Hummus (with tahini and olive oil): While this food is not part of my family traditions, I like hummus and use it as a spread on crackers, or a dip for carrots or other raw vegetables. The basic hummus is made by blending together chickpeas, sesame seed oil/tahini, olive oil, lemon juice and garlic (optional), and salt to taste. One of my new favorite side dishes is a salad made with sliced and cubed cucumber, hummus, and seaweed mixed together for a creamy salad. For extra color, I sometimes add a shredded carrot. Hummus adds a distinct creamy flavor to an otherwise bland vegetable such as cucumbers. High amounts of water in cucumbers, however, makes this vegetable one of the best foods for rehydration and getting a good supply of potassium, which is a healthy electrolyte that supports normal blood pressure as it regulates the amount of sodium retained by the kidneys. I make my own hummus when I can find all the ingredients at local food stores. If not, many food stores now sell ready-made hummus. With olive oil and sesame seeds (or tahini) added to the chickpeas, hummus provides both fiber and beneficial fat.

Olive oil: This prized oil most popular in Mediterranean diets has become a regular oil I use for salad dressing, stir-frying vegetables and cooking other foods. I have been using it regularly for nearly two decades now, since I learned of its heart-health benefits in early 2000. Olive oil is also rich in antioxidants and has anti-inflammatory properties, according to Joe Leech in his 2018 blog post. I have adjusted my use of this oil when I learned that it does not withstand heat as much as I used to think. Therefore, I now avoid cooking foods on high heat and instead, when I need to cook anything on high heat, I heat up the pot first, then add the oil and then immediately I add the onions, start stirring, and lower the heat to medium heat. Within a few seconds, I also add a tablespoon or two of water to prevent the oil from overheating and changing its chemical composition, turning a naturally healthy source of fat into one that can be harmful. I have also developed the habit of cooking most of my foods on medium or medium-low heat.

Pumpkin seed oil: I have become adventurous in finding newer and more flavorful sources of healthy fats, such as pumpkin seed oil that I use as a base for a healthy homemade salad dressing. This cold-pressed pumpkin seed oil is quite expensive at around $24 for an 8 ounce bottle, perhaps one of the most expensive oils I have ever used. So, I reserve it for special occasions, using it occasionally as a treat for my family or special guests. It is sold in dark bottles, and it has a deep dark green color and a flavor that is so rich, I would describe it as a blend between high quality cold-pressed olive oil with high quality cold-pressed avocado oil. In my opinion, it is one of the best oils I have ever tasted. Even a little bit enhances the flavor of a dish in ways that I rarely find in other types of oil. I love it in a cold-potato salad as a gut-healthy resistant starch snack or a side dish. If you have never used it, I highly recommend it! Pumpkins are really one of my favorite foods that I rely on both as a replacement for high-carb grain-based starches and also to make pumpkin pie, usually around Thanksgiving in the United States. When I can trust the quality of the pumpkin, I roast the seeds and eat them as a snack, or I toss them into a salad along with adding some pumpkin seed oil in the salad dressing.

Hemp seeds and hemp protein powder: This is the most recent addition to my diet. I discovered hemp seeds randomly in the nuts and seeds section of a local health food store in Rockville, Maryland. I bought whole seeds once there but when I ran out and went back to replenish, I could not find the seeds. I searched other health food stores around and could not find them either. What used to be sold as whole seeds, is now sold in components as hulled seeds, with little fiber, or as protein powder with a good amount of fiber but less fat. While I use both, I prefer the whole seed over these other components. The nutrients in these are watered down. Hemp seeds supply one of the highest amounts of magnesium, fiber and protein I have ever found in one serving of seeds. Magnesium supports sleep, which can be challenging during the transition into menopause, as I explain further below in Chapter 8. Hemp seeds are also a good source of dietary fat. Sometimes, I now add the hulled seeds and/or hemp protein powder to my morning cereal made of quinoa, ground flax and almond butter whenever I can access these ingredients. I add them to a smoothie when that's what I am in the mood for.

WHAT ARE THE SIGNS THAT FAT HAS BENEFITTED ME?

Within a few weeks of consuming fats regularly, I could tell that my memory was improving. I had noticed that I was becoming more and more forgetful, something I did not think I should be experiencing in my 40s or 50s. My skin also became less dry. My legs and elbows no longer looked cracked and lifeless, as was the case early on in my transition to menopause. In addition to maintaining a healthy weight, I lost an inch around my waistline. At that point, the only additional change to my diet and other lifestyle habits was adding fat. I am happy to report that I am no longer losing weight. Instead, I am maintaining it, staying in the range of 127-132 lbs when I am in the US and between 125-128 lbs when I am in Africa. I continue to fit in size 4 dresses as well. Therefore, good fats have helped in weight management and maintenance.

When I add seeds and nuts or an avocado to my meal, I tend to feel satisfied longer, easily going for four to five hours without the urgent need to eat. I mentioned earlier that with carbs, I tend to eat more than I need, and overconsuming carbs leaves me feeling more tired and sleepy than energized. Fat does the opposite. I have clearly benefitted from this improved way of eating, and these signs of change are what has convinced me to continue adding healthy fats to my diet. I hope that you too will no longer shun dietary fat, and instead, recognize that good fats offer a critical nutrient for health, hormonal balance, and a healthy weight. All cells in your body require good fat for proper function and fat-burning, as Mark Hyman reminds us in the 2016 blog post referred to earlier in the chapter.

CONCLUSION

Fat sources were not on my list of priority foods to be consumed regularly. For years, I could not picture fat sitting alongside fruits and vegetables or brown rice, or even the long list of many other foods I considered healthy. I expected that all I did to limit fat consumption would keep me in good shape even as I aged. I had assumed, like many other consumers around me did, that if dietary fat had been the answer to people's quest for health, including a healthy weight, then food stores would not have had any reason to continue selling so many low-fat or fat-free options for us to choose from. If it had been the answer, food suppliers would not have had to go the extra mile as to label their lean meats, separating them from the rest. If it had been the answer, they would not have had to remove fat from milk to create reduced fat, fat-free and skim milk versions. The market must have spoken, and food producers responded to the demand. I too was part of this target market.

Yet, what I associated fat with was as irrelevant as it was to think that I could eat ice cream during pregnancy and at the same time avoid high fat foods to keep myself and the growing fetus from gaining too much weight. The problem is that once you consider yourself knowledgeable or smart enough to make your own sound judgements on matters of diets and even other areas of life, you do not intuitively seek alternative points of view. You think your knowledge is enough to keep you on the right path.

In the area of dietary fat choices, I lacked sufficient knowledge to help me distinguish one source of fat from another.

Looking back, my consumption of fat evolved in four distinct phases. Initially, I consumed it without thinking about it, just as I did many other foods I ate as a kid and young adult, when I relied on the food that was provided to me at home or at school. As my level of awareness increased, I avoided most sources of fat I knew of, associating them with health risks such as heart disease, high cholesterol, and excessive weight gain. At my next level of awareness, I reintroduced some fats whose health benefits I was convinced that I needed. Eventually, I came to realize that not all good fats are good for me, and I became more selective. I now find whichever of these sources of good fats and oils that work for me and I include them in my diet intentionally and consistently. I have come to realize that it is not fat *per se* but the kind of fat I should worry about. I had to admit that I had been following outdated eating habits that shun dietary fat while indulging in other foods that lacked the necessary balance.

I also had to admit that avoiding fat did not help me keep my weight in check, especially when I entered midlife. On the contrary. Therefore, to redress the damage caused by years of misinformation that led to my aversion to fat, I needed a new definition of what a balanced diet exactly looked like. Turning to dietary fat for body fat loss required twisting my dietary muscles harder than perhaps most of the other changes I had to make to adjust my eating habits.

Informed by those who had been studying the impact of dietary fat on weight, metabolism, and heart-health, as well as those who analyzed fat's role in appetite control for overweight and even obese people, I too was enticed to consider fats as a macronutrient I should not ignore if I wanted to reach my weight goals.

Many experts referred to in this chapter helped me question my thinking and convinced me that perhaps I did need dietary fat all along. Belly fat is one of the many manifestations of imbalances that take place in midlife among those who avoid dietary fat, even if they generally follow a healthy diet. Clearly, my eating habits did not work and the layer of fat around my middle was a manifestation of imbalances that took years to build, until they showed up very visibly around my waistline in midlife. The foundation was laid through misguided eating habits as my diet was as healthy as my understanding of what a healthy diet looked like. It did not include fats as an important macronutrient to be consumed intentionally and regularly.

After trying many other types of dietary and some lifestyle changes and even reaching close to my ideal weight, I still was not happy with my waistline. I had to remain open and flexible and figure out what I was missing. Those from whom I learned that "fat does not make you fat" enticed me to give fat a chance and see how integrating it in my diet would work for me. Adding good fats to an otherwise healthy diet has not added inches to my waistline. Instead, it has helped me shrink it better and brought me a few other health benefits. However, it is important to keep in mind that fats are high in calories, and therefore, they can easily contribute to weight gain if not consumed carefully, as part of well-balanced meals. Doing it right requires paying attention to serving sizes and the amounts of calories per serving so as not to exceed your caloric threshold. I had to learn to better digest fat as well, given that I had shunned it for so many years and increasing fats initially caused me to get constipated.

Nevertheless, I no longer see fat as detrimental to health as I had previously assumed. Instead of avoiding it, I now know to separate the good from the bad and enjoy heart-healthy fats to support my body to restore hormonal balance, without which I could not lose inches around my waistline. If I had embraced Hippocrates' wisdom to "Let food be thy medicine" earlier, I surely would not have removed fats from my diet in the first place. Instead, I would have sought to distinguish one source of fat from another and enlisted the good ones for my own health. I hope that this chapter compels you to give good fats their rightful place at your dinner table and in your diet. I promise that if you follow some of that suggestions shared in this chapter regarding dietary fats, your waistline will thank you for your actions!

PART THREE

INTEGRATE THE LIFESTYLE TRIO

CHAPTER 6:

EXERCISE TO LOWER STRESS AND BUILD MUSCLES

"Regular exercise can ... help you sleep better, reduce stress, control your weight, brighten your mood, sharpen your mental functioning, and improve your sex life" in "The secret to better health – exercise", Harvard Health Publishing

I remember going to a health fair nearly a decade ago and one of the organizers was checking people's body mass index, commonly known as BMI. I stood in line, thinking for sure that mine was normal. I looked at other women around me and was already guessing and placing them in different categories based on what was obvious. Well, you are right if you guessed that I, too, was overweight. Anywhere between 18.9 and 24.9 is considered normal. Mine was at 25.9. Not too far off, but I had already crossed the line. With my lifestyle habits, I had failed to notice that my weight was no longer where I thought it was. I never kept a scale to monitor my weight. Even when we had one, I did not use it much, except to check the weight of our luggage before we had to fly out. I have no doubt that the sedentary lifestyle that started as I entered midlife precipitated the weight gain, putting me on a path that seemed to be common among many other women around my age. This path to weight gain created physical strain on my body, especially my lower back, as well as mental stress. Excess weight built up after I had spent the previous five years without doing much exercising. I did nothing on a regular basis to keep myself even minimally fit.

The healthcare workers at the health fair advised those who were overweight to exercise more. Advice on diet was not something that they discussed with us then. But wherever else I looked, diet along with exercise were and still are included on most prescriptions for what we must do to lose excess weight. Eating less and exercising more, following the "calories in and calories out" paradigm, was the dynamic duo recommended for achieving and maintaining a healthy weight. So, when I heard "exercise," I knew that to reverse the weight gain trend and trajectory I was on, I had to re-establish the habit of moving around again, something that I had abandoned when my responsibilities led me to think that I had no time for it.

Little did I know that what I did not have time for then,
I would have to find time for when I got sick.

Since I thought my diet was healthy, exercise seemed like the next best thing to work on to better manage my weight. I needed to adjust my daily routines and add exercising to my schedule. Walking regularly was

BELLY FAT IN MIDLIFE

the simplest and easiest form of exercising that I felt ready to engage in. And when done mindfully, walking can reverse the harmful effects of a sedentary lifestyle, which as I will explain further below, is detrimental to health, and is linked to weight gain. "Exercise is a definite plus in overall body fitness and health, especially if done regularly and in moderate amounts" (Steward, Bethea, Andrews and Balart 12-13).

To succeed, I needed a mindset shift to allow myself to stop finding excuses not to engage in exercise and instead to make time for it in my busy schedule. I had to push myself and believe that I could do it. I had to act on this belief and exercise regularly. This initial push or motivation is common among people who have not exercised in a long time. However, as Shawn Stevenson encourages: "... [I]n the beginning, if you have to push yourself a little more to exercise, have the courage to do so, knowing that eventually you won't have to *push* because the vision of a better life and the way you feel [and look] will start to *pull* you" (92). I certainly can attest that reaching my ideal weight continues to pull me, looking always and anywhere for opportunities to keep a consistent exercise routine.

WHAT LED ME TO A SEDENTARY LIFESTYLE?

Various responsibilities at home and at work led me to believe that my priorities were right and that there truly was no time left for regular exercise.

Responsibilities tend to increase in midlife for many, with aging parents, kids' events and activities, various duties in the home and at work.

In midlife, we tell ourselves that we no longer have or can afford the luxury of playing ball, tag, or even jump rope. We believe those were things we did in our childhood and younger years, the time when play was exercise and exercise was play. Then, for me, exercise was even part of my daily chores. It was part of my daily walk to school or Sunday walks to church. What I did then enabled me to retain many health benefits of exercising, including managing weight naturally.

Exercise continued to help me when I was a young adult living away from home. Then, my daily routine involved trekking across the campus grounds, as a high school, college, or graduate student, moving from one classroom to the next, or from the dormitory to class or bus stop, to get where I needed to go each and every day. These activities counted as exercise. When I started teaching, I added a stop to my office as I walked to and from different buildings where I taught my classes. At the end of the day, when I was teaching college classes, I also walked to the parking lot where my car was located and then drove home, after having logged at least two to three miles of walking each day.

What happened when I left academic life was in part to blame for my sedentary lifestyle. I was entering midlife and my excuse was that I was too busy to include leisurely activities such as exercising in my schedule. I could not think of a better way to fit exercise into my schedule without making sacrifices I was not ready to make at the time. Then, my body changed gradually but consistently, as a layer of fat started building around the belly, along with all the other changes that were taking place in my midlife body. Through it all, I was mostly oblivious to these changes. Over a period of five years, I spent my workdays primarily sitting down in my workspace or travelling to wherever work took me.

When I was in another country, I was mostly sedentary as well, either sitting at meetings and interacting with an audience, or giving a presentation; and travelling by car, from one town to another, one village to another and eventually back home by road or by air. My work was intended to change lives and contribute to building healthier and more resilient communities. I thought that by giving all I could, I would ensure that those communities would also get what they deserved, and their lives would change for the better.

Taking time for myself seemed selfish. Adding exercise to my busy schedule would have meant taking time away from the greater good.

And because I am not one of those people who cannot sit still, people who are constantly moving their feet or legs around while sitting, there really was very little movement in my body when I was sitting day in and day out, for months on end and for most of my waking hours over five consecutive years. "Western culture is full of laborsaving devices, thus reducing exercise and energy expenditure and creating an abnormal energy expenditure", writes John Lee with Victoria Hopkins (227). I wish I naturally had the habit, like my husband does, of getting up frequently throughout the day to stretch and move around to prevent getting stiff and improve blood circulation. I wish I had internalized the message that doing so would have helped me focus better when I returned to my seat.

Getting up and moving around does add up and can count as exercise, when done mindfully. After all, isn't exercising about moving around intentionally? "The impact of movement — even leisurely movement — can be profound. For starters, you'll burn more calories. This might lead to weight loss and increased energy. Also, physical activity helps maintain muscle tone, your ability to move and your mental well-being, especially as you age," writes Edward R. Laskowski, who warns of the dangers of a sedentary lifestyle in an answer to the question, "What are the risks of sitting too much?".

What's unfortunate is that even when I had embraced, like many of my colleagues, a sedentary lifestyle, I knew that exercise was needed and that it would benefit me. I just was not ready, nor could I convince myself that I had the time for it. I had other more important priorities to occupy my time. After all, didn't my kids, my family, and the communities whose lives I believed my job intended to change deserve all of it? I could not imagine any better way to share valuable time. So, at home with my kids, I aimed to give them undivided attention. If they wanted me to read a book for them, I read. If they wanted a snack or a full meal, I prepared it. If they wanted to play outside, I went out with them, but most often I did it to keep them company, rather than actually allow myself to play like a kid again. After all, I was a parent and not a kid, and an African mother for that matter.

At work, I sought to learn and grow and contribute in a meaningful way. During the day, once I was in front of my computer working on a project, I barely moved. Those who know me well know I can focus, for hours at a time. When I am fully zoned in, I think I even forget to breathe, or at best, my breathing is too shallow to count. At times, I even tried to delay going to the bathroom until I could not hold it in any longer. Sitting in front of the computer, hunched over as I read and wrote might have helped me to get more done, but it came at a cost to my health. The consequences were diagnosable: I became overweight, my BMI was above normal, and my blood pressure was rising. I did not need any diagnosis to confirm my stress overload as well.

Through it all, I knew that exercising was (and still is) critical to losing weight, boosting energy and health. In the rest of the chapter, I will explore what makes exercise beneficial and how it impacts weight, as well as what types of exercises are required to lose belly fat. I will also share how my exercise routine evolved to support my goal of shrinking belly fat, a difficult task indeed. As part of what I refer to here as the lifestyle trio, I look at exercise in the broader context of a lifestyle balance, which also includes stress management and adequate sleep, as the key factors needed to maintain a healthy weight and lose belly fat.

To make exercise work for me, the initial step was to shift my mindset and stop believing that I had no time on my busy schedule to dedicate to exercising.

I had to stop thinking that the better time will be when my kids are older, or when my aspirations to climb the professional ladder have subsided, perhaps in retirement. I had to stop believing that my time was too important to waste it on myself instead of serving others.

I had to start believing and owning my time to include self-care as a critical component of what I needed to better serve others. I had to embrace what gender expert and author Shelly Zalis shares with us, that self-care is not selfish. I had to convince myself that taking the time to exercise as part of self-care is the right thing to do if I wanted to be healthy and strong enough for long enough to be of use to my children and others who wanted to see me around and strong even in old age. I knew that I had at my disposal a set of options to create a customizable plan that I could rely on to make exercise a lifestyle priority. Changing my mindset allowed me to open up to the idea that I alone held the key to making exercise a habit that will work and benefit me in the long run. I hope I will convince you to make it a priority, as well.

WHY MAKE EXERCISE A LIFESTYLE PRIORITY?

"As a matter of fact, it's [exercise] essential to being the healthiest version of yourself. You get so many positive benefits from improving insulin sensitivity, to boosting hormone health function, to enhancing your metabolism", Shawn Stevenson, *Sleep Smarter: 21 Essential Strategies to Sleep Your Way to a Better Body, Better Health, and Bigger Success* (82).

The list of exercise benefits goes on and on for anyone willing to listen, hear, and act. In fact, there are so many articles written on the benefits of exercise that a Google search on this topic yields as many as 1.4 billion results! Sifting through all of these to gain a full picture of the types of exercises that will yield the intended health benefits would be a monumental, if not impossible task. Yet, one does not need to read through even a small portion of these articles to be convinced that exercise is important and that certain types of exercises promote body fat loss better. Knowing where to find reliable information is important, but it can still be overwhelming. A search on the same topic on Harvard Health Publishing, an online newsletter of the Harvard Medical School, for example, yielded 1,362 results in February 2019. Let me quickly highlight just a few of the topics they cover:

- Five ways exercise improves the quality of your life;
- Regular exercise changes the brain, to improve memory, thinking skills;
- The secret to better health – exercise;
- Benefits of exercise - reduce stress, anxiety, and helps fight depression;
- 5 of the best exercises you can do;
- Exercise and weight loss: the importance of resting energy expenditure; and
- Natural "exercise" hormone transforms fat cells.

With a consistent exercise routine, it's possible to lower the risk of major diseases because "[e]xercise decreases blood pressure, decreases serum lipoproteins, especially the bad cholesterol components, decreases obesity, decreases insulin resistance by increasing insulin sensitivity, decreases basal insulin levels, stimulates clots resorption, and reduces the tendency for clot formation" (Steward, Bethea, Andrews and Balart 100-101). In this context, the authors recognize that "estrogen and exercise both decrease insulin resistance and are known to have a beneficial effect on the cardiovascular system in retarding the arteriosclerosis process."

In an article summarizing the "5 Surprising Benefits of Walking", Harvard Health Publishing concludes that walking "counteracts the effects of weight-promoting genes." Researchers found that study participants ... who walked briskly for about an hour a day, the effects of those genes were cut in half." Others have also found that walking can lower the risk of Type 2 diabetes as well as dementia and Alzheimer's with a "remarkable effects on cognition and brain cell regeneration" as Joseph Mercola states in his blog post on "Strengthening Your Body Strengthens Your Mind." Mercola highlights further many other benefits of exercising and advises the best way to enlist them to our advantage. For example, when done consistently, walking can benefit those with hormonal imbalances, thyroid disorders, varicose veins, depression and anxiety, arthritis, PMS symptoms, fatigue, constipation. Some of these are common problems among women, especially after the age of 50. "Walking is powerful medicine," writes Maggie Spilner, walking editor of *Prevention* magazine. Weight loss and weight maintenance can improve sleep and fend off diabetes by "improving the body's ability to use insulin" (3, 7).

The benefits of exercise are often placed against the risks of a sedentary lifestyle that tend to cripple many as weight gain and other aches manifest themselves in those who have convinced themselves, like I used to, that they have no time for exercise. In response to the question: "What are the risks of sitting too much?", Co-director of the Mayo Clinic Sports Medicine Center Dr. Edward R. Laskowski points to research that has linked "sitting for long periods of time with a number of health concerns. They include obesity and a cluster of conditions — increased blood pressure, high blood sugar, excess body fat around the waist and abnormal cholesterol levels — that make up metabolic syndrome. Too much sitting overall and prolonged periods of sitting also seem to increase the risk of death from cardiovascular disease and cancer."

And it does not matter whether we are sitting in front of a computer working, watching our favorite shows on television, or sitting behind the wheel while driving to or from work. Sitting anywhere is still sitting, and it impacts our health in ways we only wish we had avoided, in hindsight.

Most often, we do not take action because we do not have the capacity to monitor how a sedentary lifestyle taxes our health gradually but consistently. Engaging in exercise is therefore a health-promoting habit.

"I have found that it is a great-stress reduction technique. It also helps to increase your levels of dopamine and increase your metabolism, giving you the extra energy you need to keep up with your busy life. Even 15 minutes a day can make a profound difference," Eric Braverman states.

The type and amount of time we spend exercising enables us to achieve many health benefits, over and beyond a stronger physical body. Working out long enough and with some moderate level of intensity to allow the skin, a major detoxification organ, to break out in sweat will lower overall toxic load in our body. In a blog post on the benefits of sweating, Joseph Mercola refers to an article published in the *Journal of Environmental and Public Health* that confirms that "an array of toxins is excreted in sweat including arsenic, cadmium, lead, mercury, flame retardant chemicals and bisphenol-A (BPA)." The article recommends that "sweating should be the initial and preferred treatment of patients with elevated mercury urine levels." Elevated heavy metal toxicity is also a factor in many cases of poor health, as well as in weight gain.

Therefore, sweating adds to the general benefits of exercising, forcing many of these toxic compounds out of the body. One such compound, bromine (found in some flour and baked goods, soft drinks, pesticides and fire retardants), competes for the same receptors used in the thyroid gland to capture iodine. Bromine actually is all around us. It is added to many sodas including Mountain Dew and some Gatorade products in which it is disguised as "brominated vegetable oil." Deli meat, peanut butter and fish may also contain bromine. It is also a compound in many household items including furniture, clothing, mattresses, and computers.

Could the bromine found inside cars be the reason why I get headaches every time I go on long trips with the windows closed and air-conditioning on? Headaches are one of the symptoms of bromine overexposure. My headaches often come gradually and after sitting for at least an hour in an air-conditioned car. It gets so bad that I have to get out and get some fresh air. My family knows this, and we alternate between air-conditioning and keeping the windows open to get some fresh air in, whenever we can. We stop regularly to stand up, stretch, and use the bathroom as needed but for me, getting fresh air for even five minutes often clears the headache. So, in my opinion, there is no doubt that there is something in the enclosed car that triggers my travel-related headaches. Other places we should all pay attention to are swimming pools as bromine is used as a more stable compound than chlorine in warmer temperatures. The list of where it is hiding and its side effects goes on, making it hard to avoid completely. However, anything we do to minimize exposure will help us prevent long-term health risks. Given its ability to block access to iodine receptors, bromine can contribute to thyroid hormone dysfunction.

Regular exercise, and sweating in particular, is one easy way to lower bromine exposure inside the body, and at the same time, enhance thyroid function, an important step in promoting wellness in midlife.

Obviously, diet does play a role in enhancing hormone function, and for this reason, I try to avoid soy products, especially unfermented soy. I avoid drinking water straight from the tap as it is most likely treated with fluoride. Both soy and fluoride are known to impair thyroid hormone function. Keep in mind that the two main thyroid hormones, triiodothyronine (T3) and thyroxine (T4) are responsible for regulating body temperature, heart rate and even your metabolism. A dysfunctional thyroid is a factor in weight gain. Therefore, any form of exercise that pushes out more sweat reduces our overall toxic load, enabling our bodies to hold onto iodine, which supports a better functioning thyroid and a more efficient metabolism. With all the hormonal changes that occur in midlife, including those that manifest themselves through thyroid dysfunction, maintaining a regular exercise routine that allows us to sweat contributes to improving thyroid function and weight loss.

John Lee and Victoria Hopkins concur that exercise benefits every system in the body and improves hormonal balance.

> …. [F]rom your organs, circulatory or lymph systems, to your muscles and bones, performs best for you when it is moved and stretched regularly. Estrogen is made and stored in fatty tissue, so obesity is a major cause of estrogen dominance. Women who are obese also tend to become insulin resistant, which means sugar isn't being removed from the blood and utilized properly. This sets up imbalances in the adrenal glands, which affect the reproductive organs. Your body works as a unit - when one part of it is out of balance, the rest tends to follow (293-294).

Others link exercise to the ability to lower body fat specifically. Joseph Mercola notes in an article on grass-fed beef that the regular intake of dietary fat and exercise are the best ways to lower body fat. And according to a Harvard Health Publishing on exercise and fat cells, "…white adipose tissue, more commonly known as body fat, is the tissue that dimples thighs, enlarges waists and derrieres, and pads internal organs. Each white fat cell stores a large droplet of fat. Brown fat, in comparison, is chock full of energy-burning mitochondria. Its main function is to generate body heat by burning fat." This research, led by Dr. Bruce Spiegelman, Professor of Cell Biology and Medicine at Harvard Medical School, showed how "irisin transforms white fat cells into brown ones, at least in mice," adding that there is a likelihood that the same thing happens in humans. What's interesting about this finding and of great relevance here is that "you can make your own irisin today, for free, by exercising.".

Generally speaking, there are three main types of exercises necessary for losing fat: moving frequently throughout the day; strength training 2 to 3 times per week to preserve your muscles; and adding interval training to burn more calories. Interval training involves short bursts of fast cardio workouts, which can be as short as 30 seconds at time, followed by a time of rest for 60 seconds during which one slows down to enable the heart rate to go down before repeating the exercise several times, generally between 8 and 12 times. These short but consistent sessions can make a big difference in your ability to lose body fat.

A word of caution: As women enter perimenopause and estrogen levels drop, exercising too much can be counterproductive, Sara Gottfried warns. In fact, she counsels against overexerting oneself, especially when one is overweight: "Exercise helps low-estrogen symptoms only if you are lean. Women who are overweight can actually increase their vasomotor symptoms - such as hot flashes and night sweats - if they do too hard a workout. If you are overweight ... it's better to walk briskly than run, to jog one mile three times a week instead of six miles four times a week; to spin or bicycle at a moderate speed" (190). Clearly, in exercise as in diet, there is no "one size-fits all", as the saying goes.

Even too much of a good thing can backfire. This is true of exercise. While consistency is important, being too consistent without diversifying your exercise routine, can get your body in a rut and prevent you from reaching your ideal weight. Working out too much without the necessary time for recovery can keep you from reaching your weight goals, as well. This is because the real benefits of a good workout come during recovery. "All exercise has some negative effects that are usually outweighed by the many positive effects, but without proper recovery, these negative effects pile up and get you into trouble. Intense, focused exercise is taxing on your hormonal and nervous systems, so pay attention to how your body and mind feel. If your performance and energy is declining, it's time to lower your training volume or intensity until you feel strong again," writes fitness trainer Jesse Walker in an article on the "7 unexpected reasons why you're not losing weight."

These days, when I exercise, there are a few things I pay attention to ensure I get from it what I am looking for. For example, I am careful about the pace and timing of my exercise routine so as not to raise cortisol too close to bedtime. "Night time is not the right time," states Shawn Stevenson who refers to a study at Appalachian State University that compared three groups of exercisers based on the time when they worked out: 7:00 am, 1:00 pm and 7:00 pm. "What they discovered was that people who exercised at 7:00 am slept longer and had a deeper sleep cycle than the other two groups. In fact, the morning exercisers had up to 75 percent more time in the reparative 'deep sleep' at night" (82).

I also try to spend enough time exercising until I get sweaty as a way to lower toxic load. A visit to a functional medicine physician surprised me when she looked at my fingernails and bottom of my feet and was almost certain that what she saw were signs of high levels of toxicity in my body. Therefore, when I exercise, one of my goals is to sweat and lower this level of toxicity. I aim to achieve this through a sustained walk on the treadmill for 30- 45 minutes or mixing this time on the treadmill with some other muscle-building, strength training exercises on different exercise equipment. Going for a walk outside up to one hour allows me to break in sweat as well. Doing this increases the potential to make my own irisin and increase brown fat cells. The benefits of exercise in lowering stress often drive me to keep a consistent exercise routine as well. Nonetheless, it is important to recognize that not all exercises have stress-lowering effects or are beneficial for shrinking belly fat in midlife.

"Exercise can reduce stress; however, exercise can also increase stress on the body because it increases cortisol. The goal is to exercise in a way so as to not raise cortisol too much. This would mean keeping your pulse rate low during exercise. Weight training is resistance-type exercise and increases cortisol unless you do fewer repetitions and rest between them. You also would not want to exercise over soreness", Eric Berg, *The 7 Principles of Fat Burning: Get Healthy, Lose Weight and Keep It Off* (141).

In the next chapter on stress management, I discuss the interaction between exercise and stress further, to help shed some light on what to do to enhance the benefits that each offers. For now, I will focus on how adjusting my exercise routine has helped shrink my waistline, as it continues to lower my risk for type 2 diabetes.

Taking action sooner rather than later was no longer an option because an over-expanding waistline was a sure sign that I was headed in the wrong direction, laying the foundation for diabetes and poor health as I aged.

Over the last few years, I have decided that I must find time for exercising regularly, as a preventive measure for the health risks I saw in my parents and in many other aging relatives.

Once I was ready to fit exercise into my schedule and I was able to get into the habit of exercising regularly, I learned in the process that with exercise, like with many other types of activities aimed at helping to improve my health, doing some was better than doing none. Walking and aerobic workouts through dance were the main ones that I engaged in at first. They helped in losing some weight, but not enough to reach the fat inside my belly. The types of exercises I engage in have continued to evolve as I feel prompted to test myself to see which will bring the benefits I am most looking for. I have also come to realize that not all help reduce the waistline. Let me share what I learned from the different types of exercise I have tried and how they have challenged or benefitted me – and my waistline.

WALKING

When I returned to exercising, this time doing so intentionally in midlife with the goal of losing weight, I was totally out of shape. I could not keep up with others. My husband had to slow down for me. Colleagues had to slow down for me. My kids did not know what to make of me, but they knew I was slower than they preferred. I will never forget one time when I joined colleagues for a march to support the "end of gender-based violence" activities in town. I was based in Kigali, Rwanda at that time. I was in my late 40s. My fitness level was mediocre. I realized that I had to take action to get myself back into better shape. The little bit of walking I had done in Lilongwe, Malawi did not prepare me for hiking up the hills of Kigali. However, I knew that even there, with commitment, I could move as fast as some of my colleagues who looked heavier than me but were faster. I saw others who walked so smoothly as if they carried no weight on them. I envied them. I wanted to be as fit as they, because that is how I used to be. I used to be a fast walker without even trying. I inherited this trait from my father. He was tall, relatively slim, and fast. When we were kids and walked with him to church, there was no excuse for not moving fast enough to make it there in time. After all, how could we be late when he was the one to play the church piano?

Walking had been a daily routine for most of my life. Walking regularly had been beneficial in ways I had taken for granted. Then, there was nothing about my physical shape that I thought needed to change. In fact, in my teen years and through my 20s, I would have been happy to add a few more pounds. Though I had different stressors then, I walked and played and danced regularly. This helped me feel normal, happy, and refreshed on most days, as I moved around freely without thinking about what I was doing. Then, it was not about exercising. It was about living a normal life that required movement as part of life. That continued until later, when my professional career took me to a job that required being more sedentary and less active, as mentioned above.

When I decided to start walking again, my midlife crisis continued to hit harder on my body with heavy periods and eventually insomnia as added problems to the excess weight I was experiencing. With a renewed sense of determination, I developed a new walking routine that I maintained even after we moved from Rwanda and back to the US. I made it a habit to go out at least three times a week, even when the weather was not conducive to spending time outside. I was so determined to exercise that at one point, to prevent the excuse of not wanting to go out in winter cold, I used our open floor design on the first level of our house that allowed me to go around in circles, walking from the kitchen through the family room, the living room, and the dining room that were all connected without an actual door in between. This kept me walking through the winter months until spring came again.

I walked any time of the day whenever I could find some free time, but I aimed for a morning walk as often as I could, when I learned that this is the best time to exercise if getting a good night sleep is one of the goals, as Stevenson recommends. If I could not find time to walk during the day when the weather was pleasant, I would walk in the evening, usually before dinner. As time is always of essence, walking seemed to be the simplest and quickest form of exercising that required no costly or complicated equipment, and I could fit it into my schedule without having to rely on the schedule of a given class at a gym or the additional time it took to get there and back. The other good news about walking is that as long as your legs are strong enough to move, and your mind is alert, you can do it and gain many health benefits that many other types of exercises offer. All that is needed are comfortable clothes and walking shoes and you can get going. I aimed for an hour of walking.

I took it slowly initially, but it did not take long before I was able to regain strength and stamina and start moving fast enough again. I continued to push myself to stay consistent with my walking routine. I was happy with the results, feeling less tired and more energized with each subsequent walking session. I knew I was doing something good, an investment into my physical health. I felt that walking helped to release stress, which is good for my mental health as well. I sometimes brought music along. However, for me, music can be distracting when I am exercising. Listening to a song that's not moving along the rhythm of my feet can be a bit frustrating. Sometimes, listening to music can push me to move faster than I intended in order to follow the rhythm of a song. This is not always advisable, as fast-paced workouts can negatively impact stress hormones and low estrogen, as Gottfried reminded us above, especially when overweight.

"Exercise, especially intense exercise such as weight training as well as short, quick intense types of sports are the types of activities that help growth hormones. The problem is that exercise can trigger cortisol release and cortisol inhibits growth hormones. The trick is to trigger growth hormones without triggering cortisol. This means you need to do high-intensity, short-duration exercise with lots of rest in between," notes Eric Berg (110).

Music also creates emotions that are not always in line with what I need at the moment, bringing back certain types of emotions I'd rather not focus on when I am trying to take a pleasurable, focused walk. So, while it may seem strange to millions who keep music on in their ears anytime they're working out, I prefer to be able to control my moods and my pace, especially when I'm walking. I sometimes also like it quiet not having any noise but the sound of birds, frogs and crickets while I walk. Keeping a walking routine did help me lose an initial 10 lbs. So, I knew it worked. But why did I hit a plateau at 147 lbs even when I continued walking off and on for nearly three years? There was still 20 lbs more that I wanted to lose and I wanted to wear size 8 dresses again. What was keeping me from losing these additional pounds? This was the question I had to answer before I could reach a breakthrough. I continued searching for ways to improve the effectiveness of my work out routine.

When I hit the plateau, I thought that perhaps I needed to push myself harder. I tried to walk faster, off and on during the duration of the walk, to get my heart to pump harder and my body to burn more calories. Sometimes I would find hilly trails instead of flat sidewalks for harder walks to see if I could improve results. Walking longer and faster was not the answer, I eventually learned. Walking however does benefit health in many other ways, as noted earlier in this chapter. For this reason, it is definitely one form of exercising that I continue to engage in, and I think you too should consider it or continue to do it if you already walk regularly. In my case, I tried a different form of exercise that increased the intensity of the workout: dancing!

ZUMBA AND AEROBIC DANCE

In 2011, I joined a free Zumba class immediately after work. I was based in Kigali, Rwanda at the time. I attended a few sessions but then stopped going because the timing did not fit with the schedule of my ride back home. But I was determined to improve my exercise results, and it gave me the idea of continuing with aerobic exercise through dance that fit better with my schedule. I found a few CDs I could dance to and with the help of my husband, who set up the music system in our large master bedroom, I hit the dance floor and was able to do some heavy-duty dancing with as many styles as I chose. I would sweat it out, usually as soon as I got home from work and before dinner. I was often done between 6:30 and 7pm. Thankfully, I had enough help in the kitchen, and my kids were both teenagers by then. So, I did not have to be the one managing the kitchen all the time. After the workout, I thought I had burned enough calories to deserve a big plate of pasta or brown rice or whatever starch we chose that evening as the main portion of the foods on my plate, in addition to all the other food choices and fruit for desert.

Between the timing of exercise and the high carb diet I was on, I can now understand why I was not losing weight fast enough. I was certainly not shrinking my belly fat. Working out harder and faster when I was already overweight, as Sara Gottfried reminds us, was not benefitting my efforts to keep my hormones in balance. Moderate exercising would have worked better for my hormones. Some even recommend less to no exercise when already stressed, which I was. While dance can raise mood, high aerobic exercise, in the form of fast dancing, also raises cortisol, and therefore, did not help much either. As I discuss further in the next chapter on stress management, high cortisol is a detriment to shrinking belly fat. Over the following 6 to 8 months, I lost another three to five pounds, but even then, my weight fluctuated, and it did not take much for me to go back to the plateau at 147 lbs, which happened especially when I travelled and skipped exercise for even one week.

I remained disappointed with my results. I had assumed I would benefit a whole lot more from eating healthy foods and exercising than I experienced. What I ignored then also is that not only does stress dictate the results of intense aerobic workout, but high cortisol impacts sleep as well. I will discuss in the next two chapters how stress negatively impacts sleep and how poor sleep quality prevents body fat loss. This will help you understand why my workout routine was setting me up for failure and why I could not shrink my waistline by just exercising harder.

When the body is in a state of homeostasis, "intense anaerobic (higher-pulse-rate or resistance-type) exercise triggers several fat-burning hormones - growth hormone, testosterone, adrenaline and glucagon," writes Eric Berg (140). Otherwise, you are working against yourself when you engage in intense exercise with exhausted adrenal glands. Berg therefore recommends that "if your adrenals are stressed, only do light aerobics (low-pulse-rate endurance-type), if any at all, until you get your energy back and your sleep is improved" (140).

I wish I had read Eric Berg's book before I tried to lose the extra 20 lbs or so. As I learned more about the most appropriate exercise for shedding those unyielding pounds, and as I understood better the interaction between exercise, stress and sleep, I changed my workout habits once again to focus more on building muscles. I sought the help of a fitness trainer as well. It took some time, but I did eventually convince myself that perhaps joining a gym was not a bad idea after all.

BUILDING MUSCLES AT THE GYM

Once I had finally joined the gym, the next challenge was to learn how to use the exercise equipment and to use it consistently to improve results of my work out routines. With time, I switched from the routine treadmill to other equipment that allowed me to better build muscles of my upper body and my legs.

Gym in Maryland, USA

Going to the gym on and off in 2012 and 2013 was the first time I learned that my weight was about 37% body fat. Ideally, the coach told me, that the fat needed to be around 25%. So, what was I to do? I learned a few tips from him and I tried a few of them, but I did not feel motivated enough to continue. Hiring the personal trainer to coach me regularly would have cost more than I could afford at the time. So, I found myself using mostly the treadmill or the elliptical machines. These turned out to be just like another walking routine, only that this time I was using a moving machine, instead of walking on the ground inside my home or outside. I felt de-motivated after a few months, and eventually I decided it was a waste of my money. I did not renew my membership after one year because I was not getting the results I wanted during the time I went there, or at least not fast enough. I also realized that I enjoyed walking outdoors more so than inside the gym.

I tried to do a half hour full body workout on YouTube that was easier to follow on my own, and I maintained this routine for at least a full year, committing myself to doing it four to five times per week. Although this did not bring me to my ideal weight, the workout which involved several moves to tone my body allowed me to lose another 10 lbs. This brought me down to about 137 lbs. I was able to keep this weight for a while. At this point, I could no longer assume that as some of the excess 20lbs melted away, my belly fat would also follow along. My waistline remained bigger than the rest of my otherwise slimming frame.

As I continued to search, this time for what would bring my body fat to fall at least to 30 percent, my husband was offered a position in Liberia. We sold our house and moved overseas again. This was my first time living in West Africa and only my second time travelling to the region. I lost quite a bit of weight, getting down to 125 lbs, with the hard work that comes with packing dozens and dozens of boxes, and often skipping meals as we prepared to move yet again during the fall of 2017. I was still not pleased with the fat around my belly, but my dress sizes were smaller, between 4 and 6. My sleep improved during this time as well, reaching close to five hours of sleep on most nights, better than the two to three hours of my early experience with insomnia. I will provide further details on my struggles with midlife insomnia in chapter 8 below. When I checked my body fat at the gym, before I moved to Liberia, it had fallen to 32 percent. Not bad!

I had to continue learning and applying different techniques until I found the best formula for my own midlife, a strange and exciting, but also confusing phase, I must add. I wanted to live a long and healthy second half of my life. So, the search continued. Once we were settled in our new home away from home, I decided to give the gym another try.

Gym in Monrovia, Liberia

A combination of being in a new country and working from home in an apartment building with little access to colleagues and my usual communities of friends made it even more enticing to join the gym again. The few pounds I had lost during the move did not take long to return. Fortunately, the new gym that I joined this time had a few fitness coaches available all the time to help clients reach their goals without an additional charge. I took advantage of this. My older son who had used a personal trainer before gave me ideas on what I should ask the trainer to focus on. I was specific about my goals: Lose belly fat, strengthen my legs and tone my arms in particular. ".... [S]trength training ... increases your insulin sensitivity as lean muscle is highly sensitive to insulin, which helps restore metabolic flexibility. By using insulin more efficiently, your body also ends up using more glucose, leaving less to circulate in your bloodstream - hence the improvements in glucose control," states Joseph Mercola in his online article on "The Most Effective Forms of Exercise for Diabetes: Strength Training and High-Intensity Exercise."

The trainers and the additional research I did gave me more tips that helped me diversify my workout routine even more. "...[I]f you've thought of yourself as 'skinny fat', try increasing your protein consumption and focus your fitness on lifting weights and high intensity interval training," recommends Jesse Walker. I started lifting weights and using the steps, in addition to a treadmill or elliptical for warm up. I spent the last ten minutes on a stretching machine that allowed me to improve muscle flexibility. I gave myself one hour each day, four to five days a week to do these exercises. Over three months of doing upper body and leg work, building and strengthening muscles, I reached a weight breakthrough, moving below 130 lbs and hovering between 125 and 127 lbs, while also eating three regular meals each day. My waistline was smaller as well as my size 6 dresses became loose around the middle. The challenge was to never lose the gains and to continue moving forward as I kept track of my diet and exercise routine as well.

Over a period of two years, I was able to keep my weight at 130 lbs or a bit below. I stayed closer to the shape of my younger years, able to fit better into a couple of favorite dresses I had kept for posterity, like the little red dress I wore as a newly-wed, when I welcomed our first guests to our apartment. And I am confident that no one would mistake me for being pregnant! I continue to pay attention to my exercise routine to include those that enable me to build muscles, as I also pay attention to the other elements of the lifestyle trio, namely stress management and sleep because they too can make or break our exercise routines, making it nearly impossible to reach or maintain our belly fat loss goals, when ignored.

STRETCHING AND STRENGTH-TRAINING THROUGH YOGA AT HOME

I had tried yoga classes a few times but was never consistent enough to get many of its health benefits. Often, I stopped attending a class after just a few sessions or a few weeks, feeling unmotivated to continue. I know myself better now and going to an exercise class is not my thing, even when I know it would benefit me to stick with it. With yoga, I have never been able to find a trainer for beginners where most students are truly what I consider to be beginners like me. Therefore, I find myself a bit frustrated when I cannot bend enough, twist enough or curl enough. Working with a personal yoga trainer would cost more than I am ready to pay. However, because I believe in the power of yoga to transform body and mind, and YouTube has a range of self-taught and self-paced yoga videos, I decided to give yoga another try. There are three YouTube videos that I have been following consistently for nearly one full year now and interestingly, doing yoga and exercising three to four times a week has increased my weight by a couple of pounds, still keeping me around 130 lbs. I continue to wear a dress size 4. Recent blood work confirmed also that I am no longer on the trajectory of muscle density loss as I was two years earlier. I can only hope that as I keep on building muscles, I will also continue burning fat efficiently. Three yoga models that I follow are:

15 Yoga Poses That'll Change your Body in Less Than a Month, offered by Bright Side: What I like about this video is that I can do it in a little less than 20 minutes. It provides guidance on how to do each yoga pose properly. It is slow-paced so that I can follow instructions and do as directed without too much strain, and I have been able to do most of the poses. The instructor provides warnings about which poses to avoid for specific conditions such as low or high blood pressure, asthma, monthly cycles where that applies, insomnia, or frequent migraines. I have not been in a yoga class where we were advised not to practice any yoga move based on specific health issues. So, I do appreciate this video for this reason and the other benefits I can gain from regular practice. This has also helped me strengthen different parts of my body, including the arms, the core, and legs.

10 Minute Morning Yoga Full Body Stretch with Kassandra: I like this yoga routine because it is easy for me to follow her guidance. Kassandra requires few poses, and I have even memorized them so that I can now do them even when I do not have access to Wi-Fi. The routine helps to stretch the full body and it is only slightly challenging. In fact, after practicing the yoga poses Kassandra teaches in this YouTube video, I feel fully awake and ready to get going with a busy day of work. It's also an easy and restorative ten-minute break in between projects.

Morning Yoga for Weight Loss - 20 Minute Workout Fat Burning Yoga Meltdown Beginner & Intermediate, posted on Psyche Truth and called

Yoga with Erica: This is more challenging and when I am done, I really feel it. It even makes me sweat. So, I feel like I just did a combination of strength training exercises and stretching, giving me a real workout that makes me feel energized in the morning. I skip a few of the steps that are too hard for me, but I continue to challenge myself to work on improving my flexibility and strength as much as possible.

I appreciate yoga and continue to check out other videos to keep challenging myself and learning new poses that help reach all parts of my body. Yoga makes it easy to practice any time, alone or with others. Yoga is important as we age. "If people don't stretch their bodies as they age, their legs stiffen up, and they tend to shuffle," explains Suza Francina, a certified Iyengar yoga instructor who was interviewed by Maggie Spilner of *Prevention* magazine. Spilner's advice is to aim for the ideal, which is to " stretch at least once every day, for 5 to 10 minutes .... Whenever you stretch, listen to your body and concentrate on working those parts that feel most uncomfortable or stiff." Spilner also offers some tips on yoga poses that you can do almost anywhere and anytime, provided you have a flat and non-slippery surface to practice on (132-138).

When done properly, yoga exercises can help you lose weight, and "improve digestion, relieve back and neck pain, and stretch your hips, thighs, and ankles. They are also great at relieving stress," states the yoga instructor on the *Bright Side* yoga video mentioned above.

CONCLUSION

Exercise is beneficial. There is no doubt about it. What was not always clear to me and to many other exercisers I observe, including some of my clients, is that not all types of exercise will bring the health benefits that we want to achieve.

Knowing what is going on in the body that has created an imbalance and has resulted in weight gain is an important step in creating an exercise routine that is targeted and will enable you to reach your intended goals.

As I continuously searched for the most appropriate types of exercises for someone with my profile, as a woman in midlife, I could not ignore the fact that my estrogen levels were dropping, that my sleep was no longer restorative, and that my body shape was changing with more fat accumulating around the belly.

All these shifts in my body were reminders that exercising had to be beneficial and not make matters worse, as I was visibly changing and aging. Therefore, my exercise routine evolved as I learned what might be most beneficial in supporting my efforts to revitalize my changing body and shrink my waistline in midlife. Targeted and strategic exercises that keep stress hormones under control, that are timed properly so that they do not interfere with the right conditions the body needs for quality sleep, and that enable you to build muscles that burn higher amounts of calories, are what a woman needs to shrink belly fat in midlife.

CHAPTER 7:

RECOGNIZE YOUR STRESSORS AND MANAGE THEM CONSISTENTLY

"...The mind that harms the body can help to heal it", Walter McQuade and Ann Aikman, *Stress, What It Is, What It Can Do to Your Health, and How to Handle It* (Foreword).

I did not grow up around people who recognized the impact of stress or proactively did anything to mitigate its effects. Stress was a part of the ups and downs of life. We did not even talk about being stressed. It would have been a sign of weakness of mind and spirit. I even remember the first time I mentioned to a friend in graduate school that I was stressed, she giggled, saying, "Oh Rose, you've become American!" We had met initially when I was still back home and had spent a lot of time together. In fact, I was her research assistant at the time. She knew then that stress was not part of my vocabulary.

It did not take long for me to embrace the "American" way, stressing over what I now consider as some of the small stuff, as well as more serious issues. But had I lived a sheltered life before? Not exactly. I had experienced stress for a long time, even before I understood what is was! For example, my immune system seemed to be weaker than that of some of my siblings who rarely complained of constipation or heartburn, things that I experienced from a relatively young age. These were early stressors on my body that evolved until I understood what they were, recognizing that what I felt in my physical being had an emotional impact on me, as well.

There is a saying in *Kirundi*, my mother tongue, that can be translated as, "when you 'brag about a disease', you will eventually find a cure for it." In other words, the more people you tell about what aches, the higher the chance of finding someone who knows the treatment for it. Without knowing that what we feel emotionally has a name and that it can be treated or handled productively, we would not know how to "brag about it" and allow others in our lives to help us find a solution or treatment. When we don't know how stress is harming us, we continue to go along, not looking for alternative solutions or approaches that can help us minimize its impact. When eventually I had a name for stress, I started identifying its causes, and there seemed to be many. Some were preventable, such as avoiding foods that I did not digest well and caused acid reflux. Others were manageable, such as changing my schedule so that I did not have to stay up late to finish an assignment because I had procrastinated. The stress of hanging around negative people is also manageable. I stay away from them as much as I can.

There are stressors we cannot control or avoid, however. Every parent knows how it feels when a child is sick in the middle of the night, and neither the parent nor the child are able to sleep through the rest of night. That parent is stressed if he or she has to go to work in the morning, despite the lack of sleep the previous night. Another unavoidable stressor is if violence breaks out in your home country, leaving in its wake the loss of hundreds of thousands of lives, including friends and relatives. This was a major stressor for me, especially in 1993, and throughout most of the rest of the decade because of the civil war in Burundi. The stress left me feeling hopeless during this period. Therefore, we cannot assume that stress and the weight gain that follows, come with the territory of moving into our 40's and 50's. Actually, problems start much earlier and build up gradually until we reach breaking point, often in midlife, as stress continues to intensify.

"Stress can be physical, emotional, psychological, environmental, infectious, or a combination of these. It is important to know that your adrenals respond to every kind of stress the same, whatever the source", James L. Wilson, *Adrenal Fatigue: The 21st Century Stress Syndrome* (11).

Below, I provide a quick review of what I learned from experts who have researched and written on the way that stress affects our health, and specifically, how stress affects our ability to lose weight and belly fat, despite our efforts.

STRESS CONTRIBUTES TO WEIGHT GAIN

Much has been written on the dangers of chronic stress and the interaction between stress and weight gain. Chronic stress disrupts homeostasis, forcing the adrenals to work overtime. The adrenals control many functions in the body, including metabolism. According to *The National Institutes of Health* (NIH) website, hormones released by the adrenal glands perform many functions including:

- Maintaining metabolic processes, such as managing blood sugar levels and regulating inflammation;

- Regulating the balance of salt and water;
- Controlling the 'fight or flight' response to stress;
- Maintaining pregnancy; and
- Initiating and controlling sexual maturation during childhood and puberty.

The NIH adds, "the adrenal glands are also an important source of sex steroids, such as estrogen and testosterone."

As chronic stress disrupts these adrenal functions, the consequences are felt throughout the body. They are not just limited to the site of the two small organs on top of each of your kidneys. One of the consequences is unhealthy weight gain. The other is worsening sleep. "Stress isn't just mentally and physically taxing, it can also confound your weight-loss efforts. Chronic stress can lead to an unbalanced hormonal state that keeps your body from growing stronger and/or shedding weight. Stress also disrupts your sleep cycle, which limits recovery and dampens energy levels," writes fitness trainer Jesse Walker in her blog post that summarizes 7 unexpected reasons why we do not lose weight. In fact, both persistently low and high cortisol are problematic for the adrenal glands. Low cortisol has been linked to low sodium and potassium, the electrolytes that are critical for mediating water retention and blood pressure. Low cortisol has also been linked to a higher sensitivity to pressure, rapid heartbeat, and similar to high cortisol, to sleep problems as well (Gottfried 71).

The adrenals perform so many functions that we tend to ignore as we fail to protect them from use and abuse with stress overload. Perhaps if we all had the opportunity to read James L. Wilson's book, *Adrenal Fatigue: The 21st Century Stress Syndrome*, we would know that the hormones secreted by the adrenals are not just supporting our response to stress, they also "closely affect the utilization of carbohydrates and fats, the conversion of fats and proteins into energy, the distribution of stored fat (especially around your waist and at the sides of your face), normal blood sugar regulation, and proper cardiovascular and gastrointestinal function" (4).

As if these were not enough, "the adrenal glands gradually become the major source of the sex hormones circulating throughout the body in both men and women. These hormones themselves have a whole host of physical, emotional and psychological effects, from the level of your sex drive to the tendency to gain weight," particularly after mid-life, Wilson adds (4).

While a little bit of cortisol, like cholesterol and insulin, is necessary and beneficial (7), it becomes harmful when allowed to keep rising. Stress is stress, regardless of the cause. The stress hormone cortisol that is released each time one feels stressed, must be dealt with swiftly and efficiently before it becomes damaging, both physically and emotionally. Adrenal fatigue is what chronic stress brings as "the amount of stress overextends the capacity of the body (mediated by the adrenals) to compensate and recover from that stress or the combined stresses. Once this capacity to cope and recover is exceeded, some form of adrenal fatigue occurs," adds Wilson (11).

Midlife seems to be a prime time for stress overload as a survey of more than 300,000 Americans looking at their state of mental health revealed. Out of this group, "those with the worst mental health scores were between ages thirty-five and fifty" (Gottfried 79), perhaps a bit younger for those still in their thirties in the United States, but otherwise, this is prime time midlife. Stress is so prevalent that a HBO documentary, "One Nation Under Stress" featuring CNN commentator Dr. Sanjay Gupta, points out that in the US healthcare costs for stress-related diseases are staggering, representing as much as "seventy-five percent of our health-care costs." At the same time, Gupta adds, "our life expectancy has fallen three years in a row." One of the reasons for these, as Gupta points out, is a drop in "... our ability to take care of ourselves and our loved ones. It's about our definition of success and how we pursue a life of purpose. And it's about the future of our country."

While it may be comforting to know that the stress I failed to manage is common in millions of others, the responsibility for self-care lies in each of us. We owe it to ourselves first, and then to our kids and spouses. We owe it to loved ones who see us as a resource, a mentor, a friend, or a teacher. In my case, I owe it also to those who will learn from my experiences and become inspired to take better care of themselves. You will offer the best of yourself to the rest of the world as a result. That is what the world needs. Not a lesser you. Not a stressed-out you! Nonetheless, not all stress is bad. In fact, a little cortisol is necessary. There are many pathways through which a little cortisol is beneficial as Shawn Talbott explores in his book *The Cortisol Connection: Why Stress Makes You Fat and Ruins Your Health and What You Can Do About It*. Talbott explains that cortisol's many functions include: 1) to stimulate the breakdown of glycogen into glucose in the liver; 2) to stimulate the release of fatty acids stored in the adipose tissue; and 3) to promote the release of amino acids in the skeletal muscles (8).

In addition, cortisol "governs your hunger cravings, digestion, blood pressure, sleep/wake patterns, physical activity, and capacity to cope with stress," Gottfried adds (72). Cortisol can also be useful as a mechanism for instant response to a threat, such as being chased by a predatory animal, increasing the body's fuel to feed the muscles and brain to help us run till we're safe. The problem is that often the reasonable amount of stress that was meant to be beneficial becomes chronic, because what gets us stressed is no longer the tiger that might kill us if we don't run fast enough. It can be as simple and as frequent as our normal response to "an angry boss or gridlock on the freeway," as Sarah Gottfried shares in a blog post on stress-induced belly fat by Jaime Osnato. Whenever cortisol levels are elevated, blood sugar rises to help your body escape what it perceives as danger. This is why cortisol is in the family of glucocorticoids, which includes substances that are known to raise blood glucose. The constant reliance on insulin to handle the excess glucose in the blood in turn inhibits fat-burning.

Whenever sugar is available, the body stops burning fat and instead it stores it especially in the liver, through a process called glycogen storage. This is what makes a high sugar/high-carb diet one of the greatest contributors to belly fat, as we discussed in Chapters 2 and 3. This is also why stress must be carefully managed because it raises blood sugar in the same way that dietary sugar does. Glucose is your body's preferred source of energy. And because in most situations, we do not move to run away from the daily stressors of life but instead "we sit at our desks, [which means that] the glucose released by our body to prep the muscles to run gets stored as fat by insulin" adds Jaime Osnato.

Therefore, while a healthy amount of cortisol will provide the body with the necessary support it needs to function properly, helping you to act quickly in response to a threat or to run fast away from danger, chronic stress does more harm than good. Gottfried describes chronic stress using the analogy of the pendulum on the alarm system that never gets turned off (72-73). Chronic stress, for example, no longer results in fat breakdown as would happen under normal stress conditions. Instead, the fat is stored and leads to weight gain. The same applies to the release of amino acids. They are " either used directly by the muscles for energy or sent to the liver for conversion into glucose. The main problem with this last scenario ... is that if it continues for any prolonged period of time, a significant amount of muscle mass may be lost (bad for long-term weight maintenance)" Shawn Talbott adds (8).

In excess, cortisol inhibits growth hormone and destroys collagen, which makes the proteins we need to help tone the body. Growth hormones help to regulate fuel between meals (the pancreas regulates fuel while we eat). Collagen helps to hold us together instead of sagging. Excess cortisol will "eat up your thigh muscles, making it difficult to climb stairs or get up from a chair. In many cases, it's not growth hormone that is the problem but the cortisol that inhibits it," writes Eric Berg (132). And because the body does not distinguish one stress trigger from another, sometimes even activities that were meant to benefit us, such as exercise, can trigger a stress response when done at the wrong time and with the wrong intensity. As I explained in the previous chapter on exercise, high intensity workouts can exacerbate stress in an already stressed body, making it difficult to lose belly fat, since stress releases more and more glucose in the blood. Any unused glucose turns to fat and congests the liver, causing other negative side effects. A congested liver blocks the production of growth hormone whose many functions include:

- Regulating the size of your organs;
- Decreasing fat;
- Increasing lean body mass;
- Controlling sleep cycles during the first half of the night; and
- Rebuilding body tissue (including joints, bones and muscles). Other hormones break down these proteins - for instance the adrenal stress hormone cortisol (Berg 141).

Toxic load in the body contributes to stress as well. These include medications which, as Berg notes further, "can be big barriers to losing weight" (108). He includes the following drugs and medications on the list of factors that put stress on the liver and prevent weight loss:

- Recreational drugs;
- Psychiatric drugs (they deplete hormones and make it hard to lose weight);
- Prednisone (an anti-inflammatory and a fattening steroid);
- Insulin (also a fat-making hormone);
- Anti-cholesterol and blood pressure medications, which impact the liver;
- Diuretics (which deplete minerals and affect the adrenal glands); and

- Antibiotics (which kill your friendly bacteria along with the harmful ones, putting stress on your liver because of stress on digestion).

Blood pressure medications, diuretics, and antibiotics are the ones that apply to my particular situation. These are meant to help manage disease, but they too continued to be barriers to the ideal weight I wanted to reach as they contributed to overloading the liver. A stressed liver cannot perform its main task of detoxification. Excess toxins from drugs and medications, waste matter, or water retention as well as fat build-up under the skin and inside the organs contribute to stress and weight gain. Therefore, to manage weight in midlife, we must pay attention to the routines of daily life that may include a full-time job, child-rearing and care giving for aging parents, along with environmental toxins that end up in our bodies, triggering a stress response and resulting in weight gain when poorly managed.

While I adopted a diet that has kept my blood sugar in check before the need to take diabetes medication, I am still looking for strategies to naturally prevent hypertension. This is my biggest health challenge to date. Once you are on high blood pressure drugs, which I was for at least four consecutive years, it is very difficult to get off of them. Yet, I know that taking medication to control blood pressure is causing both harm and good. It certainly is not helping to protect my liver from toxic load and the one I take impacts the kidneys as well. Besides, while I had stopped relying on antibiotics before I reached midlife, some of their side effects stayed with me, and I continue to be extra careful to manage the skin rash I mentioned in Chapter 2. It continues to be a challenge when I live in a hot, humid, and moldy area such as Monrovia, Liberia. This is an environment that is conducive to its growth. Thankfully, my current diet and lifestyle enable me to keep it in check without requiring medication for it. Generally, I am at a point in my life where I do the best I can and no longer stress over what I cannot control. Also, I no longer allow the ideal to prevent me from enjoying other positive outcomes that I have achieved. My waistline is normal. My weight is healthy. I am able to protect myself from diabetes with a proper diet and lifestyle that keep my blood sugar stable.

I continue aiming for normal blood pressure, without putting pressure on my heart. God knows I need it for as long as I live! I continue searching hard, both within myself and from outside sources, to understand what else I can do to protect myself from whatever continues to predispose me to high blood pressure. As I continue to do what I can, based on the knowledge I have, including taking medications when that is the best option I have, I do believe that God sees my efforts. He sees my persistence, determination and faith. I have placed my health into His hands and I know that He still performs miracles in the lives of those who believe. He even does it for unbelievers and causes them to believe. Getting off some of the blood pressure drugs I was taking is already an answer to prayer. Living free of hypertension will be my miracle!

Managing stress therefore, brings many health benefits including weight management. It is a matter of balance as cardiologist Dean Ornish notes, having pioneered a program that integrates dietary changes with a social and psychological stress management component. This program is intended to prevent "loneliness, isolation, depression, and anger ... because a lot of 'bad' behaviors such as smoking, drinking, and overeating are actually people's attempts to self-medicate emotional pain," summarizes Monique Tello, a contributing editor of *Harvard Health Newsletter*, in an article on the need for lifestyle change beyond diet and exercise.

Managing stress is a must for anyone looking to get leaner, targeting specifically the waistline. In the rest of the chapter, I will focus on the different stressors I ignored, not knowing until more recently, that they too had something to do with my over-expanding belly. A big waistline is a threat to the health and balance we seek in midlife and beyond. It is a precursor to diabetes and a signal that other imbalances of the metabolic syndrome may also be on the way, as I explained in previous chapters. I will close this chapter by sharing tips on what I do to manage stress better, and how these steps continue to help me maintain a healthy weight and a normal waistline among many other benefits to my emotional and spiritual health.

THE BLESSINGS THAT TURNED INTO STRESSORS

Many of my stressors are common among women in midlife. We tend to experience more stress than other age groups for reasons I explain further below. Some of these stressors were meant to be blessings, but they end up being part of the stress equation when we are unable to manage them adequately. In hindsight, I can easily see how, when I was stressed, I was not always successful at separating my stressors from my blessings. Let's look at how some of these blessings turned into stressors.

Work

Women who, like me, follow a traditional career path after college or graduate school, have a higher level of responsibility by the time they reach midlife, managing not just their own specific daily tasks in the workplace but also overseeing the work of other members of our teams. These additional work responsibilities leave us feeling appreciated for our contributions and potential. However, issues do come whenever two or more people have to work together on any given task and in the process, they reveal their different viewpoints and approaches. Working out these differences can be sources of tension and stress in the workplace. Besides, not everyone manages time or people in ways that minimize stress. And not everyone takes feedback productively, either. Stress can result from, or become an emotional response to these differences in approaches or attitudes. Additionally, stressors from outside work can interfere with one's ability to manage work-related stress effectively.

I am blessed to have had rewarding jobs throughout my professional career. I am thankful for every job opportunity I have held since I started working as a research assistant for an American Fulbright scholar doing research in Burundi when I was preparing to graduate from college in 1988. After my work with the Fulbright scholar ended, I taught high school for another year until I left for graduate school in the United States in early 1991. I resumed professional life with a teaching career in college first, led a Women's Resource Center, conducted research as a Visiting Scholar at a university, and eventually moved on to do international development work. While in development work, I moved into management roles until I left it all to pursue what I now feel to be my calling. I enjoyed each position I held, learned so much about myself and others while working and interacting with my students and colleagues.

Within a few years of my academic life, I started to feel unfulfilled. I joined the world of international development while looking for a better way to connect with the communities that I had been researching to build my academic career. Each of my publications left me with a feeling that I was getting credit that was due to those communities, while also keeping me at some distance from the subjects of my research. When I moved into international development, I thought that I would find the answer to that initial search for work that was more meaningful and purposeful. And I enjoyed my time at the firm Geneva Global, my entry point to a post-academic career. It was meaningful and brought a quantum leap in my understanding of international development. I learned about the different players: the implementers, the donors, and of course, the beneficiaries.

The two job opportunities that followed continued along the same line of managing development projects and working with a diverse team with different skills and backgrounds. I enjoyed my work, and for a while, I felt relevant. Over time, liking the job I had was no longer sufficient for me. After nearly a decade of involvement in international development,

I felt stretched to the maximum and started feeling out of place. So, I returned to soul-searching for a better fit—again. The push to follow my passion got stronger than the pull to stick with the bird in hand.

At that time, it was no longer so much about stress as it was about questioning the relevance and efficacy of international development. Were we making a difference? Were we listening enough and hearing the cries of the people ready for and needing change and transformation? Was I a part of the problem, or was my role, even in some small way, contributing to a solution that would change lives in a positive and lasting way? If not, was there any other type of work I could do that would be more meaningful? I felt more frustrated than stressed, but both were there. They were there for different reasons and I had limited tools to address either of them productively. Why was it so challenging for me to manage stress at this time?

Recurring deadlines: There is a certain amount of stress that is associated with deadlines, even when you enjoy your work very much. Stress comes when others depend on, and are waiting for you, to complete a task or an assignment for them to complete theirs. Stress comes when you depend on others to meet your own deadlines. Actually, there is nothing in international development work that allows you alone to suffer the consequences of missing deadlines. Having supportive and equally hard-working and committed colleagues and managers can help, but this is not enough to prevent stress when a deadline is fast-approaching.

Deadlines also take place in the context of our individual lives that can add to the stress as well. Obligations at home that include kids, a spouse or partner, aging parents, and sometimes friends and neighbors, often require our time. And each of us has to bear our own individual stress burdens, based on our own circumstances and the life stages we are in. Parents of newborns or young children have particular stressors, while those who are grandparents are in a different phase of child-rearing and often have a different set of stressors.

Those with children that are settled and independent, and who are themselves in good health, most likely have less stress than those who maintain responsibilities for children or grandchildren. Those who are single and "free" may have more time to enjoy themselves, taking time with friends after work to relax if they choose to, which can help to lower stress. In my opinion, the ones who suffer most from recurring deadlines are those who are simultaneously climbing the professional ladder while raising younger children and providing social, emotional and/or financial support to aging parents. This was my situation.

The opportunity to climb the professional ladder: As much as I saw it as a blessing, climbing the professional ladder meant additional job responsibilities. These can cause or lead to stress when strategies to manage it productively are not in place. I spent more and more time working to keep up or catch up, often taking work home with me, working during my evenings and weekends. My workdays rarely started at 9 am or ended at 5 pm, a normal workday in the United States. I often arrived earlier and left later. And I was never the last one to leave the office. I did not mind the extra effort, even when I was stressed. I sacrificed many vacation days to keep moving projects and reports forward, all for the greater good.

Gradually however, stress pushed me to unhealthy limits. I reached rock bottom with both stress and unhealthy weight gain. I did not have the knowledge and awareness that my lifestyle was slowly killing me, one extra pound at a time, combined with rising blood pressure. And I did this until I was able to internalize better what my mom said to me once while she was visiting us in Malawi, as I explain further below. What I ignored then was that by failing to manage my work and the stress that came with it proactively, what I was doing would eventually lay the foundation for poor quality sleep, a few years later. I will discuss sleep and its impact on weight in the next chapter. Needless to say, suffering from insomnia when one feels exhausted, is risky to one's survival.

Marriage

Let's face it, marriage is not just about living happily ever after. It takes a lot more effort to make marriage work than we imagine when we first begin this journey. My husband and I had dated for four years before we got married. That seemed to be more than enough time for us to get to know each other before tying the knot. We are both reasonable, well-educated, caring, compassionate and hard-working people. Did we have any reason to expect surprises in our personalities, preferences, and habits that would become stressors in our relationship? Did we have any reason to expect any issues to emerge that we were not aware of already after four years of dating? Even if issues emerged, with the love and commitment that brought us together through the marriage covenant, were there going to be any we could not handle? We have remained committed to making our marriage work, not without stress though.

Some of the differences between us were quite mundane, but others were not inconsequential. Among the mundane, were things like making the bed in the morning or before leaving the house for the day. It turned out to be my habit, not his. We assumed that after using the toothpaste, or a jug of milk, we would close it tightly before putting it away. It turned out to be my expectation, not his. We assumed that each of us should clean every single dish in the sink before leaving the house for work or school or before going to bed at night. His habit, not mine. We assumed that everybody must naturally love singing and dancing to the groove and not just learn about and listen to music. My assumption, not his. Don't ask me how I failed to notice all these when we were dating.

And there is one more, we assumed that every adult, male or female, should know how to hold and feed the baby by the time they have their own. This one especially surprised me, as much as it annoyed me initially. Having been raised with 10 younger siblings, I had more than enough experience with babies before my own came. He, on the other hand, is the youngest of three and there were no young children around him growing up. He came into fatherhood with zero experience in child-rearing. So, I had to teach him my way. Clearly for us, as I assume the same applies to other couples, routine behaviors in our always and forever (we hope) shared space revealed our distinct differences and preferences that we had to learn to live with.

Some of the preferences and inclinations were rooted in different personalities showing up through natural inclinations and tendencies that we most likely overlooked when we were dating or as newly-weds. However, when you are married to someone who does not freely express the full range of emotions you expect in any given situation, and you happen to be someone who was raised in a family that is very emotional and very expressive, it can be quite difficult to reconcile differences in this area. I grew up in a family that sang together, laughed a lot, prayed together when I was young, cried when we were sad (even my dad could not hold his tears in), and danced when music was playing on the radio or cassette player. We enjoyed the boys' jokes. Girls did not seem to have many. Perhaps we were too busy with chores that we had no time to learn or tell jokes. We took this characteristic for granted until we brought friends home, and they would tell us that compared to theirs, ours was a happy home. We must have managed stress well then!

My husband, on the other hand, is less expressive. Perhaps it's not fair to compare his family to mine, but I find his, especially his parents (dad and late mom) to be generally less expressive and just doing what needs to get done with less emotions brought into the mix. To be fair however, I did witness the whole family's deep sadness at the loss of his mom. Other than that, we express our joys of living and the excitement that various moments bring into our lives differently, and my husband tends to turn mostly inward instead of expressing freely the full range of emotions that we are all capable of. Therefore, where we came from is what we brought into our marriage.

There are also differences that are innate, engrained in our genetic or physiological make-up, and we had to accept them for what they are as we cannot control them. For example, that I am a light sleeper and he falls asleep easily and snores at night, are not things one can easily change. While I could cope better before we had kids, a different time in our relationship, I know, it became more frustrating when I was trying to get some shut eye after nursing a baby for the second time in the middle of the night. I took it personally especially when my husband fell right back to sleep and started snoring while I was still listening to be sure our son was asleep again after waking us because he was hurting with an earache. When that happened, I questioned the depth of his love for his son and for the mother of his son, and on and on. In fact, I questioned his sense of fatherhood. What irrational thinking comes with being sleep-deprived or stressed, in the middle of the night! I certainly cannot claim to have been objective then. And by the way, his snoring has gotten better with a better pillow and weight loss.

There was also the bigger issue of racism and the rejection I experienced on his side of the family early on. We learned to live with it—*bon gré, mal gré*—but eventually, his parents and I did reconcile, and I am thankful for that.

Based on this experience, I will tell you now and without an ounce of doubt in my mind, that forgiveness is one of the best gifts you will ever give to yourself. It's a monster load off of your mind and off of your heart. And your healing is dependent on your letting go of the anger, bitterness, frustration or the stress that comes with holding a grudge against someone who hurt you. The grudge only compounds the hurt on you. Letting go and truly forgiving is healing. I speak from experience!

Coming from different cultural backgrounds, nationalities, and races (the human race - smile!) therefore, my husband and I were bound to continue uncovering differences that we had to work out, to prevent our egos from getting too much in the way. It seemed like the right sacrifice to make in a marriage. This is what my mother did, sacrificing for her family even when things were unfairly difficult for her, often for reasons beyond what she or my father could control. So, she took life as it came, and did the best she could with it. There is a lot I learned from her and my parents in general. Theirs seemed like a happy marriage, and it was in many ways. And so is ours in many ways as well. Similar to my parents, there is no abuse, neither physical nor verbal, in our relationship and interactions.

We have had to balance our differences, trying to remind ourselves that we now have a responsibility towards our kids, and what we want is the best of both worlds in them. And this works so long as the kids are home and we can focus on them. But they too eventually do leave and we become empty-nesters. Those differences that we used to tolerate come back to "haunt" us. We continue to manage them and I see great improvements from where we started out as I explain further in the section on what helps us manage the stress in our marriage better these days.

Child-rearing

Let me start by assuring you—and my kids—that being a mother to these most wonderful children (young men now) has brought the greatest joy I have ever and will perhaps ever experience. Being a mother was not only a test to my ability to love another person in a pure and profound way, but it also tested my patience, helping me to practice what it means to start each day every day with a clean slate and anticipation, building memories to cherish as I love them unconditionally and without effort. It taught me that mothers (and fathers too) have the ability to not ever hold anything against childish behaviors. This is a gift of the spirit inside of us, and exercising it with our children can train us to be more patient and forgiving. With them,

I have experienced the love of another to a degree I never knew I could reach and had never experienced before, as well. I want you therefore to put the stress that came with parenting in proper perspective.

Child-rearing has many requirements that go beyond the love we have for our kids. There is a time commitment in a world that increasingly wants more from us, and getting things done faster (not necessarily better) comes at a cost.

The simple task of driving back from work after a hectic day, to pick up the kids during rush hour each day of the week, is enough to keep the adrenaline going and the cortisol high until the kids are finally sitting in the car and you are ready to drive home with a sigh of relief! When already stressed because of the impending deadline, any traffic jam on the way to your kids' school only keeps the cortisol rising. Perhaps you can relate if you have ever driven on busy highways and neighborhood streets while preoccupied with how long it will take for you to make it to the school and with the report that is due very soon, and when you finally make it to your destination, you are thankful that you made it without causing an accident. With each day, month, or year that I kept stress unmanaged, I was only building a higher wall of chronic stress and with it, a thicker layer of fat around my belly.

Balancing family and professional duties, when both are time-consuming, is not easy. It was not for me, and it is not for millions of other full-time professional moms (and dads) of young children. Any of you in this group, can certainly relate to a daily routine that requires getting up early whether fully rested or not, getting the kids ready for daycare or school, taking them either to school or the bus stop, driving or riding to work, staying busy throughout the day, taking work home (often), driving home after work, stopping to pick up the kids, getting dinner ready, eating quickly - not mindfully, doing the dishes, getting the kids ready for bed which may include helping them take a bath when they're not old enough to do it on their own, getting ready for the next day and eventually going to bed. It is hard to avoid stress, when your day starts at 5:30 or 6: 00 am, if not earlier, and it is a non-stop race until the kids are in bed between 7:30 (when they are younger) and 9:00 pm (you hope).

Your day may extend even further as you plan ahead for the kids' lunches, making sure you do not miss anything they may need, including snacks or other tasks that require parental consent or involvement, before the kids leave home the following day. You will, if you are fortunate, end up sitting in a recliner and relaxing before your bedtime. Watching TV is an option but not the healthiest, especially when you are already stressed. There seems to be something gloomy out there all the time, and it ends up on the TV screen for our indulgence, especially if you like to catch up on the evening news. You may also still have to finish that report that you brought home with you, because there won't be enough time to finalize it before you have to pass it on for review the following day. These additional duties are reasons why parenting as a busy professional comes with its own stressors, even for someone who truly enjoys what parenting normally requires when the hassles and bustles of modern lifestyles are not in the way.

With the trend for women to wait until their 30s or even their 40s to have children, women are increasingly entering midlife both with younger children and the added responsibilities that come with climbing the professional ladder. For those who have children at a younger age, midlife may be a time when they re-evaluate their careers and may decide to go back to school. They realize that, without improving their knowledge and skills, limited education (where this applies) may not allow them to go any further than where they are professionally. Some may enroll in evening classes or go back to school full-time, which means that they sacrifice income at a time when they may need it, especially with kids who may be on the way to college. Either way, children are still part of the equation, and though they are usually not the cause, stress can overshadow the appreciations and joys that come with parenting.

Menopause

Midlife is a prime time for women to experience changes associated with a drastic drop in estrogen levels. Here come hot flashes and night sweats, and you guessed it, insomnia, low libido and belly fat! As natural as this sharp drop in estrogen levels is in midlife, it is a cause of stress on the body. Insulin levels rise to deal with the excess glucose released when the body feels stressed due to lack of sleep. I will discuss sleep further in the next chapter. For now, let us keep in mind that when left unaddressed, high cortisol from lack of sleep, and low estrogen in midlife, are both contributors to weight gain. Excess body fat is a good hiding place for cortisol as well. This is a dangerous combination for anyone trying to shrink her waistline.

Taking care of aging parents

In addition to taking care of children, many women reach midlife with higher levels of responsibility to take care of aging parents. When our parents are in good health, we are thankful. When they get sick, we worry. Eventually, sickness does take their lives. I recall the day and time when I received a call informing me that my dad had just passed away. This was May 26, 2006. I was in the office, still early in my workday. The news, as you can imagine or perhaps relate to, shook me to the core. I lost my bearings. The feeling of sadness was too strong, too deep, too unbearable, too different from any other feeling of sadness I had ever experienced before. It was too painful to describe, worse than anything I would even wish on an enemy, and I don't have many. In fact, I have come to believe that we are our worst enemy. That my dad's passing followed a few months of sickness in a hospital bed did not prepare me enough. What increased my stress was a realization that I did not have the opportunity to spend quality time with my parents before their health started deteriorating.

"Time heals," the saying goes. Time was perhaps what I needed to move on from the devastation that I felt after that phone call. However, I don't necessarily believe that time heals the scar that the loss of a loved one causes.

What I believe, depending on the circumstances, is that time can lead us to a different place and space where we are able to cope better, accepting what cannot be changed in a way that enables us to maintain some sense of emotional integrity.

My husband and I had made it our duty and responsibility to take care of my parents, at least financially, making sure they received a regular contribution from us to help them live a relatively comfortable life as they got older and the cost of living increased beyond their means. In their last few months, we agreed to take a major chunk of their medical bills as well. They had sacrificed for me and my twelve siblings. It was my turn to express appreciation for what they did to keep us alive, sending us to school and encouraging us through difficult times while also celebrating our successes. Financial support was the only way I could be there for them as I could not offer any social or emotional support, living so far away for at least 15 years by the time my father passed away. With an equal sense of duty towards my parents, I considered working hard and being professionally successful as my way of making them proud and happy as well.

I put so much value and energy into my career and was proud and thankful for my professional achievements. And for nearly ten years before both my parents passed away, I gave them the support I felt they needed the most, which was financial. It never occurred to me that being with them would have benefitted them and me emotionally, then and into the future. When a loved one is no longer around, all we have left are memories of them. There are a few more I could have created, but I did not think I could because I was focused somewhere else.

With my husband, we focused primarily on our kids, a sensible priority, and gave them any time we could spare from our jobs. This is how I perceived things, and I made priorities based on this principle. This is how I spent valuable time until my mom, who was visiting us then in Malawi, said something that really woke me up from my sleep. She had gone to bed at around nine thirty that night, as usual. When she woke up to use the bathroom, it was nearing midnight and there I was, still sitting in the corner of the large wicker dining room table, where she had left me before she went to bed. I was still working. She said, "My goodness, you are still up? This is not a job!" That really got me thinking and rethinking about what this life on the edge of recurring deadlines and stress overload does to us. As I reflected on that question, I imagined the following conversation with my mom.

Mom: This is not a job
Me: So, what is it, Mom?
Mom: This is not a job. You should be in bed right now, like the rest of us
Me: I know, but I still have this part of the work to complete before I go to bed
Mom: This is not a job. It is causing too much stress on you!
Me: I know, but that's life [...as if she didn't know!]
Mom: This is not a job. Perhaps you should consider leaving it and finding a better one
Me: Are there better ones out there? You realize that the one I have is a great job
Mom: This is not a job. It is slowly killing you
Me: It's not that bad, Mom! There will also be a time when I can slow down and go to bed   earlier. Until then, I have to do what I have to do. Right?
Mom: What can I say? Take care of yourself
Me: You, too, Mom....

I rationalized my attitude so that I did not have to change my habits. But I often reflected on what she said to me then. She stayed with us for nearly three months and then went back home. I needed that time with her, because I had missed many other opportunities to be with my parents. I needed that time with her to offer some emotional support as I think she was not equipped to live without my dad at home. She had dedicated her life to serving as his true soulmate and a helpmate. That she got very sick shortly after he died was a clear sign that their lives were so intertwined that one without the other was unbearable. Her declining health soon after my dad passed away was another cause of stress for me.

Having her with us was our small way of supporting her by giving her a break away from the familiar environment that was a constant reminder of the absence of my dad: around the house; in her bedroom; around the compound under the mango tree where they used to sit together to relax in the afternoon, at the end of a busy day or anytime on the weekends; around the table at mealtimes; on Sundays going to church, and on and on. Giving her a break was also helpful for me since I had the wonderful opportunity to have some meaningful conversations that we never had in the past. Could this have been another cause of stress for me? Most likely, consciously or subconsciously. At home her attention was always divided between all her kids. Though I cannot recall any time when all thirteen of us were living at home at the same time, and being one of the oldest, there were always younger ones who needed her attention more than I did for as far as I can remember! So, that time with us in Malawi was precious to me.

After a couple of months in Malawi, my mom seemed to be coping better, and she even admitted that she did not think she would ever get better again. Then she started insisting on going back home. After all, didn't she have other kids there who needed her attention as well? My mom felt a sense of maternal duty towards all her children, especially those who were still living at home with her. She also felt a sense of duty towards the home that belonged to her and my dad. She could not spend too much time away from this home. That seemed like betrayal to her life partner. So, after nearly three months with us, she returned home. In my opinion, she was still fragile and needed to be handled with care. Back home, even though she had several adult children with her, I do not think that any of them was well-equipped to provide exactly what she needed to move through the grieving process in a way that was not self-defeating. They were also still coping with grief and the loss of our dad. It did not take long for her to fall apart again, and about three months after she returned home, she too passed away.

In a period of 10 months, I lost both of my parents. They had known each other most of their lives, having grown up in the same village. They had been committed to each other, based on what my mom told us, for a number of years prior to getting married, when she was 20 and he had just graduated from a teacher training school at around 22. He had lost his own parents while still in elementary school. My mom became his most dependable and loving female figure as well, filling a hole left by his own mother. They were soon to celebrate their fiftieth wedding anniversary when my dad passed away. My mom had been looking forward to that moment and so were we, their children. She said with sadness when she was visiting us, that she would not have a companion at her church to celebrate this monumental milestone in life. She succumbed less than four months prior to that coveted anniversary date.

I continued to reflect on what she told me that night on her way to the bathroom, however. My stress levels must have been at their highest then. Seeing my mom looking so frail while I was still mourning the loss of my dad, combined with moving to Malawi and helping the kids adjust to a new environment, and sometimes questioning whether our move was a good decision or not, especially for our kids, all required a level of resilience I did not have at the time. I was in the thick of my midlife years, but not yet concerned about the changes that my body would soon experience. I had no idea that such changes worsen under conditions of stress. My waistline was already expanding to proportions I ignored. I had also not paid attention nor managed productively other stressors in my life as mentioned earlier.

Losing my parents before I had more time to return home and give them the opportunity to watch my kids grow and be a part of their lives left a gap that is not easily filled. Offering support from a distance was meaningful for them and for us, but it did not replace the need to be with them in person. It's never easy to fully recover from the grief that follows the sickness and loss of a loved one. Although stress can be subtle, it still is destructive when not dealt with effectively. With this stress linked to loss and grief along with all the other stressors in my life, many of which came in my younger years, is it possible that I reached a point of *adrenal dysregulation* by the time I entered midlife? Most likely. Adrenal dysregulation, as Gottfried explains, happens "... when psychological stress is incessant, or when you perceive that life is incessantly stressful, [and in such a case] you move progressively from healthy adaptation to toxic, stress-related harm to your body" (93). Then, I did not know the difference, but my body knew. It was building a layer of fat around my belly. It just took years for me to notice.

My body was changing as I developed a sedentary lifestyle so that I could stay on top of tasks at work. My body was changing as I drove home day-in and day-out, stressed from a hectic day, and worried that I might miss the next deadline. My body was changing as I kept checking the clock when traffic slowed down, which pushed me closer and closer to closing time at the after-school/day care program for my kids. My body was changing as I stressed over my parents' declining health. My body was changing as I continued to ignore that the grudges I held against those who had hurt me, were also biting back at me. My body was changing every time I went home stressed and frustrated about what I was not happy about in our marriage. Through it all, I became an expert in stress, ignoring how damaging it can be not just in the way I felt it through my emotions, but also through physical pain and changes inside my body.

Failing to manage stress left me with real symptoms. Stubborn belly fat that became especially obvious in midlife was one of the manifestations of the stress I held inside for years. Even my kids mentioned in passing once that they noticed my belly had gotten really big. My body was coping with chronic stress from various unresolved stressors of the past and present. I had not started experiencing sleep disturbances then and I was not even aware that insomnia is a common symptom of perimenopause. And I did not know yet how difficult it can be for a woman in midlife to lose belly fat. Now I know without a doubt that managing stress and giving self-care the place it deserves is required for anyone who wants the energy required for taking care of others.

One cannot give what one does not have. With stress, one gives from a place of stress and not one of peace and balance.

I realized also that if I left stress and weight gain alone and allowed them to continue to own me, I might not even make it to 70, the age at which my parents passed away. So, something had to change. And something did change. I resigned from my job to take care of myself first. I needed a break. I needed time to properly grieve the loss of my parents and my stress overload, before I would feel ready to find another job. My husband was supportive, and so were our boys. It was bittersweet. Part of me felt a sense of relief. But I also grieved. I had never imagined ever leaving a job without another offer in hand. I would not have and could not have imagined doing this when my parents were alive. I certainly would not have found words to explain it nor expected to gain the approval of my dad if I had asked his opinion. This was a no-no behavior in his time! But my husband and kids were game. We played soccer afterwards in our backyard! The load was off. I did some volunteer and short-term consulting work while waiting to be ready to go back to formal employment again. I joined a women's prayer and support group in town. The group included spouses of international development professionals, independent business owners, missionaries, and short-term consultants. We kept each other inspired. I had more time to engage with my kids' extracurricular activities as well. I was happy about that.

It was also a very much needed time of reflection on what I should do next. What's interesting is that ever since that moment, my relationship with work changed. I have never again allowed it to be a source of stress. Even when the job had higher expectations, I learned that in life, I can only do the best I can, and that there is a lot I can and should control without stressing over it. Anything else is beyond my sphere of influence, and therefore, fussing over it is a waste of valuable time and emotional energy. I learned also that my feelings and attitudes do not need to depend on nor be influenced by external factors. The pressure to meet monthly targets was still there at my next job, and to an extent, it was even more intense as my days were generally longer. What had changed was my attitude toward it.

I worked harder, but I knew my boundaries as well. I knew that taking short breaks and stepping outside to get some sunshine on my skin was no reason to feel guilty, and that it was not a waste of time. I knew that resting in between assignments or in between phases of a project throughout its life cycle was a healthy way to refresh and return better equipped to pick up where I left off. I was working smarter, aiming for balance beyond the immediate short-term goals. I continued to pay attention to my diet as well, even though my understanding of the right diet for a woman in midlife was quite inadequate. Looking back in fact, my intake of sugar from fresh fruits was particularly excessive. And although I tried to maintain a healthier bedtime routine, I was often working on the computer until late in the evening. Nonetheless, my mom's voice remained a constant reminder that I should never allow my job to be a sleep robber.

Therefore, midlife showed up according to how I handled my life before I reached this stage. And I was not alone. Belly fat is a common characteristic of women (and men) in midlife. I see it all around me. If my situation had been unique or unusual, I might have noticed and taken action earlier. Not having the right role models to inspire us is never helpful. As I started looking around to see who I might get wise counsel from, what I saw instead was that I was in good company. There is nothing worse in changing a behavior than waiting to be inspired by those who find it normal to do that which you may need to avoid. So, I decided to trust my gut, and without delaying any further, I searched far and wide for techniques that are known to help with stress management and I applied those that resonated with me.

SIMPLE TECHNIQUES I APPLY TO MANAGE STRESS

The first and most important change I needed to make in the area of stress management, as was the case in the other areas discussed in this book, was a mindset shift. I realized that outside stressors do not have to control my emotions and actions. I started developing and applying habits and practices that helped me maintain healthier boundaries around my life, my health, and my work. I learned to be intentional to calm myself down and not get stressed even when work-related stress was affecting others around me. I did not allow myself to get stressed, especially when the cause of stress was nothing that any of us could control. Controlling my response to stress was my choice. I learned specific stress-management techniques that I continue to implement on a regular basis, sometimes daily. These steps include maintaining a consistent sleep schedule, as I discuss further in the next chapter. Together with targeted exercises that do not raise cortisol too much while I am working out or even afterwards, as discussed in the previous chapter, I am able to maintain a healthy weight and keep the lost inches off my waistline.

Some of the stressors I experienced years ago are no longer relevant today. However, knowing that stress is part of life, the techniques below are more general and beneficial in any given situation that I encounter today, helping me prevent stress from getting a stronghold into my life and my health again. We must all find what works for us and apply it. Living with chronic stress is not how life was meant to be. By managing stress better, we can experience the many positive health benefits that such a step offers.

Listening to instrumental music while working

When I am working on the computer, instead of forgetting to breathe normally, especially when I am fully zoned into my work, I keep instrumental background music on. I have found a few selections on YouTube that do not distract me when I'm focused. Instead, the music reminds me that I am not alone, giving me a little boost of the "feel good" hormone, dopamine. This is the hormone that is released when we experience pleasure and reward. This release is not limited to tangible rewards such as sleeping, sex, or eating. *PsyPost* founder and editor Eric W. Dolan summarizes new research findings that link the act of "listening to the music you love ... [to] your brain release [of] more dopamine."

Why is dopamine important in stress management, and what does this have to do with belly fat? According to Robin Wood-Moen, "[e]xcess stress depletes natural dopamine." Wood-Moen includes excess blood sugar, digestive and sleep disturbances among the many side effects of chronic stress and depletion of dopamine.

Let's keep in mind that cortisol and dopamine interact in interesting ways that do not benefit fat loss efforts. Renowned expert in brain-based diagnosis and treatment, Dr. Eric Braverman, has an equation that speaks directly to this interlinkage between cortisol, dopamine and belly fat. He calls it "The Cortisol Equation: Low Dopamine = Bigger Belly Fat = A Heavy Burden to Carry for Both Brain and Body." As discussed earlier, cortisol increases blood sugar and "prompts your body to store this fuel in places it can be used easily, as fat, such as at your waist," Braverman states. There are different mechanisms through which this happens, "[w]hen you have a dopamine deficiency, the body naturally increases production of the hormone cortisol ... the backup energy hormone [to enable] the brain and body to continue to function ..." Braverman adds that when you're stressed, you naturally burn more dopamine, which is why the cortisol is released.

Over time, consistent high cortisol levels lower dopamine further, which in turn "forces your metabolism to slow down because when brain energy falters (low dopamine), the body is forced to send up to the brain its reserve units to pick up the slack, in the form of steroid hormones (cortisol) from the adrenal glands." This is meant to be a temporary solution because "when your brain is continually turning to cortisol for energy .... In the end, you get puffy, round-faced, blood-pressure rises, your appetite increases, and you experience weight gain (especially around your midsection) ... It causes fat to be deposited in the abdominal area where there are the most cortisol receptors" Braverman notes further. I have therefore learned that anything I can do to boost dopamine will counter the effects of cortisol and protect me from continuous fat accumulation around the waistline. Listening to pleasurable music while I work helps me achieve that.

Keeping lines of communication open in my marriage

My husband and I have agreed to improve communication about what affects each of us, trying to limit unnecessary stress as much as possible. We have greatly improved in sharing what's on our mind. Even when we get annoyed or frustrated with each other, we do not let our emotions get out of hand to the point of getting abusive. We listen to each other's concerns even when we cannot come up with an immediate solution or a way out. We keep doors open, share ideas, and are committed to managing issues as best as we can before they get out of hand. We support each other with our different duties and responsibilities, outside the boundaries of our respective jobs. We have always shared family responsibilities as a dual professional couple. We were and still are equal partners in decision-making, raising our kids, and doing housework. We have always co-managed financial resources regardless of who brought in the bigger paycheck at the end of the month. We accepted the added financial responsibility of taking care of my aging parents, even when we had our own financial burdens. And I consider any time or resources we spend with and on his dad (and his mom when she was still with us) to be worth it!

What continues to help is that my husband and I have many things in common. We share a commitment to raising our kids and helping them in the best ways we know how, so that when they are out in the real world, they know how valuable they are, at least to us and to God. What helps also is that we share academic and real-world interests and experiences. We spend hours reflecting on our roles in international development. As former academics, we are good at analyzing and overanalyzing topics of interest. We can sit around the table and debate issues until we know we have to stop. We enjoy these conversations that continue to teach, grow, and expand our knowledge and awareness of many current affairs in politics and culture as well as historical issues. And I make sure that he knows my latest discovery in diets and wellness and that we apply whatever may benefit us.

What helps is also that now, we both believe and practice self-care, having learned the hard way that if we do not take care of ourselves, no one else will, and our health can easily slip out of our hands.

We enjoy going for regular walks in our neighborhood and have even started doing yoga together a few times a week (You're never too old to start learning yoga!).

That's why we get along. That's why my husband and I are still together. That's also why we continue to stretch ourselves to learn from each other the best way to help each other become the best version of ourselves, as we aim to reach our potential and pursue a life of purpose. We both know that we are slowly approaching the end of midlife and entering our senior years sooner than we may wish to believe. In spite of a few aches here and there, we are blessed with relatively good health at our age. Other than our grey hair that I can hide sometimes (he doesn't try to), we feel younger than we are in reality. We are eager to learn new skills and habits that will benefit us. And we seek to remain relevant in the lives of others. That's why we continue to do all that we can to make our marriage work and after twenty-five years, we have reached a comfortable zone, and the stressors in our relationship have become less over time. And what we went through is nothing extraordinary, I believe. We have never reached a point where we would consider separation as the best option. It helps that we are aware of some challenges we have handled successfully together.

I am glad we are where we are today because in this journey, he remains my best partner, dependable friend, and best source of encouragement.

In fact, he continues to surprise me with small acts of kindness that I appreciate a lot. Let me share a note he gave me about a year ago, while I was struggling with what some call "the writer's block." He brought me home an inspiring book by former US First Lady, Michele Obama. I simply admire her. She models love, fun, authenticity, adventure, focus, excellence, and dignity. These are qualities that we aspire for. Her book *Becoming* was one of the fastest reads I have ever completed. I could not put the book down. I have so much love, respect and admiration for her. When my husband brought me the book after returning from a trip abroad, he inserted a note saying that when he saw Michelle Obama's book, he immediately thought of me and the important work that I am doing on my course and book. He wrote, "I hope that the book by the former First Lady will inspire you to continue to aim for the stars, share your message of health and wellness, and make an impact on more and more people that need to hear your message..." The message on the front of the card read: "Follow Your Dreams." Needless to say, I have always felt encouraged and appreciated along this journey that has taken much longer than I intended when I set out to create an online course and write a book building on my experiences and the lessons I have learned that I consider worth sharing. And that he is paying my bills as I write this book is a testimony that he's got my back. And I am still hoping that one day, he will take me dancing and enjoy it as much as I do!

Letting go of past hurts

When I started searching for a way out of stress and a healthier relationship with myself and others, I read a book on boundaries. I do not remember the exact title but it spoke to me. A lesson from that book allowed me to consider what it means to create a clean and clear line between the hurt caused by someone else and the way I reacted to it. The book taught me to detach myself, my thoughts, and my actions from how someone else treated me. It taught me that one can only control or change oneself and that when someone else does wrong to me, they are the ones in the wrong and not me. It was then that I also started applying helpful skills such as resilience and forgiveness, repeating to myself quietly with a little voice inside my heart, "I do not need to allow someone else's wrong doing to live inside of me." It worked and changed my attitude tremendously. It allowed me to live at peace with myself knowing that when I have nothing to blame myself for, I have no reason to feel bad about myself or keep the hurt alive inside of me.

I learned to let others live as they see fit. I no longer wish I could fix other people's flaws either. I have my own to deal with. Eckhart Tolle's *The Power* of *Now* truly deserves a mention here as well. One of his key points in the book is that when we live in the moment, we can easily catch ourselves before we drift too far away into a place where we are no longer able to see clearly how stress is holding us hostage. When I started paying attention to how the stress of life and the emotions tied to the hurt of the past were still with me, I wanted to let them go. Without accepting rejection or hate, I have learned to live with it when it happens and maintain inner peace with myself. Leaving the baggage of stress behind and to never pick it up again is what living in the moment promises. Whenever I choose to focus on the "now" and let go of the past that hurts, the load is relieved. It puts me in a much better space. The peace in me intensifies. I know that forgiveness is a real stress-buster.

Meditation and deep breathing

When I am busy behind the computer, I forget to breathe normally. When I eventually tune in to myself, I realize that my stomach is tight and needs to loosen. I have developed the habit of taking short deep breathing breaks throughout the day. Laying on a yoga mat in child's pose is always helpful, giving me a deep breathing break. Intentional deep breathing helps even in the middle of the night when my mind starts wandering off in a hundred different directions, instead of peacefully slowing down to allow me to go back to sleep. It works; I am convinced of that. I continue to practice deep breathing as my mind calls me back to it.

Similarly, I have adopted the habit of looking for words to live by, to guide me throughout the day. I look for inspiration in Christian podcasts as well as from other inspirational speakers and leaders that I respect, including current and historical figures such as Martin Luther King, Oprah Winfrey, Michele Obama, Brené Brown, Joel Osteen, and more recently Priscilla Shirer. Listening to these podcasts allows me to start my day thinking positively and with a thoughtful message to reflect on throughout the day. I sometimes do a quick check on Facebook for inspirational messages that some friends like to post. My sister Goretti's posts often speak to me and inspire me as well. She seems to be on a mission to encourage others, almost daily!

Keeping realistic and reasonable daily goals

I believe that part of the challenge of wanting to do it all and be it all, is that we either set no goals and just keep doing whatever comes our way, or we set unrealistic goals. Taking on more tasks than can be accomplished by any normal human being can leave us feeling frustrated, stressed, and unhappy with our inability to live up to our desires, wishes, and sometimes promises. Nowadays, I have learned to set realistic goals. I have given myself permission to get at least one important goal achieved each day, and I add a few additional smaller tasks that must be done but are less time-bound or time-consuming. I get a sense of satisfaction when I check things off my list, even though I rarely need to write down my tasks on a list because I no longer plan to do more than I can remember in my head. Thankfully, I can still trust my memory, for the most part. I have been able to avoid the stress that comes with a long list that leaves me feeling like I barely scratched the surface by the time the day is over. So far, so good!

Diet

My diet is carefully selected based on my current health goals, which include weight maintenance, blood sugar stability, and boosting my immune system, which declines as we age. Maintaining healthy eating habits with the goal of keeping blood sugar stable instead of leaving it unmanaged helps to prevent the pressure on the body from fluctuating blood sugar. Since Chapters 2 and 3 discussed in detail the importance of maintaining stable blood sugar and the steps I took and continue to take to achieve this goal, I will not repeat myself here. I will add however, that I pay attention to foods rich in Vitamin C as these foods are needed to boost the immune system, preventing the stress of getting sick often and when I do, vitamin C rich foods help me recover faster. Vitamin C also holds tissues together instead of sagging, hence taking us beyond our weight loss goals and helping us to tone our body as well. This is why I keep lemons in my pantry and add them to my water regularly. This is also why I eat kiwi and broccoli often. They are all high sources of vitamin C.

WHAT ARE THE SIGNS THAT I AM MANAGING STRESS BETTER?

I am compassionate again, caring about other people's needs in a genuine and proactive way. I had slowed down on this when I felt like the world was using and abusing me instead of appreciating the contributions I was making to improve the lives of others by sharing my time, skills, and resources.

I take time to take care of myself. I pay attention to my diet, I take select supplements off and on, I exercise regularly, and I practice yoga and meditation. I no longer believe that it is my job to control every situation that impacts me. I worry less about the things I cannot control. And when stressed, I take action faster to not let it linger. I know to calm myself down effectively in situations that would have worried me for long in the past.

My faith is stronger. I pray and meditate regularly. I have returned to an old principle I had applied for years before, trusting that the same God who has always taken care of my needs, will continue to do so, not because I deserve it but by His grace and mercy.

Sleep has improved from two hours at my worst to six or seven hours with less trips to the bathroom in the middle of the night.

I am less forgetful.

I am optimistic about my future.

My weight is consistent, where I need to be. While I do not have the flat belly of my teen and twenties, my waistline is normal and I continue to fit well into size 4 outfits. That is a major improvement from my old size 14.

CONCLUSION

Stress is part of life. How we handle life stressors is our choice, even though we often forget that we have this power within us to make this choice. There was a time when I had given that choice and power away to outside forces that controlled me. Instead of managing stress productively, I rationalized it. My thinking was that, being a professional woman in midlife, with many responsibilities and expectations at home and at work, there was more than one reason to be stressed. It's a matter of perspective, the lens through which we approach or perceive our lives. The challenge often is that we overlook what we have, turning even blessings into life stressors at times. Stress from one situation can also be compounded and magnified to proportions beyond what it really is or needs to be.

The stressors I experienced were real, but so were my blessings that I did not focus on. I did not believe that I could handle either of them more productively. I could have been more patient, shown more care, enjoyed the moment better, appreciated what I had more, or spent more time with those I cared to be with more, if my priorities had been in the right place and stress had not been in the way. As I allowed stress to build a stronghold around my life, it took a toll on my health in ways that I ignored until my rising blood pressure forced me to recognize that I, too, was as fragile as my parents. The difference between their situation and mine was that my kids were much younger when I was diagnosed with hypertension. I needed to take care of myself. They needed me.

When I decided to do a bit of soul-searching to understand better my real life-stressors so I could call them out by name and separate them from my blessings, I wanted to stop handling those blessings as a stressed freak.

This exercise led me to a realization that separating stress from blessings in all situations is a tall order to ask of us human beings, definitely a tall order to ask of me. Looking around, I find few who are able to handle the present with a level of calm and care, regardless of the level of stress in their lives. Yet even in those moments of hardship and stress, we do not have to let stress control how we handle ourselves and others. This is what I failed to recognize when I allowed stress to dig deep roots on the inside, making it harder to see a way out.

What I did then, prior to midlife, built the foundation for how I have experienced midlife. Belly fat was one of the physical manifestations, which came as a result of my mishandling stressors along with other areas required for a balanced life. Belly fat can start building up at any age, but in midlife hormonal changes, as well as dietary and lifestyle choices, are major contributing factors to its most prominent manifestation. Stress is one such factor. I needed to find a solution to my stress that would not only restore some level of balance but that also would build resilience. My attitude needed to change. I needed to recognize as Richard Blonna advises, that my "stressful thoughts ... and painful emotions [can remain] as pages in [my] scrapbook from an earlier time ..." but that they do not have to control how I live my life in the present. I needed to believe that by adding new pages with more helpful thoughts and emotions, I would be able to experience the fullness of life as I want to live it, recognizing my value, while also striving to bring value to others (150, 151). This too is about living a life of purpose.

CHAPTER 8:

BREAK AWAY FROM YOUR SLEEP ROBBERS

"Unless you give your body the right amount of sleep, you will never, I repeat *never*, have the body and life you want to have", Shawn Stevenson, *Sleep Smarter* (2).

I was not doing anything different, or so I thought, but something was changing on the inside. Perhaps it had already changed, but it took some time for me to see the visible signs of this change that had been taking place gradually. Menopause was knocking on my fertility door and with it, insomnia. When I thought that insomnia could not get any worse, it knocked me down harder each night. What started out as a sleepless night extended into weeks, then months, then years. It was nearly a couple of years before I could experience what I would call a gradual sign of recovery. I could not believe a human being could survive with so little sleep for such a long time. But I did, not without frustration or stress, though. It was tough.

This is the symptom I was least prepared for and the most challenging of all perimenopause symptoms. I had not been around women openly discussing menopause and its many symptoms, particularly hot flashes or insomnia. So, I had to learn about them through first-hand experience. When hot flashes came, they were never as extreme as what some have experienced. They are not painful; that's the good news. They can be embarrassing, though. They come without a warning and will hit you even while in the middle of the most important meeting of the season. Before you know it, you get this quick surge of heat and your face starts dripping in sweat, just in time for your turn to speak. You cannot hide it. You wipe your face and proceed as if nothing happened. And it is true. Nothing major happened. You are not nervous. It was just a little sweat. No details needed. This happened to me once. I was at a networking event, meeting with a middle-age gentleman, which made it a bit more embarrassing. Had it been a woman, I might have said something—but a guy? You just have to keep going until it's over. Perhaps he knew what was going on. Perhaps his wife had gone through the change, and he might have guessed what was going on in my life. Or perhaps he was confused, wondering why in the world I would start feeling nervous when we had been chatting for at least half an hour. No, it was not something he said. It was just me and he had to just let me be, and soon enough the storm cleared.

If you have not yet experienced hot flashes, there is no need to sweat over them. They come quickly and, in my experience, each surge dies down pretty fast as well. It is most bothersome at night because it will likely wake you up from your sleep, feeling too hot and uncomfortable to stay asleep. Other than that, they are more of an inconvenience than anything else. When they hit while you are asleep, however, hot flashes can worsen symptoms of insomnia. This is the bad news. Whatever keeps you awake at night is bad news. Midlife just seems to be a sensitive time when it comes to insomnia triggers, and there are quite a few of them that we'll discuss later in this chapter. Some of these triggers can be managed and controlled relatively easily. Others are much more challenging, but there are still things you can do to lower their frequency. I will share the steps I follow to protect myself from known triggers of hot flashes, one of the factors that interferes with quality sleep – the focus of this chapter. I will also share some practical steps to help you lower incidences of insomnia and improve sleep quality in midlife.

You cannot leave insomnia alone to end on its own. I can tell you from personal experience, this does not work. It is your job to pay attention to all of the triggers and manage them effectively so that you can improve your ability to fall asleep and stay asleep at night. If you take no action, insomnia can ruin your life. In fact, I compare insomnia to an invisible guest in your bed, who does everything to keep you awake, even when the last thing you need is a chatterbox in your bedroom. Insomnia does not care whether you have a job interview the following day or have been invited to give a keynote speech at the most important conference you have ever attended. It does not care if you need to drive your kids to school or your husband to the airport the next day. It does not care if it has kept you awake for a month or six consecutive months already. What is most disturbing is that this type of insomnia can come anytime in midlife. For some, insomnia comes when they are in their early 40s while for others, they are anywhere in their 50s. In my case, midlife insomnia came in my early 50s.

I had already been working on improving my diet, minimizing consumption of foods and drinks with artificial ingredients, and choosing organic foods when possible. I had also started limiting sugar as I understood it and I was in the process of reducing dairy and removing gluten and many other food choices known to trigger reactions in sensitive individuals. I had started exercising several times a week to stay physically fit, as well. I did not consider myself stressed, but I had not taken the time to manage previous stressors that left a scar on the inside which did not allow me to relax enough to lower cortisol consistently. Attempting to lower it when I was not able to sleep was a real challenge.

I needed sleep to lower cortisol, just as I needed to lower cortisol to be able to sleep better.

Without sleep, my healthy diet and regular exercise continued to bring suboptimal results in my attempts to lose weight. Therefore, insomnia won't spare you, even if you feel generally healthy but continue to ignore habits that negatively impact your sleep.

Sleep is essential for giving you a body that feels and looks good. "Sleeping well is the first step to living well," notes the UCLA Sleep Disorder Patient Education page. When sleep failed me, I wanted to try anything that would help me recover, except for sleeping pills such as Zaleplon, Eszopiclone, Ambien or Lunesta, known to be effective in treating acute insomnia. I stayed away from these medications when I learned that "…tolerance, withdrawal, dependence, and rebound insomnia" might be the end result after discontinuing them, according to Martica H. Hall, Christopher E. Kline, and Sara Nowakowski in a 2015 article on "Insomnia and Sleep Apnea in Midlife Women". Insomnia affects as many as fifty percent of midlife women. How fortunate are the other half spared of this disaster?

A February 2019 WebMD article that provides "An Overview of Insomnia" identifies significant life stress, environmental factors, some medications, and interferences in our normal sleep schedule as some of the main causes of insomnia. Insomnia has many side effects on physical, mental and emotional wellbeing as well. Midlife insomnia is the most challenging perimenopausal symptom, in my opinion. Unless you learn to tame it, it will always ignore the clues that you are ready for it to go and leave you alone. In fact, if I were to rank wellness enemies from the riskiest to the most benign, I most likely would put insomnia on top. You cannot talk yourself out of it nor can you make any plans with it. It will not share its schedule with you, and it may be around for a while. So, you wonder, what does "a while" mean exactly? A week? A month? A year? Longer? There is no easy answer, but what I do know is that with midlife insomnia, anything is possible. It can last a year, or five, or even longer. "... [H]ot flashes occur in 60-80 percent of women during the menopausal transition and persist for 4-5 years on average. When hot flashes occur during the night, they frequently but not invariably awaken women from sleep," say Martica Hall et.al. in the online article referred to above. My doctor told me that some women still suffer from night sweats and other menopausal symptoms through their 70s. I did not want to ask if that meant that insomnia could also continue until then as well. What if it did? I did not want to hear it! My hope was that this would not be the case for me. Oh, how I wish I had inherited my mom's genes! She once told me that she never had any trouble sleeping through the night. Her belly fat in midlife must have been caused by other factors, not lack of sleep.

In my case, because I was aware that the change that was taking place was part of the natural process of aging, I waited with the hope that in due time, my body would respond naturally to the diet and lifestyle changes I continued to make, and eventually reach some balance even in the area of sleep. Until then, I chose to ride it out as I tend to do, to see how much my body would use the tools I was giving it to heal itself naturally. So, I continued to educate myself and to apply whatever I learned that appealed to me without the need to rely on pharmaceuticals. Not doing anything was only going to compound the many side effects of insomnia on me, just as it does on millions of people who are sleep deprived. The National Sleep Foundation states on its website that "nearly 40 million American men and women suffer from sleep disorders." This means that nearly 10 percent of US population is not able to get proper sleep on a daily basis. The National Sleep Foundation adds that "sleep problems affect more women than men" in an article on "Women and Sleep." On the extreme end of sleep disorders is insomnia, which affects many social groups, but is especially common among midlife women as they enter the perimenopause phase. Insomnia is "an extremely common symptom of perimenopause", writes Cathy Garrard in a 2018 article on "10 Ways to Beat Menopausal Belly Fat."

In his book, *The Sleep Doctor's Diet Plan: Lose Weight Through Better Sleep*, Michael Breus writes: "The reality is that women face different situations in life that cause their weight gain - ranging from ongoing family or career stress to ignoring the importance of daily exercise to hormonal changes at midlife that pack on the pounds - and most will have a hard time reversing that weight gain .... I have discovered that there is a 'missing link'. ***That missing link is proper and adequate sleep*** [emphasis in original]" (4-5). Shrinking insomnia-induced belly fat requires approaching the task from many angles. It requires an appropriate diet that meets your nutritional needs. It includes exercising right so as not to interfere with sleep or increase stress on the body. It requires managing stress effectively, as we discussed in the previous chapter. Results will remain less than optimal if you neglect these three areas. Without addressing sleep and removing your sleep robbers however, you will not succeed at losing the bothersome fat around your belly either.

And losing inches around your waistline with sustained action, can help you get back on track of sleeping better again - hopefully most of the nights.

Once you take action and experience improved sleep, it becomes a motivating factor to continue implementing the other actions that your body needs to return to homeostasis, a state of body, mind and spiritual balance. It is possible even in midlife. Yes, it is possible to feel free and to enjoy this phase of life. I can say this because in an informal survey I did with women in my social media network, out of the 19 women in midlife who responded to my survey, most define this time in their lives in terms of freedom. Midlife is a time when you finally learn that living your life as you understand it, and not according to existing social pressures and expectations, is what matters most. It is a time when you can mix and match the colors of your outfits and not worry about impressing anyone. It is about feeling comfortable in your own skin. It is a time when your true self shows up. It is the time when many respond intentionally to the wake-up call that self-care must be a priority if one wants to live a purposeful life, giving one's best to others.

While focusing on our jobs and taking care of our children and aging parents is a noble and necessary cause, it can come at a cost to our health and wellness if we forget to take care of ourselves first. Midlife is therefore a time when many realize that the time for self-care has come and can no longer be ignored. With adequate sleep, our true selves show up more beautifully as we wake up feeling energized and we go out into the world to serve others and make a difference in their lives, freely and gratefully. While intuitively I would not have associated midlife as a time of freedom, given the inner turmoil that showed up as insomnia, among other signs of imbalance, I now recognize that out of that turmoil came the freedom that many women, including those I surveyed, associate it with. Out of it came an appreciation for the little details of my life, including a good night's sleep that I had taken for granted until I experienced insomnia. Out of it came an understanding that we have so much power to influence where we go with our lives than we give ourselves credit for. We need to take the time to listen to our bodies' cries for help and then to respond accordingly. I am not so naive as to expect that when I take action, everything will go according to my wishes and desires all the time. However, I do believe that we can do so much more to influence the direction of our health when we take informed actions.

The steps I took to recover from insomnia, while still having hot flashes, taught me that even in hopeless of situations, there is still room to improve our health and wellness. We all desire optimal health. We all desire the ideal, but the ideal is just that. When insomnia hit, I came to appreciate any additional hour of sleep beyond the two to three hours that I relied on every night during the early months of perimenopause.

As I continued researching what I could do to cope with insomnia, I stumbled on an advertisement for a new book, *Sleep Smarter* by Shawn Stevenson. I liked the "smarter" in the title. It caught my attention, just as I listen when someone wants to teach us how to work smarter, and not harder. Both save time and energy. Even though *Sleep Smarter* was not targeting women in midlife, my hope was that it would include tips that would work across life's stages, and that I could apply these tips to my situation. This turned out to be the case. I applied many of Stevenson's recommendations as best as I could. What I learned was that despite my efforts to improve my health and wellness, I was not focusing my efforts on doing what would enable me to protect my sleep. I did not even think that I, or anyone else for that matter, could do much to influence sleep. Avoiding noise pollution was as far as I had taken it. And since I lived in a quiet neighborhood, I could not blame insomnia on noisy neighbors.

In the rest of this chapter, I summarize some of the key points that sleep experts like Stevenson raise, tying lack of sleep and poor sleep habits to weight gain, and belly fat in particular. I then discuss how I undermined my sleep through dietary and lifestyle habits that were not conducive to healthy sleep and a smooth ride through midlife. I will also share my ongoing strategies for promoting better sleep. Although I do not always sleep through the night like I did prior to midlife, I sleep much better now. My sleep has improved because I know what to do throughout the day and into the evening to support my sleep at night. My sleep has improved because I now prioritize sleep as I understand better its implications for my overall health and wellness, and for losing some of the stubborn deposits of fat inside my belly.

POOR QUALITY SLEEP AND BELLY FAT

"One of the things that truly combats the menopot is high-quality sleep", Pamela Peeke in Cathy Garrard, "10 Ways to Beat Menopausal Belly Fat".

Lack of sleep, or inadequate sleep, can inhibit fat-burning hormones and instead promote fat-storage hormones, particularly insulin and cortisol. "Getting enough sleep ... triggers growth hormone and for this reason fat burning occurs during sleep (110)," writes Eric Berg in his book, *The 7 Principles of Fat Burning*. Berg adds that the "... [f]at-burning growth hormone is active throughout the night while you sleep; however, it increases during the first two hours of deep sleep especially between midnight and 4:00 am. Omitting this sleep can prevent the fat-burning effect" (142). Could this be the reason why I could not lose fat until I fixed my sleep problems? There was a time when, no matter how hard I tried, I could not fall asleep before 2:00 am or even 3:00 am. What was most frustrating was that then, when others were getting ready for bed, I became so alert and felt so awake that had I chosen to make this my most productive time of the day (or night should I say), I could easily have worked through the night, awake without trying. The longer it took for me to get into deep sleep, the greater the challenge of missing my ideal time for growth hormones to do their job of shrinking belly fat.

Poor sleep triggers an insulin response and as discussed earlier insulin is a fat-storage hormone. This is most likely what made it hard for me to lose belly fat effectively, even when I started losing some of the excess weight, thanks to the diet and exercise habits I had adopted. My sleep was inadequate. My results remained suboptimal. My body was stressed, even when I was doing everything to lower stress and manage it better. Without sleep, success at managing stress is another tall order. In Jaime Osnato's 2019 blog post that I referred to above, she summarizes key points in Natasha Turner's book *The Supercharged Hormone Diet*, specifically highlighting that quality sleep is a factor that counters stress effects on the body. Without sleep, metabolic syndrome follows, and this almost always includes visceral fat. Without adequate sleep, the body is in a state of chronic stress with high amounts of circulating cortisol, a condition known as hypercortisolemia. Turner considers sleep as an essential best fat-burning activity.

As we learned in Chapter 7, stress impacts weight because cortisol triggers the release of sugar in the blood, which under the right conditions would make it possible for us to run away from danger. Bedtime is nobody's ideal time for running away from danger of any kind. Therefore, this sugar is quickly stored as fat when not required to help us use it urgently. When you experience spikes in blood sugar, you will inevitably also feel a sharp drop, whether asleep or awake. When you are asleep, this sharp drop in blood sugar will wake you up. The more sugar is in circulation when you go to bed, the sharper the drop as well, and the greater the stimulation to your brain. You cannot achieve restorative sleep under such conditions. Hypoglycemia - which is when the sugar crash occurs - also raises cortisol, the stress hormone which is a sleep robber. Cortisol suppresses melatonin, the hormone that helps to control the daily sleep-wake cycles.

There are several linkages here that we must keep in mind if we want to achieve quality sleep and shrink belly fat. One of these linkages is between high sugar consumption and raised insulin levels, which we must prevent. If we don't, a sharp sugar drop will follow and wake us up from sleep. A high sugar diet and high insulin levels and poor-quality sleep all contribute to belly fat. The other linkage is between low blood sugar and increased cortisol, which reduces melatonin, a necessary sleep hormone. Anything that keeps cortisol elevated contributes to belly fat as well.

Cortisol has the same effects whether released in response to stress or to sleep deprivation. And as it turns out, cortisol receptors are the highest under the skin around your belly. While your body can manage a reasonable amount, cortisol will always interfere with sleep if it is elevated when you're trying to sleep. Chronic stress keeps your adrenals busy when they should be slowing down to allow you to sleep well. The dysregulation of the adrenals is what happens when your body adapts to chronic stress to a point that "over time, your cortisol surges come later and later," as Alissa Vitti notes in her book, *Woman Code* (104). If you pay attention to your sleep patterns, it's easy to know when your adrenals have become dysregulated. If you used to fall asleep easily when you went to bed, but somehow things have changed and you have become a night owl, most likely your adrenals need retuning. Dysregulation can happen both with cortisol levels that are too high or too low. Neither is good. Low cortisol can result from having chronically high cortisol levels, paradoxically.

In my case, even during the worst of my insomnia, I knew all along that I needed quality sleep. I just did not know what I could do to get it because I did not even think I was stressed then. I did not know then that what I did during the day and into the evenings could have any repercussions on my sleep at night, my stress levels while trying hard to sleep, or even on belly fat. With a choice, I would have opted for better sleep over belly fat.

Sleep supports weight management efforts and excessive weight gain negatively impacts sleep. They are a dynamic duo. You cannot succeed in one without addressing the other and moving both in a positive direction.

While existing research recognizes that we all have our individual sleep clocks, and that not everybody gets the best sleep at the same time, experts agree on the importance of sleep for weight loss. Midlife is unfortunately a time of inner turmoil, a phase in our lives that can challenge our ability to maintain quality sleep. Living with insomnia is what convinced me that I should not - and no one should - play around with sleep. I appreciate sleep so much that when I wake up feeling well-rested, I thank God for a restful night and I am proud of all I did the day before that supported my sleep. Nowadays, I pay careful attention to the details of sleep. I know too well how bad it feels to be sleep-deprived. I am convinced that whatever we do that deprives us of quality sleep, we need to address those causes as soon as possible. We need to appreciate the immediate benefits of feeling rested when a new day comes, and the long-term benefits of chronic disease prevention. Remember, belly fat is a health risk!

As mentioned earlier, Stevenson's book *Sleep Smarter* had a major impact on my thinking about sleep and how it affects other aspects of our health, including our weight. *Sleep Smarter* was my first and most convincing entry point into the science of sleep. One of its key messages was that sleep is important in supporting the body to prevent insulin resistance. It is as important as all the other factors discussed in previous chapters related to our food and lifestyle choices that affect our weight. To shrink our stubborn belly fat, we much chase away the sleep-robbers. I read *Sleep Smarter* from cover to cover, something I rarely have time for these days, especially when it comes to technical books. Reading this book turned me into a sleep advocate, convincing me that this information, even in a highly condensed form, should be accessible to all, especially women before they reach midlife, and obviously also those who in midlife struggle with weight gain and belly fat. Such information should be posted for all to see, in every doctor's office, every classroom, every bus stop, every train station, every community center, and even information corners at places of worship!

I continued to look for other resources on sleep and learned from experts, including Michael Breus and Debra Fulghum Bruce, who, in their book *The Sleep Doctor's Diet Plan*, confirmed many of the same key points that I had read in Stevenson's *Sleep Smarter*. Breus and Bruce also link poor sleep to weight gain, and more specifically to belly fat. They write that there is "a high correlation between poor sleep and weight gain (usually as belly fat) in women at midlife. The problem with an expanding waistline at this life stage is that it increases your risks of heart disease, diabetes, and certain types of cancers" (70). I am certain that nobody wants to put themselves at risk for any of these diseases. I certainly do not. In fact, this is what keeps me motivated to do all I can to give my body the sleep it needs each night.

I do so no longer because of the short-term benefits of feeling rested the following day, nor even for the aesthetic value of having a smaller waistline, although both are important and remain a priority for me. What is most motivating for me is the link between poor quality sleep and the health risks of chronic diseases associated with belly fat. I am motivated by the understanding that If I cannot prevent these chronic diseases, I can at least work hard to delay their onset.

I'll do all I can and take whatever benefits I can get from sleep. I'll do all I can to prevent or delay the onset of diabetes and heart disease, even if it may take a lifetime to reach my goals.

An expanded waistline is one of the consequences of poor sleep, and it is in and of itself a health risk that must be treated as such, notes Lisa Morrone in her book *Sleep Well Again* (44).

There is more that affects our overall health and weight when we are sleep deprived. In fact, when we are deficient in deep sleep, the production of two appetite-regulating hormones, leptin and ghrelin, are thrown out of balance (Morrone 44-45). Leptin tells your brain that you are full. It acts as an appetite suppressant. Ghrelin is the hormone that lets you know that you are hungry. It acts, therefore, as an appetite stimulant. Some people respond to this stimulation by going for more food when what they really need is better sleep (45). While I rarely turn to food for comfort, I have learned that achieving quality sleep will enable me to control these two hormones, leptin and ghrelin, better, and lose some of the belly fat as well. Perhaps sleep was the missing link to this belly fat breakthrough all along.

With sleep problems, as with many other areas of health and wellness, prevention is key. Knowing what our sleep robbers are and working to break away from them makes such a difference in the quality of sleep we get. As we improve sleep, we will also help our bodies function better, and we will have a better chance of melting inches of fat off our waistlines. So much good happens to your body during sleep. It is not a waste of your time. In fact, it is as important as the most important activities you have planned for the day, only that the best time for it is at night. It is essential because sleep "helps to repair and improve functions of our brain, our muscles are getting repaired, our hormones are being optimized and getting back on track," states Shawn Stevenson in his podcast on the "4 Hidden Things that Could Be Destroying Your Sleep Quality."

If you have not yet hit midlife, you need to make the necessary adjustments that will benefit you now, while also preparing you better for a more balanced midlife. Equipping you with the tools and strategies to manage hormonal changes when they are in full swing in perimenopause is one of my goals in this book. The insomnia that comes as you reach this phase of life is not something you can easily manipulate according to your wishes and desires. It does not respond to your pain if you have ignored the steps required to promote good sleep. Not knowing the challenges that inconsistent sleep habits will bring later in life is not enough to conquer insomnia. As with other habits, the longer you wait to make the necessary adjustments for better quality sleep, the longer it will be to restore lost balance. And with insomnia, you can forget about losing belly fat for a while.

If you apply the steps I followed and that I share in this book, and in this chapter in particular, you will be able to keep too much fat from accumulating around your waistline. If you adopt these healthier practices now, rather than later, your body will not be dealing with the many other physiological and especially hormonal changes that occur when you reach midlife. The sooner you can adjust your sleep schedule to follow the circadian rhythms, while also honoring your ideal bedtime, the sooner you will lay a healthy foundation for maintaining or restoring quality sleep. You alone know what that time is, but for most people between 9:00 and

11:00 pm is the ideal time to go to bed. I must also emphasize here that I consider the actions I outlined in the previous chapters as co-factors for what it takes to sleep better at night. I hope that by applying the tips and tools I share in this book, you will avoid the worst of sleeplessness: insomnia. You will also prevent the belly fat that builds up as a result of inadequate sleep in midlife!

Sleep is truly amazing when you know how it feels to be deprived of it. Sleep is amazing when you can rely on it to give you many of its benefits. Sleep is amazing when you're able to reach old age without ever suffering from insomnia. I hope that following the advice in this book will protect you from the risks of chronic diseases linked to insomnia and keep your waistline in shape as well. Factors that rob you of quality sleep must therefore be addressed and taken out of your life and your bed. I will share next what these factors were in my case.

THE HABITS THAT ROBBED ME OF QUALITY SLEEP

The list of sleep robbers turned out to be longer than I had imagined. I turned to experts first to understand where these sleep robbers may be hiding, assuming they would be mostly found in my bedroom. As I learned, they hide in many other places, both in the home and outside as well. They hide inside the foods we eat, including sugar and high glycemic index foods that raise blood sugar and rob us of key sleep nutrients. They hide in the environment, including places and gadgets that emit artificial light such blue LED lights from TVs, smartphones, lamps, computers, radio clocks, and even lamp posts that dimly shine through the windows of your bedroom. In the environment, the sleep robbers hide in the noise around us, the poor quality of our bedding (such as polyester sheets that do not breathe, trapping heat and moisture), as well as various beauty products. They also hide in the lifestyle habits we adopt and that may be healthy but are poorly implemented. Which of these sleep robbers applied to my case?

Diet

Sugar and highly processed foods: I have already said enough about the impact of sugar and starches on my weight and belly fat in previous chapters, but to summarize my point, I was ignorant of the amount of sugar I was consuming. I was not aware that it is not just the sugary foods such as cakes, cookies and ice cream that impact blood sugar, but also the unsweetened carbs such as oatmeal, pasta, rice, potatoes and bread. For a long time, I did not see myself as someone who needed to change my habits around sugar or carb consumption. What I ignored then also was that the packaged cereals I ate, including the organic ones, had natural or added sugar in them even though I did not always recognize it. The hidden sources of sugar, especially those added to processed foods, act as some of the worst triggers of insulin resistance, and they affect sleep when blood sugar drops quickly at night. Limiting the amount of sugar that I added to my foods was good, but not enough to prevent troubles with maintaining stable blood sugar and quality sleep in midlife. I needed to pay attention to all the foods and some of the habits that triggered elevated blood sugar and insulin release. In a blog post focusing on "8 Easy Ways to Boost Nutrient Absorption," Juliette Steen writes about practices that can affect nutrient absorption and indirectly affect sleep. They include a diet high in sugar, which can "actually rob your body of nutrients, particularly magnesium," according to nutritionist Fiona Tuck interviewed by Steen for this blog. Excess sugar in all its form is bad news for sleep.

A number of other sources confirm the link between sugar consumption and poor-quality sleep. Marie-Pierre St-Onge from the Department of Medicine and Institute of Human Nutrition at Columbia University was principal investigator for a study that demonstrated that "a higher percentage of energy from saturated fat predicted less slow wave sleep. Greater sugar intake also was associated with more arousals from sleep". This research was summarized on the American Academy of Sleep Medicine, which also includes a link to the study. In addition to sugar intake, Tuck identified highly processed flour foods, salty foods, fried foods, sugary foods and drinks, caffeine, alcohol, and refined vinegars that are generally low in nutrients to be among nutrient robbers that negatively affect sleep. Other nutrient robbers that also impact sleep include "certain medications such as antacids, blood pressure medications, antidepressants and hormone medications." She also emphasized that stress "increases our nutrient requirements – particularly vitamin C, the B vitamins and magnesium". We need these nutrients for quality sleep. We need them also to decrease the body's acidity. Highly processed foods are low in nutrients, they are acid-forming and they deprive us of quality sleep.

Donna Gates and Linda Schatz remind us that when you eat an acid-forming diet, "your body is constantly trying to return to a more balanced state by calling on your stored reserves of alkaline minerals: sodium, potassium, calcium, and magnesium," leading to deficiency in these, which can become severe over time (35). A deficiency in calcium and magnesium as well as the D and the B complex vitamins are linked to sub-optimal quality sleep. Shawn Stevenson refers to several studies that demonstrate this correlation between nutrient deficiencies and poor-quality sleep. Calcium is one of them, but he also points to others including potassium, selenium and vitamin C. Deficiency in vitamin C is associated with waking up during the night and not being able to fall asleep quickly again. Melatonin deficiency is well-known to impact sleep and melatonin supplementation (in small doses only) is well accepted for helping to boost sleep quality.

In the Stevenson podcast mentioned earlier, he identifies three sleep robbers that are related to our diet. They are monosodium glutamate (MSG), caffeine and sugar. Alcohol consumption is also "linked to a reduction of digestive enzymes, so people who drink heavily may not be able to break down the nutrients from the foods in the first place" states Jayta Szpitalak, another nutritionist interviewed by Juliette Steen in the blog post referenced above. I have already discussed how my regular consumption of sugar (many from hidden sources) contributed to some of the challenges I experienced in midlife and even earlier. Below I share a bit about my short-lived experiment with alcohol.

Alcohol:I tried red wine in my mid-twenties, often when I went to formal events where everyone seemed to enjoy a glass of wine to celebrate the occasion. I hated how I felt afterwards, and eventually I gave it up, resorting to Fanta Orange or Sprite. As we know by now, these were not good choices either, given the high amount of sugar added to most soft drinks. It took some maturing for me to reach a point where I felt comfortable enough to insist on having no other drink than water or soda (sparkling) water at a formal event or as a guest in someone's home. Nonetheless, perimenopause opened a can of worms, filled with health discomforts that forced me to try anything that would ease the pain of erratic cycles and the heavy bleeding that caused me to become anemic. I felt dizzy quite often while walking around the office and even at home.

A colleague suggested red wine. She seemed knowledgeable and in good health herself, and she had had similar heavy bleeding that she associated with perimenopause years before. I did not know then, what else was coming, but I was ready to try anything to prevent anemia triggers. We started buying red wine at home and knowing my low level of alcohol tolerance, I would have about half a glass in the evening with dinner. Even this amount made me feel uncomfortable and disoriented. I used to joke about being drunk, something that seemed absurd to those who felt more at ease and comfortable even after their second or third glass of wine. My kids got a kick out of seeing their mom behave drunk. That experiment failed. Bleeding got even worse, and it affected my sleep as I had to wake up at least a couple of times in the middle of the night to change my pads. I was looking forward to real menopause and to being done with it! I gave up wine once and for all, and I am glad I did then. When someone at a woman's health conference in Baltimore suggested red wine to help with my perimenopausal insomnia, I thanked her, knowing that never again will I go near it! There is enough evidence to link alcohol with sleep disruptions, and if I had continued drinking red wine, it might have made my sleep problems even worse. Somehow, I cannot imagine sleep getting any worse than how I experienced it, however! Alcohol is not only addictive, it also affects hormones elevating cortisol, a known sleep disruptor. And both alcohol and cortisol are known to create conditions that build a layer of fat around the belly as well.

I am not here to judge nor to imply that wine is bad for everyone. I respect every person's dietary and lifestyle choices. I realize that not every diet is best for everyone. In fact, during my studies at the Institute for Integrative Nutrition, we were reminded of the importance of "bio-individuality," recognizing that one person's food can be another person's poison. For a perfectly healthy person, a glass of red wine a few times a week can be a healthy complement to a balanced diet and lifestyle. It was never for me, and it is not worth my money as I think about it even today. And because it raises cortisol, a known sleep-disrupter, and lack of sleep triggers insulin, it is not on the list of what I would recommend to anyone looking to lose belly fat either. This is also the reason why I avoid caffeine. Both caffeine and alcohol are known sleep disruptors. Avoiding them within several hours of going to bed is what sleep experts recommend. Knowing your level of tolerance of these stimulants will help you to decide if you should avoid them completely to protect your sleep. For some people, even caffeine ingested at 10:00 am can be enough to affect their sleep at night. Alcohol affects Rapid Eye Movement (REM) sleep. Avoiding it for a week or longer can allow your body to reset its sleep clock and to determine its effects on your sleep. Anyone with sleep issues is better off avoiding alcohol and caffeine altogether until sleep is improved. But even then, one must be vigilant to prevent sliding back.

Environmental factors

I never paid much attention to several environmental factors that are now well known to negatively impact sleep. The ones that apply specifically to my case both before and as I entered midlife were increased cell phone use, watching some television shows or entertainment videos, and working on the computer in the evening, in particular.

Increasing cellphone use: I enjoyed the freedom that cell phones gave me, allowing me to keep in touch with family and professional colleagues and partners. I assumed that cell phones were better and more efficient versions of landline phones. Overtime, it became almost a requirement that one keeps a cell phone for work. In fact, for one of my jobs, Blackberries were issued to all full-time employees, and the expectation was that they be returned only upon resignation or termination.

Electromagnetic fields (EMFs) from cell phones has REM suppressive effects, and they reduce the percentage of REM sleep we get. This is the phase of sleep that occurs several times throughout the night and can last anywhere between ten minutes to as long as an hour. During REM sleep, you have vivid dreams, your brain is more active, your heart and breathing rate quicken, according to a WebMD article focusing specifically on the importance of both REM and non-REM sleep. We need both types of sleep and we get different benefits from each. Unfortunately, EMF suppresses REM sleep. "We are more permeable and conductive entity than floors and walls. We are electromagnetic beings ourselves. They [EMF] interact with our cells. They can cause issues with cell communication and hormones and neurotransmitters and how your body functions," states Stevenson in the podcast referred to earlier in this chapter.

There is still a lot I do not understand about how cell phones work, but the little bit I have read scares me. And when it comes to my own health, I often err on the side of caution, until I have enough evidence that I have no reason to worry. Stevenson recommends getting cell phones and other electronic gadgets out of our bedroom to promote better sleep quality, but he goes further in expressing concerns that EMFs could be "cooking up cancer." This is based on his review of research that links EMFs to "Leukemia, brain tumors, and breast cancer. " He adds that even the World Health Organization has now classified cell phone radiation "as a group 28 carcinogen" (Stevenson 95). Therefore, cell phone radiation may not be as benign as some marketers may want us to believe. For sceptics, cancer specialist Siegal Sadetzki will perhaps convince you to not just dismiss this information as irrelevant to your health. Sadetzki "testified at a United States Senate hearing that cell phones were identified as a contributor to salivary gland tumors. The report states that your risk of getting a parotid tumor on the same side of your head that you use for listening to the cell phone increases" by 34 percent if you are a regular cell phone user and have used a mobile phone for 5 years, 58 percent if you have had more than 5,500 calls in your lifetime, 49 percent if you have spoken on the phone for more than 266.3 hours during your lifetime" (Stevenson 95).

How did blue light and EMFs apply to my case? As I explain further below, I suspect that both impacted me in ways I may never be able to prove. Before I moved to "the field" (a term used in international development to distinguish "the home office" or headquarters, usually in a developed western country, from offices based in developing countries where program implementation takes place) in 2006, I used cellphones only sporadically. As a family, we relied mostly on our landline and in the office, we also had landlines that we used for making calls and keeping in touch with partners and team members in other countries. When I moved to Malawi, I started using my new cellphone every day, sometimes for short calls, other times for calls as long as 1 hour at a time. There were several reasons why I used it more frequently. I did not have access to a landline, and the process and cost of acquiring one did not seem to be worth it. Cellphone calls became the main mode of communication with my managers and other team members both in the field and in the home office. By then, almost every professional staff I knew who worked in international development had a cell phone.

Being based in the field required keeping my cell phone on all the time, expecting calls whenever people in the headquarters arrived in the office in a completely different time zone. While those in the home office could be sitting in a conference room, using the landline to make the call, I was hooked to the cellphone attached to my ear. I never paid attention until one time I felt the cellphone heat getting intense around the left ear, which is the one I used often for listening. It got so hot that holding it became uncomfortable. I did not have enough knowledge to question whether this could be damaging my body, my hearing, my left side of the brain, not to mention my heart, in ways that were not well known at the time. Hearing decline happens gradually with age. Could mine have been precipitated by cell phone use?

Because I needed the cell phone to keep in touch with my family when I was working away from home, which I did more regularly after I left Malawi, I am hoping that I am an exception to the rule and will live against all odds. In addition to the heat radiating from my cellphone to my left ear, I did eventually hear a little crackling inside my ear at one time after being on the phone for a while. I remember just thinking, "This heat going straight into my ear cannot be inconsequential." But I did nothing to mitigate the effects, whatever those might have been, as I was doing what I had to do for my job and for my family. With each call with my family, I was speaking with my husband and our two boys. Depending on what was going on, and on how many updates they wanted to share with me, I listened and enjoyed the conversations. I did not have a headphone then. I did not even know that I needed one or that it would have made any difference either way.

Could the times I spent on the cellphone have set the stage for hormonal imbalances, elevated cortisol and poor-quality sleep that I experienced in midlife? I cannot establish a causal link, but research does show that EMFs do impact the quality of sleep. Stevenson refers to a study published in *Radiation Protection Dosimetry* that found that "melatonin secretion is significantly disrupted by exposure to electromagnetic fields." Melatonin not only regulates sleep, but "it's also an important anti-cancer hormone" (Stevenson 96). This is not to say that we should go out and get a melatonin supplement if we cannot make enough of our own. Even when needed, experts recommend only a small amount to allow the body to make its own naturally.

Can anything be done to lower the risk of cellphone radiation? Keeping the cellphone away from the bed is one easy solution I wish I knew then, but one that I hope you will adopt. Turning wireless routers off at night is another good practice, and that is exactly what my husband and I do these days, especially when we are alone in the house. I hope that you too will turn yours off at night as well. Can we do anything to counter the damage already done to our bodies? I would like to know. Nonetheless, I do believe that proper nutrition, accounting for individual optimal dietary needs, as well as having a mindset and lifestyle that promote health, can support the body to reach a level of healing that is still possible. Even if it means living with some irreversible damage, not stressing over it can be beneficial in the end. Not doing anything only compounds the harm, because we know that EMFs are a real problem and they do affect sleep. And poor sleep habits and suboptimal sleep quality in one way or another, is a factor in building a layer of fat around the belly. And belly fat is a risk factor for many chronic illnesses including diabetes as mentioned earlier.

Watching television: My husband and I used to have our favorite shows that we watched until it was time for bed. We watched CNN evening news as well. My husband still likes to watch the news on TV regularly. Later on, as the kids got older, we had favorite shows that we watched together as well. These were shorter, time-bound shows, usually comedies such as *Seinfeld* or *The Cosby Show*. We did not watch much TV news with the kids. Overall, even when I had no trouble sleeping through the night, I never spent too much time watching television. Perhaps this is because I did not have a television at home growing up. Television did not make it to Burundi until 1987. Also, although I do not remember who the presenter was at one of the schools that my kids attended, the advice then was to limit the amount of time kids spent watching television, linking too much TV to trouble concentrating at school. I extrapolated and decided that it most likely applies to adults as well. Even though I limited the amount of time I spent watching television, I did watch the news or the entertainment videos at night and often it was before I went to bed.

Working on the computer in the evening: One of the habits I adopted to keep up with recurring monthly deadlines was an inconsistent sleep schedule. In the chapter on stress, I made reference to the time when my mom visited us in Malawi and she found me still behind the computer screen in the middle of the night. While I recall this incident very well, perhaps because of the emotions attached to that time of loss and grief in my life, working on the computer in the evening was more of a rule than an exception for me. I had the habit of turning the computer back on and working after the kids went to bed. The problem with computers is that, similar to other electronic devices, they emit artificial blue light that "triggers your body to produce more daytime hormones (such as cortisol) and disorients your body's natural preparation for sleep," writes Stevenson (19).

Blue light from TVs, computers and other electronic devices do affect sleep. There is accumulating evidence that blue light suppresses melatonin production. A Rensselaer Polytechnic Institute study cited in a *New York Times* article by Anahad O'Connor showed that "exposure to light from computer tablets significantly lowered levels of the hormone melatonin, which regulates our internal clocks and plays a role in the sleep cycle." The study showed that "two hours of exposure to bright tablet screen at night reduced melatonin levels by about 22 percent." A University of Basel study cited by Ferris Jabr in *Scientific American* found that "volunteers who were exposed to an LED backlit computer for five hours in the evening produced less melatonin, felt less tired, and performed better on tests of attention than those in front of a fluorescent-lit screen of the same size and brightness." In another study cited by Jabr, those who "read on an iPad for four hours before bed reported feeling less sleepy, took an average of 10 minutes longer to fall asleep and slept less deeply than those who read paper books at night."

I know that not everybody can make the drastic career changes I have made, but in my opinion, any job that requires compromising your health and your sleep on a regular basis was not meant for you, even if it is a job you love. Anything that interferes with sleep must be moved out of the way to enable the body to produce melatonin, which controls your sleep-wake cycle naturally. Computers and cellphones are guilty as charged! Not managing their effects on sleep means not taking all precautions needed to trigger shrinking your belly fat either.

Lifestyle factors

Poor management of stress: I discussed earlier what my stressors were and by now we know that poor management of stress contributes to weight gain and a resistance to belly fat loss. But stress makes it harder to sleep as well. And lack of sleep is another factor that keeps cortisol levels high, as they play yo-yo with each other. Embracing a lifestyle that respects sleep, which helps to lower the stress hormone cortisol, sets the stage for a more balanced transition through midlife. Looking back, I did not keep my stress levels in check, but then again, what did I know? I was stressed in my younger years, and my stressors changed, but they did not go away through midlife. Life is full of stress. It is unavoidable. The only choice we have is to change our response to it and our attitude towards it. This is what I do now and it helps tremendously, both with weight management and with sleep. Effective management of stress for better sleep means addressing unresolved traumas and stressors of the past as well.

Poor sleep habits: We all intuitively know that we need sleep. I know now that sleep matters much more than I had imagined. As a result, I have become a sleep advocate in my own home, seeking to inform and hopefully influence my kids and my husband to also take sleep seriously. For my kids, I hope they start sooner rather than later. I want them as I want you to give up your poor sleep habits that will affect the quality of life and your sleep, both now and in the future. Let me share how some of the habits I developed long before I entered midlife came back to haunt me. I developed some of these bad habits when I was in high school, but most especially later in college and in graduate school.

Interestingly, by the time I read *Sleep Smarter*, my older son was himself a junior in college. He had already missed many hours of quality sleep, not just as a college student, but a high school student, too. At least in high school, he could take a nap after school. And he often did. My younger son was a freshman in college at the time, following in his brother's footsteps when it came to sleep habits. In fact, my younger son told me several months ago that he stayed up for 48 hours straight, with a few short naps thrown in here and there, when he was studying for his Statistics final exam. Thankfully, he did well! And while he is proud of his overall college experience and the opportunities that come with a college degree from a top university, he is willing to admit that this experience has also taught him how to stay up all night. Could there be a better way to ride through college without sacrificing sleep? College students know what boundaries they can draw. They also know which, in their opinion, are beyond their comfort zone and that is what they do.

I was a bit encouraged, nonetheless, when I confirmed that at least one of them still has his copy of *Sleep Smarter* that I had given to each of them with a note saying, "You will never think about sleep the same way after you read this book" or something like that. When I gave my kids this book, they warned me with a simple statement: "Not now, Mom!" I should, of course, understand that college is a different beast altogether, and few college students in the US are inclined to go to bed early (which would mean by midnight, by the way). I understand. I too have been there, in a different country and decades earlier, though. Then, I was able to control my schedule somewhat better, and my roommate was one of my best friends since high school. We respected each other's bedtime. We are still friends and stay in touch, nearly forty years later!

There was more that worked in my favor when it came to sleep. We had no phone in our dorm rooms—not even a public phone in the hallway. There were no social media distractions, and not even internet. This made it easier for me to go to bed between 10:00 and 11:00 pm almost every weekday. My schedule even then, however, varied greatly on weekends. Often, my roommate and I, along with several of our friends would be up past midnight, chatting away about life's trivia. None of us had any grand vision of changing the world to keep us awake, that's for sure! The black tea with milk and sugar that we drank any time of the day, including the evenings, helped. It was also on weekends that we went out dancing when we had the opportunity. Then we could be up till the early morning hours the following day.

When we returned to our dorm rooms after dancing through the night, hoping to get at least a few hours of sleep, before each of us had to do what we had planned for that day, quality sleep was not a guarantee. In fact, I felt as if the sound of music from the dance club continued bouncing off my inner ears even once back inside the quiet four walls of my dorm room. The adrenaline that kept me awake at the club did not leave me alone just because I was finally lying flat in bed. It was hard to get restful sleep when I had just spent the night bouncing up and down to the beat of contemporary African music. I still want to get up and dance when I hear some of the favorite songs they used to play at the club then. Sam Fan Thomas, Kassav, Yvonne Chaka Chaka, and a few others were the popular artists we danced to then. We danced to our favorite Rhythm and Blues and disco music of the 60s, 70s, and to popular music of the 80s as well. This was the type of music that kept us awake and entertained then.

These days, our kids and many others, including busy professionals (some of whom are women in midlife), no longer require the slowing down of academic schedules on weekends to keep themselves up at night, however. Constant and instant connectivity and messaging, whether inside homes, in classrooms, in offices or on the go, along with access to social media gadgets and other tools and technologies that allow us to interact remotely, have overhauled traditional approaches to social interactions and our sleep habits as well. While I hear from some people that it does not matter when they go to bed, they still sleep well and wake up rested, I am not convinced that the quality of sleep they get is as good as it could be, if they followed their circadian rhythm and all that sleep experts recommend. I have learned important lessons about why I should respect sleep. I have learned it the hard way, unfortunately. Perhaps you can learn it the easy way.

A sedentary lifestyle and Vitamin D deficiency: With my work habits, spending entire days indoors behind a computer without direct access to sunlight, I should not have been surprised when my blood tests came out showing Vitamin D deficiency. The neurotransmitter serotonin is one of the powerful compounds that is affected by the body's exposure to sunlight. I wish we all learned from a younger age that "our eyes have special light receptors that send information to the center of the brain [hypothalamus] to trigger the production of ... serotonin" (Stevenson 11). I wish we learned as well that without serotonin, there will be no melatonin, the sleep hormone.

Serotonin is indeed the building block of melatonin, but serotonin production cannot happen when we deprive ourselves of natural light.

Working in well-lit buildings is not a suitable replacement for natural light. Apparently, working near a window that allows the sun to pierce through can even make a difference, according to a study that compared those with and without direct access to windows at work. Those who did not have access to windows "got 173 percent less exposure to natural light and, as a result, slept an average of 46 minutes less each night," Stevenson adds (11). The irony is that there are many hard-working professionals based in tropical environments who are not taking advantage of this precious gift of nature, sunlight. Vitamin D deficiency is more common than it needs to be, but it should not surprise anyone who works indoors day in and day out, all year round. It should not be a surprise that this deficiency will negatively affect their sleep either.

Others

Beauty products: Many skin care and other beauty products are endocrine disruptors. This means that they contain "chemicals that interfere with the production, release, transport, metabolism, or elimination of the body's natural hormones" (Vitti 35). I started paying attention to the skin care products I used when I noticed that whenever I applied some of them, I had more frequent hot flashes throughout the day or at night than when I avoided these products. As usual, I started educating myself on the link between beauty products and hot flashes and learned about which are safer to apply. Just as with most highly processed foods, skin care products have so many ingredients that it is nearly impossible to know which among them must be avoided. I will share below which skin creams I apply these days.

Bed sheets and clothing: Most polyester sheets and outfits cause me to sweat too much, and I often cannot even tell whether I am having hot flashes or just poorly breathing because of the quality of the material I am wearing or sleeping on. Polyester does not breathe and wearing polyester clothes or sleeping on polyester sheets will affect normal breathing and trap the heat inside our bed, making it uncomfortable for us while we sleep. Trapped heat often wakes me up from sleep.

PRACTICES THAT HELP ME SLEEP BETTER

The good news is that there is a lot we can do to influence our sleep and that help us to recover from insomnia and many of its side effects. Having taken the time to uncover my sleep robbers, I proceeded to deal with them one by one, while adopting behaviors that helped me achieve better quality sleep. Below, I share some of these habits and behaviors. They are informed by experts including Michael Breus, Shawn Stevenson, Eric Berg, Chris Idzikowski, Paul McKenna, Lisa Morrone, and others who agree on several general principles and make specific recommendations regarding what we need to do to prevent sleep robbers from interfering with the quality of our sleep.

I tried many strategies. I considered any habit that seemed practical and realistic and without known long-term side effects to be worth a try. Hence, the habits I adopted since midlife insomnia hit continue to help me improve the overall quality of my sleep. I share below what I try to do on a daily basis to promote better sleep.

Diet: What I drink and what I eat

Water: Water is a source of life. In fact, we can live a bit longer with water than we would if we had food but were deprived of water. Fortunately, drinking water has never been an issue for me. What has changed however, is knowing the optimal amount of water my body requires to feel hydrated and to sleep well. There seems to be no general rule for everyone to follow when it comes to how much water we need. I hear often that we all need 8 glasses of 8 ounces of water each day. The University of Missouri System offers the following guidelines:

Body weight (in pounds) divided by 2 = minimum ounces of water to drink per day

Generally, by listening to our body, we will know when we need to rehydrate. In my case, I aim for not less than 65 ounces of water per day. With the additional fluids that come from the foods I eat, I am sufficiently hydrated each day and I feel uncomfortable when I fail to drink at least this amount of water throughout the day.

Drinking too much water increases the need to urinate, which can help to flush out toxins (a good thing), but it wakes us up from sleep, and it also creates an imbalance of sodium and potassium electrolytes that are needed for regulating heart function and preventing water retention among other functions. This can be especially dangerous when one is on a low salt diet. Such an imbalance has been linked to hyponatremia, a condition in which sodium levels have fallen so low in the body that the sodium/potassium ratio is not in balance to help the heart function effectively. It is also linked to hypertension. Knowing your ideal water needs is therefore important, and proper hydration is key to helping you sleep well at night. The average amount of eight glasses of water per day is a safe starting point for adults. Those who are active will most likely need more. Let your body be your teacher and guide here.

On a normal day, I drink a large glass (10 to 12 ounces) of water first thing in the morning to rehydrate. I do this because we all experience nighttime dehydration. I feel much better after I drink my first glass. Rehydrating before breakfast helps improve digestion, which in turn prevents digestive discomforts that can wake you up from your sleep at night. Heartburn is not fun while you are lying down, trying to sleep. Drinking a sufficient amount of water throughout the day helps also with maintaining healthy cells, hormonal regulation, and brain function, which, in one way or another, affect sleep. The National Sleep Foundation emphasizes that hydration "plays a critical role in how well (or not) you sleep at night" in an article on its website that explores the connection between hydration and sleep. Drinking a large glass of water in the morning also fulfills one of Gates and Schatz's recommendations that "high-water content, expansive foods and drinks for breakfast" help to counteract the "more acidic, dehydrated, and more contracted" state of our body during the night while we are sleeping (73).

To manage my daily water intake effectively, I try to drink about a third of my daily water requirements by mid-morning. This means that by 10:00 am, I have already consumed at least 20 ounces of water. I then drink the other third by 2:00 pm, and I finish the rest from late afternoon into early evening. I try to avoid drinking more than a few sips of water after dinner, usually around 7:00 pm, and I go to bed around 10:00 pm most nights. Drinking less at night helps to prevent the urge to get up to use the bathroom, often from what feels like deep sleep. An article on "Sleeping Well to Live Well" posted on the UCLA Sleep Disorder Center explains why this is the case: "It takes about 90 minutes for the body to process liquids that you drink. This means that you should limit your intake of fluids for at least 90 minutes before going to bed."

My main challenge regarding the amount of water I should drink comes when I am travelling and cannot easily access safe drinking water. I face a challenge also when I do not know how long it will take for me to reach the nearest bathroom. When this happens, I tend to drink less water during the day and may drink more in the evening because, either way, dehydration keeps me awake. Trying to fit the needed amount of water in the afternoon and evening hours, however, is one sure way to set myself up for middle of the night bathroom trips, interrupting my sleep.

Eating to keep blood sugar stable: Whenever I can control my meals throughout the day, I eat three balanced meals to satisfy me without snacks between meals or before bed. Not eating enough can interfere with sleep. The UCLA Sleep Disorder Patient Education page summarizes it well: "Hunger from an empty stomach may keep you from falling asleep. It may also wake you later in the night" Others, including Michael Breus agree. In his 2017 blog post on the "Ideal Home Sleep Environment",

Breus states that "[i]f you're hungry at bedtime, you will have a harder time falling asleep thanks to the stimulating effects of the hormone cortisol, that your body will release. You're better off having a small snack ... that is no more than 200 calories .... Combine a small amount of protein ... with a complex carbohydrate."

To keep blood sugar stable, I try to eat before I feel too hungry and too weak from an empty stomach. I choose food carefully to prevent a blood sugar crash during the day and also at night. This is the reason why I manage my carb intake carefully as well. Nowadays, I focus on complex carbohydrates such as green bananas, brown rice, pumpkin, quinoa, cassava or sweet potatoes. I have potatoes with red skin as well when I can find them. They are good prebiotics used to feed beneficial gut bacteria, especially when eaten cold, as mentioned in Chapter 4 on fermented foods.

I try not to skip meals either. This is not the best way to lose weight or to sleep better at night. It can create the opposite effect in fact and contribute to expanding belly fat further. When you skip meals, your blood sugar decreases, which stimulates cortisol (from the adrenals) to increase and it "turns body tissues (muscles from legs, buttocks and arms) into sugar fuel .... if this sugar is not completely burned up, it will be changed into fat and specifically deposited around your vital organs in the abdomen" (Berg 132).

Prioritizing nutrient dense and alkalizing foods: Nutrient dense foods work better for sleep. I try to identify foods that supply me with the necessary nutrients to support sleep. Poor sleep requires a higher intake of certain vitamins that are known to either help improve sleep or protect the body from harmful side effects of lack of adequate sleep. The B vitamins, as well as vitamins C, D, and E, are among those that are necessary for quality sleep and/or for minimizing side effects of poor sleep, according to Michael Breus in his blog post on "5 Vitamin Deficiencies that Can Affect Your Sleep."

I do not take sleeping pills. I do however take off and on a magnesium supplement supplied by HormoneBalance.com and I regularly take a women's probiotic supplement that includes several digestive enzymes and prebiotics in the place of a multivitamin. This probiotic helps me digest fats better, and it supports regular bowel movements. I generally take less than the recommended dosage because I can never be certain that supplements have no side effects. Nonetheless, I know that any help I can give to my digestive system supports sleep as well. Generally, I take a probiotic only when I do not have access to fermented vegetables. Otherwise, I rely on real foods as much as I can. Kiwi for example, has become one of my main sources of vitamin C. We hear often that "an apple a day will keep the doctor away" but we don't hear as much that kiwi offers similar benefits, if not more. In an article posted on the healthline.com website, the benefits of kiwi are succinctly summarized. These benefits include supporting digestion and preventing constipation due to its high fiber content, boosting the immune system with its high vitamin C content, managing blood pressure as well as protecting your eyes from vision loss.

To promote better sleep, I try also to eat leafy greens, such as spinach, spring greens, Swiss chard, kale, arugula, or any other local greens I can find. Dark leafy greens are high in potassium, magnesium and zinc as well as several of the B vitamins, which complement each other to promote sleep. Other favorite vegetables include crucifers such as broccoli, cabbage, Brussels sprouts, and cauliflower that I have steamed or stir-fried. The crucifers are helpful for balancing hormones as well as being liver-friendly foods that support detoxification.

When I cannot have a reliable source of fresh vegetables, I have started adding green powders to my diet to increase my intake of sleep-promoting vitamins and minerals. Moringa, spirulina and to a lesser extent wheat grass, are my go-to green powders whenever I live in an environment where the local supply of fresh vegetables is limited. Moringa is a complete protein food in addition to having loads of vitamins and minerals. I add it to other cooked foods such as soups and stews. Fresh moringa leaves are cooked as a vegetable in many tropical countries and it is recognized as a super healthy food by many. Spirulina is a high alkalinizer and a potent antioxidant. I add it to my morning smoothie whenever I need to supplement my consumption of fresh vegetables, and also to help alkalize my body. Raw vegetables have their own live enzymes to prevent indigestion, which can keep you awake at night as well.

Lean proteins: I try to have a serving of protein with each meal. One to two eggs in the morning, one or two chicken legs, or a serving of a lean cut of beef (about 4 ounces) are what works best for me, especially for lunch. These lean proteins keep me full and protect me from a quick drop in blood sugar that would come from carbs. I eat beef much less frequently, limiting it to once a week or even once every two weeks because it is higher in saturated fat and it is harder to digest. I avoid beef especially at night. Generally, meat is harder to digest at night when the body needs all the energy to focus on sleep and not digestion. That is why I try to have a higher calorie lunch and a lower calorie dinner as often as I can, as well. Fatty fish such as salmon and sardines are, however, good sources of Vitamin D and Omega-3 fatty acids that promote sleep. Because I eat dinner generally early, a serving of fish (about 4-6 ounces) helps.

Vitamin D3: When I can, I spend time outside when the sun is out to activate Vitamin D, which triggers production of serotonin, a precursor for and building block for melatonin. "Vitamin D affects both how much sleep we get and how well we sleep," writes Michael Breus in his 2019 blog post on "5 Vitamin Deficiencies that Can Affect Your Sleep." I also take a liquid vitamin D3 supplement regularly to support my body's ability to produce the right sleep hormones and address a diagnosed vitamin D deficiency.

Lifestyle

Reduced calorie and intermittent fasting: I practice intermittent fasting regularly. I try to fast for three days up to one week at a time each month to maintain my weight and lower inflammation, which can prevent sleep. With intermittent fasting, when I eat dinner between 5:30 pm and 7:00 pm, I break the fast between 9:30 am and noon the following day, sixteen to eighteen hours later. The idea is to allow the body to dip into stored fat as a source of energy between dinner and your first meal the following day. This approach works consistently to keep my weight in check, and a healthy weight benefits sleep. Fasting helps me keep my waistline in check as well.

The difference between a reduced calorie diet and intermittent fasting is that with reduced calorie, I limit my overall calorie intake throughout the day. Instead of three meals I have in an 8-hour interval as I would with intermittent fasting, I have less for breakfast such as a kiwi first, then within an hour, I snack on a handful of almond or mixed nuts, and then later on, I have a boiled egg. I repeat this one more time until dinner, which I have early, between 6 and 7pm. This is when I have a regular low-carb meal such as a serving of fish with plenty of vegetables.

As long as I ensure that my energy levels are stable, I am able to sleep well and I shrink my waistline naturally when I limit my overall calorie intake. My probiotic/multivitamin helps, I hope, to meet any nutritional deficiencies that may result from not eating three regular meals a day. I fast for three to five days at a time and as needed. I practice intermittent fasting as a way of life now. With this type of fasting, I have two meals a day, starting with a large lunch and a smaller dinner that I have within 6 to 8 hours after lunch. Sometimes, I skip dinner when I am still full from lunch.

The worst thing to do in the evening is to go to bed with a full or an empty stomach. When full, your body will be working on digesting food instead of focusing on sleep. When hungry, your body will release cortisol for the energy required by your brain during REM sleep.

Limiting time spent watching television in the evening: I now know that anytime spent on the screen, especially in the evening, will interfere with my sleep. So, I limit my exposure to blue light from television at night. In fact, nowadays, I avoid watching TV as much as possible and almost never watch it within an hour of going to bed when I am at home. Thankfully, my husband honors this TV curfew as well, even though he generally sleeps better and always has. As a couple, we never developed the habit of bringing a television into our bedroom, unlike many other people I know who almost always keep it on even while sleeping. They have their own reasons. I just hope they have no issue with sleep, although not having trouble sleeping now does not mean it will always be the same in the future, especially for women in midlife.

Avoiding a sedentary lifestyle and timing exercise better: Getting up frequently throughout the day and moving around promotes better blood circulation throughout the day, prepares the body for quality sleep at night, and it contributes to preventing fat build-up around the belly. I used to think that as long I exercised regularly, I would reap the health benefits that this lifestyle habit offers. To maintain a healthy weight and promote sleep, I generally go outside for a walk to get some sunshine, or I exercise inside my house creating my own routine following a YouTube video.

I no longer do any exercise that overstimulates the body and mind in the evening. I no longer ignore the importance of following the circadian rhythms even in choosing the right time to exercise. I continue to focus on building and strengthening muscles, a sure way to help my body to burn more calories and breakdown some fat even while I sleep. While I can do a leisurely walk even early in the evening, I do not do any intense workouts any time after 5:00 pm. When I can't find the time for morning exercise for reasons I cannot control, I squeeze some walking into my schedule between 5:00 and 6:00 pm, shortly before dinner. Otherwise, relaxing and calming yoga is one of the best exercises that I do in the evenings. This is another step I consistently take and that I find effective in helping me to lower cortisol as the day comes to an end, which prepares me better for sleep. Exercising, several times per week, while paying attention to its effects on sleep has helped me to maintain the gains I have achieved of a healthy weight and a smaller waistline.

Managing stress through deep breathing and relaxation: This technique is easy to apply even while in bed. It requires closing your eyes and focusing on your breathing and nothing else. If a thought comes in the way, acknowledge it but then return back to your breathing. This technique requires breathing in through your nose, to a count of four. When done properly, you will feel your belly expand as if to allow air to reach all of your internal organs. Then breathe out also through the nose to a count of eight. As the air comes out, your stomach will drop, as if to massage your internal organs as much as possible. You can also blow the air out through your mouth, with a slight opening of your lips to a count of eight, or for as long as you can do it comfortably.

I repeat this breathing technique, four to eight consecutive times. I like to do it even when lying in bed. It allows me to drift into sleep without even realizing it. This is a simple technique I use every time I am trying to get back to sleep in the middle of the night. It really works whenever I remember to do it, especially breathing in through the nose, going a little deeper and out the mouth, letting it last a little longer each time. The challenge is to remember to do it because it is not always the first thing that comes to mind when you can't fall back to sleep. If you have an active mind like mine, you probably race from one thought to another and must be intentional about deep breathing if you don't want to continue tossing and turning in frustration.

It really works because every time I turn my mind to it, within just a few minutes, I feel sleepy again, and I do not even realize that I fell asleep until I see through the windows that morning has come. I am grateful whenever that happens. This technique is adapted from the "4-7-8 breath" I learned from Andrew Weil, in his book *Spontaneous Happiness*. Weil states that focusing on breath is one of the "most effective anti-anxiety measure[s]" that we all can apply, free of charge (146). "Breath links body and mind, consciousness and unconsciousness. Working with the breath ….is a way to calm the restless mind, facilitating one-pointed attention and meditation," Weil writes (145-146). By bringing my mind back to deep breathing, sooner or later sleep follows, and while I wait, I am relaxed and not frustrated.

Emotional Freedom Technique (EFT): Also known as "tapping", this technique involves literally tapping along various energy points in your body, with the goal of restoring balance to your body's energy. It starts out on the side of the hand, and various places around the face, the collar of the neck, under the arms, and over the crown of the head. By tapping over each of these meridian points, the idea is to release stress and tension that might be hiding there, which improves circulation, promotes relaxation, and benefits sleep.

Whenever I apply this technique, it helps me relax and breathe much more normally and effectively. When I tap for 15 minutes before bed, I am able to fall asleep faster, and I feel like it helps me get into more deep sleep sequences that night. It may sound strange to those who are unfamiliar with it, but I urge you to give it a try. It really does work to release tension and to sleep better. You can check YouTube for video demonstrations of how this technique works. If you want to learn more about tapping, the book *The Tapping Solution: A Revolutionary Solution for Stress-free Living* by

Nick Ortner (2014) will teach all you need to know about it and its many health benefits.

Environmental Control

Creating a sleep sanctuary: This practice reserves the bedroom for sleep and intimacy, which creates a routine that your brain can recognize, associating the bedroom with relaxation and sleep. It also requires sleeping in the dark, hence protecting you from the overstimulation of your brain by artificial blue LEDs as discussed earlier in this chapter. I have now changed the light curtains in our bedrooms and replaced them with others that keep light out better. A sleep sanctuary requires a social media curfew as well. As mentioned above, my husband and I turn the internet router off before we go to bed at night. Access to the internet and responding to messages at night can leave your sleep schedule under the control of others. The sooner you own your own schedule, including the time you go to bed and what you do while there, the sooner you will recover from poor quality sleep.

I encourage you to experiment with removing blue light from your bedroom to see how it works for you. By creating a sleep sanctuary, reserving your bedroom for only sleep and sleep-inducing activities such as intimacy with your partner, or reading a light book that does not overstimulate your thinking, your sleep will most likely improve and you will not need any more incentives to maintain this habit. Listening to meditative music or podcasts can also help you to relax before bed as well.

Temperature control in my bedroom: Lowering the temperature in my bedroom is not something I would have intuitively thought of because I hate it when I feel cold. However, over and over again, I find myself sleeping better in cooler environments, so long as I have a blanket to keep me warm enough, but not too warm. I therefore consider controlling the temperature in my bedroom as a key strategy to sleep better at night. This is not to say that we need to sleep in freezing cold or to make it so cold that it feels uncomfortable for us. But we should not keep the bedroom hot or a thick blanket on when we feel hot and are trying hard to fall back to sleep. Layers can help. When I start feeling really hot in bed, and I don't want to get up to change the covers, I use two blankets, a thin one on top of the cover sheet and a thicker blanket on top of that, so that I can push the top one off whenever I start feeling too hot. It's like dressing in layers during the winter months. Cooling down really does help to sleep more soundly again.

When I live in a house with a thermostat, I switch it to 68 degrees Fahrenheit (which is 20 degrees Celsius) before bed. You may like it a degree or two higher or lower depending on your biochemical comfort zone. Chris Idzikowski, author of *Learn to Sleep Well*, suggests that "62 degrees Fahrenheit (16 degrees Celsius) is generally conducive to restful sleep, while temperatures above 71 degrees Fahrenheit (24 degrees Celsius) are more likely to cause restlessness" (50). When the room is too hot, the body feels the heat pressure, and this can prevent you from falling asleep or staying asleep. Idzikowski adds that the body's temperature changes throughout the day, "reaching its warmest during the early evening, before dropping again in preparation for the night and reaching its coolest at around 4 am. Ideally, then, the temperature of our room should follow this cycle" (50). In the winter months, for example, the temperature should be lower when the body is hottest and increased when the body temperature drops to the lowest.

Using breathable clothes and bedsheets: Nowadays, I buy only 100 percent cotton bedsheets and either cotton or linen outfits and support my body's ability to breathe normally without the output of materials near my skin that do not breathe. I adopted this habit when I noticed that wearing breathable clothes lowered my incidents of hot flashes.

Managing cell phone, computer and TV use: Slowing down in the evening, getting off the computer when the work day is over and generally not later than 6:00 pm, and not watching television for many hours at a time and especially not at least 1 to 2 hours before going to bed are important strategies that continue to help me sleep better at night. Not watching television before bed in particular "... gives your mind a chance to process and absorb all the adrenalin released in response to the exciting imagery, to slow down to a gentler pace that will synchronize with your natural impetus toward sleep" states Paul McKenna in his book *I Can Make You Sleep: Overcome Insomnia Forever and Get the Best Rest of Your Life* (87). I have experimented with spending less times on the screen many times and whenever I spend less time on the computer during the day, or take short breaks from it throughout the day, and refrain from using it in the evening, I do sleep better at night.

I limit most online communications, including text messages by WhatsApp, Facebook, messenger and all other forms of online communication, early in the evening. Occasionally, when I spend my day mostly offline, I can check messages quickly and respond to anything urgent and then save the rest for the following morning. With WhatsApp, I rarely receive urgent email messages these days. I have also developed the habit of dimming the light on the computer, so that it is not as bright at night as it is during the day, on the rare occasions when I must use it for deadlines that cannot wait.

Managing beauty products: The safest way is to use single ingredient or only those with ingredients you recognize and know to be safe. Since I made this decision, I apply coconut oil, pure shea butter, or argan oil to my skin as well as pure rose oil (on my face only because it's expensive). This step alone reduced the frequency of daytime hot flashes that were induced by the application of other skin creams with ingredients that most likely were endocrine disruptors.

WHAT ARE THE SIGNS OF IMPROVEMENT IN THE AREA OF SLEEP?

I measure improvement both in terms of how long it takes for me to fall asleep when I go to bed, which is now between 10 and 15 minutes. I measure it also in terms of how long it takes to fall back to sleep when I wake up in the middle of the night. Usually when I wake up within three hours of going to bed to use the bathroom, it will take less time (15-20 minutes) than when I wake up closer to the end of night or early morning hours. Sleep remains a delicate balance, but the strategies I have embraced have enabled me to recover from the insomnia of yesteryear. The good news is that what robs me of quality sleep these days is no longer the things I ignore and cannot control, but rather exceptions to my daily routines.

While I have not reached the ideal yet, my sleep has greatly improved, from two hours at my worst to six hours or sometimes seven at my best. Rarely do I get the eight or nine hours of sleep I used to aim for and achieved naturally when I could control and respected my sleep schedule and before midlife insomnia hit. I generally feel rested when I wake up. And as long as I eat a balanced diet that is low in carbs, and includes plenty of vegetables and sufficient protein, I have consistent energy throughout the day and am able to sleep well at night. I have worked very hard to achieve this level of improvement. Therefore, I do everything I can to protect my sleep. I learned how to tame insomnia and get it to a point where it was willing to cooperate with gradual improvements over a period of nearly five years. If you are only starting to experience midlife insomnia, I hope these steps will help you to tame it and recover without having to wait this long!

CONCLUSION

Ignoring sleep while trying to shrink belly fat is like omitting yeast from bread and hoping that it will still rise. It just won't happen. So, you might as well make friends with sleep and give it what it requires to give you the rest you deserve. Your waistline will thank you for it. The layer of fat that insomnia contributes to your belly with each night that you struggle to fall asleep or to stay asleep will not shrink when you are sleep deprived. Unfortunately, shrinking the waistline takes a lot of effort because what builds abdominal fat is more than midlife insomnia.

So many factors are at play when it comes to the quality of sleep we get. Following your own circadian rhythm is only one of them. Eating nutrient dense foods also helps us sleep well and so does drinking clean filtered water throughout the day. Taking short breaks in between activities to breathe intentionally, move, stand, and stretch are other important ways that make the day less sedentary, less stressed, and improve sleep quality. As I learned from personal experience, mishandling any of these factors will keep us from reaching our belly fat loss goals even when other dietary and lifestyle modifications are able to bring us to lose much of the excess weight.

Sleep quality interacts with the other lifestyle factors as we discussed earlier. Sometimes they affect each other positively, other times negatively. For example, sleep and stress affect each other positively when quality sleep helps to lower cortisol levels. They affect each other negatively when poor quality sleep keeps stress hormones elevated. When sleep and stress interact negatively, they compound their effect in building fat around the belly. Sleep works in conjunction with exercise as well. Often being well-rested creates incentives for exercising. Therefore, the lifestyle trio which include exercise, stress management, and sleep are co-factors that are as important as the right diet for achieving better fat-burning results, especially in midlife. Monitoring and adjusting caffeine and alcohol consumption, avoiding sugary foods and drinks, exercising at the right time and with the right intensity to keep cortisol low, and creating a sleep sanctuary, work together to promote quality sleep.

While this information is based on my experience and the expertise of others who informed my actions as a woman in midlife, I believe it will inform and benefit not just those who are in midlife, but also those who are younger and have not yet experienced sleep disturbances as one sign of perimenopause. It will benefit older women who are looking for tips to restore quality sleep as well. Wherever you are, I hope that what I have shared in this chapter will benefit you and spare you the worst of sleep deprivation or insomnia. I hope this information will equip you with what you need to know in order for you to plan for restful nights throughout your midlife years and also succeed at sleeping better the rest of your life. And I wish you peaceful and restorative nights, filled with sweet dreams!

FINAL THOUGHTS

You must target "the most dangerous type of fat you carry on your body, the fat that threatens your very existence. If you want to live longer and healthier, keeping that fat is simply not an option", Liz Vaccariello, *Flat Belly Diet* (325).

For many of us, the signs of declining health show more clearly in midlife, with a wider middle than we were used to in our younger years. Belly fat poses health risks that we want to avoid as we age. The fat that hides inside the belly and over key organs, especially the liver and intestines, is more dangerous than the fat that settles around the butt or other parts of the body. Knowing what it takes to lose belly fat and doing what it takes to shrink it, is a must if we want to remain healthy as we age.

As Joel Fuhrman reminds us, "[t]he longer the waistline, the shorter the lifeline." I welcome you on the journey to extend our lifeline with a shorter waistline. We can do this! You may recall that I used to wear a US dress size 14, which was my size earlier in my midlife years. You may also recall that when I embarked on this journey to wellness, I wasn't even concerned with belly fat. I did not know enough about it to make it the focus of my efforts to improve my health. I did want to lose weight. And I wanted to look and feel better. These were my simple goals. What I ended up doing in the process was to dig deeper and search wider, sometimes finding answers in unexpected locations.

This journey required stepping off life's treadmill. I needed to center and know myself better. I had never invested much energy into reflecting on what I wanted to become when I grew up. What I discovered when I finally decided to slow down was something far more profound than professional achievements and making lots of money. Perhaps this journey was to help me discover who I was meant to be all along. *We Are the Ones We Have Been Searching For*, by Alice Walker, summarizes this point well. My journey took many twists and turns and taught me many lessons along the way. I place these lessons at two different levels, one practical, the other at a philosophical, higher level. The practical level is where I applied what I learned, following the tips, tools and expert knowledge I gained to bring myself to a healthier weight, body, mind and spirit -- and a healthier waistline. Below are the key practical lessons that I learned during my journey and that I shared with you throughout this book.

LESSON 1 - CHANGE IS POSSIBLE WITH A MINDSET SHIFT

This first practical lesson focuses on the art of the possible. Change is possible if we believe it is and act on this belief. The power to change is within us and not outside of us.

Hence, when making the decision to change, what we tell ourselves is as important as the questions we refuse to ask, whether to ourselves or others.

To change requires shifting our mindset gradually and taking necessary action consistently. What motivates change is often the value we attach to the change we are seeking, including all the other benefits that we believe will follow that change.

This belief is what helped shift my focus away from the signs of poor health I experienced throughout my life, but especially those that I felt more intensely in midlife. Initially, I did not think there was anything I could do to change how I felt. After all, when nature is at work, is there much we can do to change its course of action? Not believing in change, and not acting on that belief is self-defeating. I could have also opted to stay where I was, unhappy, heavy, stressed and in pain. I could have continued to blame my nature, my job or family responsibilities for my inaction. I could have found many excuses from outside pressures and societal expectations.

Instead, I decided not to give my power away to the forces of nature to influence how I aged. I decided to keep looking for better ways to support my health as I aged, at times cooperating with nature, but other times, seeking to influence nature in my favor. I knew that I could not experience change if I continued to do the same things I had done, because my behaviors and actions were not yielding results that benefitted my weight, my waistline or my health. My desire and my goal was to see different results.

With a different mindset, I was able to move myself in the direction of a healthier goal. I recognized that in the end, I alone held the key to the actions necessary to stop the pains and discomforts I felt. A big belly was only one of the most visible manifestation of many other unhealthy changes that had been taking place inside and outside the body, many of which started years before I reached midlife. These changes would have continued and most likely evolved into other undesirable health outcomes if I did not take action to reverse them.

By now, I hope it is clear to you as it is to me that there are many health risks that inaction tends to bring our way when excess weight settles around the waistline. I decided to take the steps needed to understand my body better, increase my awareness of the changes we go through in midlife, and learn what I could do to support the change process so that it would become easier rather than debilitating. With a change in mindset, I stopped myself from standing in my way of the change I wanted to see in my body and my outlook on life.

LESSON 2 - WHAT YOU EAT REALLY, REALLY MATTERS

As I explained in chapters two through five, one set of actions I took was in the areas of my diet. I removed certain foods (all sugary and highly processed foods), significantly limited starchy foods, increased my intake of healthy fats, and introduced ferments into my diet. I also questioned some of my organic food choices as these did not stop me from gaining weight. You may be wondering why I did not dedicate a whole chapter on proteins. The reason is that I could not personalize my experiences with proteins in the same way I did with the other types of foods or food groups that I focused on in the book. However, I do recognize the importance and benefits of protein in a balanced diet and have made necessary adjustments in this area as well. In fact, one of the main adjustments I made regarding protein was to stop relying on legumes, as they too are a significant contributor to my overall carb intake. Instead, I started adding animal proteins more regularly as these have no carbs in them and therefore support my efforts to shrink belly fat better.

Also, I had to stop being complacent, assuming that the food choices I relied on in my youth, when my metabolism was much more efficient, were the ones that would continue working for me in midlife.

I had become complacent because I never had to worry about my weight until I reached midlife. And I never worried about my waistline until my weight loss did not shrink my belly despite my otherwise slimming physique.

LESSON 3 - WE MUST ALWAYS INTEGRATE THE LIFESTYLE TRIO OF EXERCISE, STRESS MANAGEMENT AND SLEEP IN OUR WELLNESS PLAN

In addition to dietary changes, I adjusted my exercise routines as well. While I almost always knew that exercising consistently is important, it became clear that not all exercises are created equal and that not all are suited to everyone regardless of age, gender, time of day, and health status. To lose belly fat, my usual aerobic exercises did not help as much as I thought they would. This is because my body was already stressed from poor quality sleep and other factors. I had to recognize, as Eric Berg notes, that: "[t]he delayed fat burning effects of exercise can be prevented if you are not sleeping or if you eat sugar before, during, or after exercise. If cortisol ... is too high, not only will deep rejuvenating sleep be prevented - which will affect the fat-burning growth hormone - but fat will be directed to and stored in the belly" (143). In both diet and exercise, there is no one-size fits all regardless of other lifestyle factors that would, under normal circumstances, benefit us.

Hormonal changes that occur in midlife, lead many to poor quality sleep, or even worse, insomnia. Responsibilities both with family and at work, seem to increase around then as well, hence increasing stress levels. The time to exercise, that were easier to find in younger years, becomes harder to find as we age. The workout routine that used to burn calories and keep weight in check seems to no longer produce intended results. Poor sleep increases stress and makes it harder to justify exercise when tired. Yet, exercise is also often prescribed for its ability to lower stress levels. Therefore, to keep a healthy weight and waistline in midlife requires approaching all these aspects of our lives much more holistically.

This interaction between diet, exercise, stress management and sleep is what I want women in midlife to focus on. Together, they affect your weight and waistline in ways that many of us tend ignore and are often surprised about. While I am not as naive as to assume that all healing is in our hands, I am convinced that our body is capable of healing itself if we give it the tools and support it needs to do the rest for us. Sometimes it is the right foods that provide the necessary nutrients required for it to restore balance. The lifestyle trio is also as important as the right diet. If we are convinced that change is possible and we supply our body with what it needs and give it time, then there is a level of balance that it will achieve and often, it goes beyond our expectations.

The second level of my learning was at a higher, philosophical level informed by the practical steps discussed above.

LESSON 4 - IT IS IMPORTANT TO FOLLOW YOUR PASSION, EMBRACE YOUR CALLING

Every single person on this planet has a role to play, a contribution to make. We all have meaning and relevance. For some, it is to develop and use the gift of entertaining others. For others, it is to restore hope, to nurture, teach, comfort, or to create with hands or with words, with a song or dance, or to mediate the peaceful settlement of conflicts, to encourage, to lead. And the list goes on and on. Whatever that place or role is, it is ours to occupy because no one else can do it without leaving their own place, or seat, unoccupied.

When we don't step into our own shoes and when we neglect our place and our space in this world, we are making ourselves irrelevant or at best, we are less relevant. We cannot, and will never become the best version of ourselves, by trying to be like someone else, as Oprah Winfrey reminds us in her podcasts. No two people are exactly the same. Not even identical twins. We each have our own unique traits, characteristics, and interests, but we also have our own unique voice and innate gifts. It is with these gifts that we can live a life of purpose, bringing the best of who we are, to a world that needs what only we can contribute.

Taking the time away from too much noise and centering ourselves, opens doors for us to discover our calling. As a part of self-care and discovering what that meant for me, my initial steps were to approach my health from as many angles as possible. This included choosing to eat organic foods, walk and dance for exercise, and tend to my garden for stress relief. In fact, it was out of my experiences in two different gardens, thousands of miles apart, one in Malawi, the other in Rwanda, that I was able to see that we can influence how the universe responds to our needs and interests. It left me also with the belief that what we truly desire can become a reality if we work hard to achieve it. This experience was humbling. It made me again appreciate the grandeur of God in our universe and the fact that what I think and how I behave matters. It left me convinced that it is not how much time we spend, but rather, how we spend our time that matters. We must remain relevant.

This new level of awareness helped me redefine my career, eventually taking me back to school to learn about health coaching, a field I did not even know existed. When I discovered the Institute for Integrative Nutrition, I was already headed in the direction the school ended up taking me. I left a full-time job and decided to focus more on my role as a mom and a wife, and on my own self-care. I spent that time learning about wellness and the many aspects required for the healing of body, mind and spirit. What I learned reinforced nascent interests, helping me to build a knowledge base that I previously lacked and placed me inside a community of others with similar interests. Eventually, I was able to carve out a little niche, and to start focusing on women in midlife.

This book is an expression of my calling. It is about how I chose to live a life of purpose. I could no longer see how I could be of help to fellow women in midlife, if I continued to hide behind a shell and refused to be vulnerable. I have shared a lot about myself, my successes and failures, my fears and my hopes. I hope you found a few areas you can relate to. This journey was therefore mine, but I hope it was yours as well. Knowing how to stay as healthy as possible during your transition through midlife is key to preventing some of the diseases of the old. For me, the expansion of my waistline was a sure sign that I was headed in the wrong direction. I realize that not everyone is predisposed to diabetes like me, but a big belly predisposes people to metabolic syndrome diseases including heart disease, for which diabetes and high blood pressure also constitute risk factors.

LESSON 5 - IF WE SEEK HARD ENOUGH, WE WILL FIND INNER PEACE

This lesson is related to the previous one. It is based on a belief that we will rarely find inner peace and contentment in the midst of noise. This is not just about the sounds that we hear with our ears. It is also about the "noise" associated with being too busy, going from one thing to the next, one task to the next, one project to the next, without taking the time to slow down, and intentionally check in. When we live like this, we will likely fail to appreciate who we truly are and how we are connected to a bigger picture in the universe. When we continuously drown ourselves in too much noise, we will miss the clues that what we do matter not just to ourselves but especially to others.

We will never succeed at choosing wisely if we do not take time to center ourselves and notice and recognize how small we are in the universe, and embrace the power of God that in the end controls it all. Slowing down, centering, reflecting, meditating, and looking deeper inside ourselves will enable us to protect ourselves from outer influences, the outer noise that drowns out our voice and keep us from becoming who we were meant to be in the first place. You do not have to be in midlife to appreciate this.

We want to be relevant, doing what truly matters and acting out of thoughtfulness, driven by the core of who we are and the spirit in us, and not out of impulse or outer pressures.

We will barely succeed at living a life of relevance when we are constantly pulled in many different directions, without recognizing that whatever we do needs to matter for someone else who needs exactly what we are contributing to the world. This is where we find ourselves. This is where we find out who we were always meant to be.

I could not find myself and reach the point of writing this book without taking the time to slow down and listen to the message that my body was sending. I needed to respond to my body's call for help so that I could be more balanced when I came out of my shell to help others in search of what I had found, the lessons I had learned.

LESSON 6 - ACCEPT TO BE VULNERABLE - THE WORLD NEEDS TO HEAR ABOUT OUR STRUGGLES AS WELL AS OUR SUCCESSES

In this book, I shared my successes. I also shared my struggles, what some would call failures. Taken together, they are part of a reality that led me where I am, healthier now than I was when I started this journey to wellness in a more focused way in 2012, wearing size twelve after having lost some weight initially through aerobic exercise. As I write, I wear primarily a US size four (or extra small) for shirts and most dresses, and a size six for some skirts and pants, depending on the brand. I am happy about my overall weight of around 130 pounds. I am happy about my BMI at 21.6. I am happy about the circumference around my waist at 31 inches (checked by using a tape measure at the level of my belly button). Keeping it below

35 inches for women, WebMD advises on its website, will lower risks for type 2 diabetes. And I am happy that my blood work indicates a low risk of diabetes as well.

The key to my success was a combination of a mindset shift, some changes in my choices of foods, and a few lifestyle adjustments that resulted in a healthier version of myself. Our bodies change as we get older. Some age much more gracefully than others, however. A closer look at the nutrition and lifestyle factors discussed in this book will enable us to stay strong and in balance when we too enter midlife and begin to show signs of aging. My belly is not as flat as it was in my teen and twenties or even my early thirties, but it is not the first thing that people notice when they see me, either. And I have come to realize that striving for the perfect, flat belly will leave me frustrated as it does many other women I interact with. Instead of being happy with who we are, with a normal weight and inches off our otherwise larger waistline, we want to continue striving for the perfect which is not always a realistic option for most. We are better off continuing to take actions that will enable us to reach healthier and healthier versions of ourselves. Isn't this what matters in the end?

Nonetheless, we must question whether the physical and mental changes we experience as we age are normal parts of the aging process or a sign of imbalance that can be corrected with informed action. To succeed, we must become experts at knowing ourselves and how our body works and interacts with foods and our environment. I have spent the last seven years taking a more proactive and comprehensive approach to self-care, paying a closer attention to how certain foods and specific lifestyle factors affect my weight and my health. In the last three years, I shifted my attention more specifically to my waistline as shrinking it became a more challenging aspect of my weight management efforts.

Interestingly, this journey took me back many years before midlife, when I knew little about dietary and lifestyle choices that impact our health and our ability to lose or gain weight. Through this journey, I learned that there are a number of "small things" we don't pay attention to and take for granted in our younger years, such as: when and how much sleep we get; spending time out in the sun during the day; moving around; lifting heavy things; stretching; limiting our sugar and processed foods intake; knowing that not all fats are created equal and that we need to consume the good ones regularly for the health of our cells and our hormones; and addressing recurring yeast infections in a holistic way instead of relying only on antibiotics that in the end have negative side effects and promote serious health imbalances. These "small things" point us in the direction of what we need to do so that we do not just survive but instead thrive in midlife.

I hope that this book will continue to serve as an important resource for you as you take steps to stay healthy and balanced in midlife. If you learned something you were able to apply and that has benefitted you, then my efforts in writing this book were worthwhile. What I shared was based on what has worked for me and I hope it will work for you as well. I relied on many expert resources and personalized their recommendations based on what seemed practical and realistic for me.

I hope that the tools, advice and guidance presented in this book will leave you feeling empowered to take action that will improve your health, bringing you back to a healthy weight and a smaller waistline in midlife and beyond.

I also hope that as you practice what I shared here, you keep an open mind. Science is not static. We must remain open to making any other modifications as new knowledge becomes available.

Together, we can hold each other accountable to do what we need to do to prepare for aging gracefully. The process is yours alone and it needs to be customized. If you have already started implementing some of my recommendations, then you are on track for a healthier version of yourself, as you revitalize your changing body. Your success is mine and so, I celebrate with you. Cheers!

ADDITIONAL RESOURCES

RECIPES
Breakfast

Power Smoothie

Ingredients:
- 1 cup of frozen blueberries
- 1/2 green apple
- 1/2 small beetroot (with skin if organic)
- 1 ripe avocado
- A handful of sunflower or pumpkin seeds
- 1/4 ripe avocado
- 1 tablespoon of ground flaxseeds
- 1 teaspoon of spirulina
- 1/2 to 1 full lemon or lime with rind in thin slices

1. Combine all ingredients in blender
2. Add filtered water to cover the mix
3. Blend together until smooth
4. Enjoy

Serves 2

Vegetable Omelette

Ingredients:
- 4 eggs (beat well)
- 1 small onion, cut in small pieces
- 2 tablespoon olive oil
- 1 small bag of frozen broccoli
- Dash of Rose's spice mix
- Sea salt (to taste)
- 1 small avocado

1. Heat a deep, frying pan for about a minute, add olive oil and heat for about 30 seconds
2. Add onions and spices, stir until they are mixed well
3. Lower heat to medium low and continue to cook onions till they turn translucent
4. Add broccoli and mix well with the onions
5. Cover pot and cook until broccoli is hot, draining excess liquid if any
6. Add beaten eggs covering the top of the broccoli
7. Cover again and cook till the eggs are fully settled and look cooked through
8. Remove from heat
9. Slice avocado and place on top of eggs
10. Enjoy

Serves 2

Variation:
1. Replace broccoli with fresh spinach
2. Follow the same direction as above or scramble the eggs separately and lightly sauté spinach
3. Slice avocado and place on top of eggs before serving.

Creamy coconut amino tempeh

Ingredients:
- Cut tempeh block in 1 inch cubes
- Coconut aminos (2 Tablespoon)
- 1 small onion
- 2 tablespoons, olive oil
- 1 tablespoon almond butter
- Dash of cayenne pepper
- 1/2 teaspoon turmeric
- Sea salt

1. Remove tempeh from casing and rinse with clean filtered water
2. Slice into 1 inch cubes
3. Cut onion in small pieces
4. In a preheated frying pan, add olive oil and keep heat on for about 15 seconds
5. Add onions and cook till they are translucent
6. Add salt, cayenne and turmeric, stirring until well mixed with onions
7. Continue to cook for 1 more minute
8. Add almond butter and 1/2 cup of water. Stir until mix starts getting thick.
9. Add tempeh cubes and keep stirring till well-mixed
10. Lower heat to medium-low and cover pan
11. Cook for 10 to 15 minutes (stirring occasionally)
12. Add coconut amino and stir till well-mixed with tempeh
13. Cover pan again and cook for 3 to 5 minutes.
14. Serve with lightly sautéed spinach
15. Enjoy

Serves 2

Lunch or dinner

Flavorful roasted chicken with sautéed veggies

Ingredients
- 6 chicken legs or thighs
- 1/2 cabbage
- 1 small bag of fresh spinach
- Medium size onion, sliced into small pieces
- 2 teaspoons of Rose's spice mix (dried parsley or oregano or basil leaves + cayenne pepper + turmeric)
- Sea salt to taste

1. In baking dish, place chicken legs next to each other
2. Sprinkle sea salt and spice mix on all sides of each leg
3. Pre-heat oven at 300 degrees Farenheit
4. Bake for 1hr 15 minutes
5. Increase temperature to 350 degrees
6. Bake for another 30 to 45 minutes based on how crispy you want the skin to be.
7. Enjoy

Serves 3-4

Spice Mix
- 1 Tablespoon of herb of choice
- 1 Teaspoon turmeric
- 1/2 teaspoons cayenne pepper (more or less depending on heat preference)

Creamy salmon tahini with mushrooms and brussels sprouts

Ingredients:
- 4 serving size salmon pieces
- Olive oil
- Sea salt
- Tahini
- Veggie choices to go with salmon:
- Portabella mushrooms, large ones sliced in 1 inch cubes
- Brussel sprouts, sliced in halves or quarters
- 1 medium onion cut in small pieces
- Rose's Spice Mix

Preparing salmon:
1. Lay salmon pieces in baking pan
2. Sprinkle sea salt (to taste), drizzle olive oil
3. Add one small scoop of tahini and drizzle some more sea salt and olive oil over each salmon piece
4. Pre-heat oven at 300 degrees Fahrenheit.
5. Bake for 20-25 minutes
6. Turn the dish around after 15 minutes, as heating may not be even on all sides of the oven
7. Remove from oven and serve with cooked veggies or 1/2 cooked veggies, and 1/2 a side salad.

Preparing mushrooms:
1. Clean mushrooms lightly on the top.
2. Cut off the ends of the stems and leave them out in a colander over paper towel to dry.
3. Slice them in long strips and then in halves or quarters.
4. Chop a medium size onion
5. Heat medium sized pot on medium-high for 1 minute
6. Add 2 tablespoon olive oil

7. Keep heating for a few seconds
8. Add onions and stir
9. Lower heat to medium
10. Add 1/2 teaspoon of Rose's Spice Mix with a little sea salt (to taste)
11. Keep stirring till the onions are well-mixed with the spices
12. When onions turn translucent, add the mushroom
13. Stir to mix, cover pot and continue to cook on medium-low heat for 2-3 minutes
14. Uncover pot and continue to cook for another 3-5 minutes, stirring until done. Serve with salmon.

Preparing brussels sprouts:
1. Cut the hard ends of the stems off of ½ pound of brussels sprouts
2. Remove outer leaves that look torn and dirty and discard them
3. Rinse the rest to remove any debris
4. Slice in 1/2 or 1/4 depending on how big they are.
5. Heat frying pan for 1 minute or till too hot to touch
6. Add 2-3 tablespoon olive oil
7. Heat for 10 seconds or less, then immediately add onions, 1/2 teaspoon of Rose's spice mix, and sea salt (to taste).
8. Lower heat to medium or medium-low
9. Stir and mix well, cooking until onions turn translucent
10. Add brussels sprouts, stirring to mix with onions
11. Cover pan and continue to cook, increasing the heat a little bit as necessary and adding a tablespoon or two of water to prevent burn.
12. Cook and keep stirring occasionally for about 10 minutes
13. Remove from heat and serve
14. For extra crispness, transfer brussels sprouts to a baking dish
15. Drizzle a little olive oil over the brussels sprouts
16. Pre-heat oven to 350 degrees Fahrenheit
17. Bake for 10 to 15 minutes (or more as desired)
18. Enjoy

Serves 3-4

Vegetarian recipes

Spicy chickpeas or black beans

Ingredients:
- 1 large BPA free can unsalted chickpeas or black beans
- One medium onion, cut in small pieces
- Rose's Spice Mix
- Sea salt
- Olive oil

1. Heat small or medium-size pot
2. Add 2-3 Tablespoon olive oil, heat for 10-15 seconds
3. Add onions, and 1/2 teaspoon Rose's Spice Mix, and sea salt to taste
4. Stir until onions are translucent
5. Drain some or all the liquid in the can
6. Add the chickpeas to pot
7. Lower heat and cook on medium-low for 15 to 20 minutes
8. Enjoy

Serves 4-6

*Serve with a mix of cooked cabbage and spinach or 1/2 cooked veggie mix and 1/2 salad with nuts or seeds such as a handful of walnuts, pumpkin, or sunflower seeds mixed in with the salad.

Spicy cabbage and spinach blend

Ingredients:
- 1 medium cabbage, shredded and chopped in small pieces
- 1 small bag of fresh or frozen spinach
- 1 large onion, chopped in small pieces
- Rose's Spice Mix
- Sea salt
- Olive oil

1. Heat large pot for 1 minute or less
2. Add 3 tablespoon of olive oil
3. Heat for 10 seconds
4. Add onions and stir to mix oil well with onions
5. Add 1 teaspoon of Rose's Spice Mix along with ¼ teaspoon sea salt or to taste
6. Mix well and continue stirring off and on until onions turn translucent
7. Add cabbage and mix well with onions
8. Keep stirring every 2-3 minutes, until cabbage is cooked enough, but not too soft
9. Add spinach and cook together until spinach is heated through
10. If spinach is frozen, after mixing with cabbage as best as you can, cover pot and let heat come through to the top
11. Stir a few more times and cover again until spinach is cooked
12. If spinach is fresh, keep stirring and mixing with cabbage but do not cover the pot again
13. You want to retain as much of the fresh green as possible
14. Within 2 to 3 minutes, it will be ready to remove from heat and serve
15. Enjoy

Serves 6-8

Creamy Coconut Amino Tempeh

See breakfast recipe above.

Green papaya salad

Ingredients:
- 1 small or medium unripe papaya
- 1/4 of roasted pumpkin seeds or a handful of roasted almonds
- One salad bowl
- Cut papaya in half and remove the seeds.
- With a sharp knife or a peeler, remove the skin of the papaya
- Hold one half papaya tightly and begin to shred it from one end to the other.
- Repeat with the other half
- Add the pumpkin seeds or roasted almonds and mix well
- Add fresh orange ginger dressing and mix well. Enjoy. Serves 4-6
- Fresh orange ginger dressing:
- 3 Tablespoon olive oil
- Juice from 1 fresh orange
- 1 teaspoon orange zest
- 1/2 teaspoon ground ginger
- 1 teaspoon of honey
- 1 teaspoon raw apple cider vinegar
- Pinch of sea salt

1. In a small jar, put all the ingredients together and shake vigorously to mix them well
2. Use immediately
3. Store leftover in the fridge and use within a week

Green bananas

Cut off the hard end of the stem but do not get too close to the flesh. Leave it covered. Steam the bananas in large pot. They should be ready in about 20 minutes. You know they are ready when the skin cracks open. You need only one per meal. They store well in the fridge in a covered glass container for a week or longer. Reheat only what you need in an open dish in a preheated oven at 350 degrees Fahrenheit, for about 15 minutes

Red skin potatoes

Clean the outer skin well. Slice them in 1/4 first the long way and then in 1/2 if large or just in 1/4 if they are small. Then steam them for about 15-20 minutes till a little soft. Remove from heat and transfer the cooked potatoes to a baking dish. Add salt and sprinkle a little bit of Rose's spice mix. Drizzle olive oil over the potatoes. With a spoon, gently mix the potatoes and the spices, making sure not to break them. Pre-heat oven to 300 degrees Fahrenheit. Set the timer for 20 to 30 minutes. Bake the potatoes in oven till time is up. Serve hot with vegetables and either chicken or fish. Cool left-overs, cover and place them in the fridge. Use as needed, either re-heated for a few minutes in the oven or cold as a resistant starch.

Butternut squash (Waltham butternut variety is the one I use most)

1 Medium size or 2 small ones. Slice them and peel skin off. Cut the slices in 1 and 1/2 inch cubes. In medium-size pot, add water and steam the butternut till soft but not mushy soft. You can serve as they are or transfer to a baking dish. Sprinkle a little cinnamon. Bake at 350 degrees Fahrenheit for 15-20 minutes to remove some of the excess water, if you prefer them a little drier. Serves 6-8.

Sauerkraut

Ingredients:
- 1 medium cabbage
- 1 tablespoon or less of sea salt
- Tools:
- Ceramic or stainless-steel bowl to hold the cabbage during preparation

Note: use filtered water to keep your hands and all tools clean

1. Remove clean outer leaves and set them aside on a clean plate or bowl. Place the rest of the cabbage on a clean cutting board and start chopping or shredding it. Add sea salt to the cabbage. Your tolerance of salt will be your guide for determining how much is enough for you. For a medium size cabbage, I use about 1 teaspoon of salt. Mix the cabbage and salt with clean hands until the cabbage looks shiny from the salt mixture.

2. With your hands or a wooden masher or pounder, press the cabbage down as you continue to mix until it releases a sufficient amount of its own juice. Salt pulls the juice out of the leaves and builds up the water content that is released as a result. Continue pressing until you see enough juice coming out of the cabbage. This amount will be as much as several tablespoons of juice that you see when you tilt the bowl you have placed the cabbage in, as you prepare it for fermentation. Pushing the cabbage off to the side will enable you to see the bottom of the bowl where the juice is settling.

3. When ready, place the cabbage in mason jars, pressing it down to leave no space for pockets of air that can form inside the jar. The juice from the cabbage should rise to the top as you press down, and it should submerge the cabbage.

4. Place the clean leaves you set aside in step 1, on top to cover the cabbage and allow the juice to rise even further on top of the leaves.

Seal shut the jars and place them in a corner of a suitable room away from direct light.

5. Check-in within forty-eight to seventy-two hours to be sure everything looks good. You should see bubbles rising up to the top of the cabbage inside. If there seems to be too much pressure inside the jar, and some of the juice starts spilling over, open the jar slightly and release some of the pressure. This may suffice. If you need to open the jar all the way to press down the top leaf again to re-submerge it, do so carefully, ensuring that everything you use is clean. You goal is to reduce pressure and resettle the cabbage. This should allow for fermentation to continue for as long as you desire up to three or even four weeks.

6. When your time is up, open the jars, remove the outer leaves carefully, and discard them. Place all the jars in the fridge. Start consuming your ferments immediately, opening one jar at a time.

*Note that you can also mix in some seeds to flavor your sauerkraut. Caraway and dill seeds are my favorite seeds to add. You can mix green with red cabbage and add other vegetables before mixing with salt if you desire new flavors and enjoy the different colors of the finished product. I have mixed green cabbage with red, shredded carrots and shredded beetroots as well. And because I now feel confident in my skills as a "fermentista", to borrow Shockey and Shockey's term in *Fermented Vegetables* (2014, 26), I allow the vegetables to ferment for longer and longer each time. When I was testing myself, I started with leaving the cabbage to ferment in a jar for three to five days. Then I allowed the vegetables to continue fermenting for a week, then two weeks, and on and on up to four weeks, the longest I have kept them to ferment in a jar, or six weeks, the longest the vegetables have stayed in a crock. I have also made milk kefir using regular low-fat milk, and I have used canned coconut milk to make coconut kefir as well.

Coconut water kefir

Ingredients:
- Young coconut water (flesh looks green or a shade of green)
- A clean stainless-steel pot
- Your favorite probiotic supplement (2 for each 1 liter of coconut water)

1. Break the coconuts and transfer the water into a clean stainless-steel pot. Warm the coconut water till it reaches the temperature of your skin. Test by placing a drop of the water on the back of your hand. It's ready if you cannot tell the difference between the temperature of your body and the temperature of the coconut water. Remove pot from heat. Open the probiotics and pour content inside the pot and mix well with the coconut water. Cover tightly and place the pot in a secure place away from the reach of children and away from direct light. Leave it there for 48 to 72 hours. Transfer the coconut water kefir to a jar or another clean container that can easily fit in your fridge.

2. Consume 4-6 ounces in the morning with breakfast and about 4 ounces in the evening before bed.

Coconut milk kefir

Ingredients:
- 3 BPA free cans of coconut milk (8 ounces each)
- Small cup of coconut yogurt with live cultures as a starter
- Pot large enough for the amount coconut milk you want to ferment

1. Open cans or containers and pour coconut milk in a pot. Place pot on stovetop and simmer till the temperature of the coconut milk reaches the temperature of the body. Test by dropping a little on the back of your hand. You should not feel the difference in temperature. Remove from heat. Open cup of coconut yogurt. Scoop out 2 tablespoons of coconut yogurt and gently drop into the coconut milk. Mix well. Cover the pot tightly. Leave in a safe and dark corner of the kitchen or other safe room, away from the reach of children or pets.

2. Within 48 hours, it should be creamy and more condensed than the milk, similar in texture to light Greek Yogurt. Whisk well to reach the same consistency throughout the kefir. Transfer content to a storage container, preferably a glass jar and store in the fridge. Use within 1 -2 weeks.

FOOD SHOPPING LIST

Breakfast

Eggs
Broccoli
Spinach
Onions
Gluten-free steel cut oats
Gluten-free oatmeal
Quinoa
Amaranth
Coconut butter
Almond butter
Coconut oil
Coconut milk
Coconut water
Beetroots
Kiwi
Green apples
Blueberries
Raspberries
Blackberries
Mixed berries
Avocados
Almonds
Almond milk (unsweetened)
Walnuts
Sunflower seeds
Pumpkin seeds
Chia seeds
Bone broth
Spirulina

Hemp protein powder
Orgain organic protein powder
(chocolate or vanilla flavor)
Ground flaxseeds
Lemons
Limes
Lemon juice
Manuka honey
Tempeh
Chicken liver
Grass-fed beef liver
Raw cheese
Chicken sausage

Lunch and dinner

Chicken legs/thighs
Whole chicken
Wild-caught salmon
Wild-caught Cod
Wild-caught sardines
Ground turkey
Ground beef
Cabbage
Brussel sprouts
Spinach
Kale
Arugula
Green beans
Cauliflower
Broccoli
Cucumber

Celery
Red bell peppers
Mushrooms (portabella, baby bella, Shiitake)
Summer squash
Carrots
Baby carrots
Green peas
Butternut squash
Red skin potatoes
Green bananas
Cassava root
Sweet potatoes
Yams
Plantains
Quinoa
Brown rice
Green papaya
Black beans
Navy beans
Cannellini beans
Chickpeas
Lentils (green or French)
Edamame beans
Tempeh
Olive oil
Palm nut oil
Olives
Hummus
Sauerkraut (raw, fermented)
Romaine lettuce
Spring green mix
Raw apple cider vinegar

Coconut aminos
Hemp seeds
Leeks
Himalayan sea salt
Iodized sea salt
Sea weed (Dried Kombu or Wakame)
Chamomile tea
Ginger tea

Herbs and spices

Ground cayenne pepper
Ground turmeric
Oregano leaves (dried)
Basil leaves (dried)
Parsley (fresh)
Cilantro (fresh)
Bay leaves (dried)
Cumin seeds
Caraway seeds
Dill seeds
Garlic (fresh or dried granules)
Ground or fresh ginger
Tahini

Supplements

Probiotics: Raw Probiotics (Women 50 & Wiser) by *Garden of Life*; Digestive Care Multi by *Body Ecology*
Vitamin D3 (in liquid form)
Moringa seeds (Private supplier)

Moringa leaves (dried and ground
- at Whole Foods Market)
Spirulina powder (on Amazon.com
or at Whole Foods Market)

REFERENCES

Introduction

Atkins, Robert C. Dr. Atkins Diet Revolution: The High Calorie Way to Stay Thin Forever. D. McKay Co., 1972.

Atkins, Robert C., with Mary C. Vernon and Jacqueline A. Eberstein. Atkins Diabetes Revolution. William Morrow, 2004.

Berg, Eric. The 7 Principles of Fat Burning: Get Healthy, Lose Weight and Keep It Off. KB Publishing, 2010.

Eades, Mary Dan, and Michael R. Eades. The 6 Week Cure for the Middle-Aged Middle: The Simple Plan to Flatten Your Belly Fast! Crown, 2009.

Gates, Donna, with Linda Schatz. The Body Ecology Diet: Recovering Your Health and Rebuilding Your Immunity. Hay House, 2012.

Gottfried, Sara. The Hormone Cure. Scribner, 2013.

Hyman, Mark. The Blood Sugar Solution 10-Day Detox Diet. Little, Brown, and Company, 2014.

Taubes, Gary. Why We Get Fat and What to Do About It. Anchor, 2011.

Weil, Andrew. Spontaneous Happiness. New York: Little, Brown and Company, 2011.

Willett, Walter C. Eat, Drink, and Be Healthy. Fireside, 2001.

Chapter 1

Adams, Marilee. Change Your Questions Change Your Life: 10 Powerful Tools for Life and Work. Berrett-Koehler, 2009.

Amen, Daniel G. *Change Your Brain Change Your Life: The Breakthrough for Conquering Anxiety, Depression, Obsessiveness, Anger, and Impulsiveness.* Three Rivers, 1998.

Ardell, Donald B. *High Level Wellness: An Alternative to Doctors, Drugs and Disease.* Rodale, 1977.

Brown, Brené. *Rising Strong: The Reckoning. The Rumble. The Revolution.* Spiegel and Grau, 2015.

Burchard, Brendon. *The Motivation Manifesto: 9 Declarations to Claim Your Personal Power.* Hay House, 2014

Carson, Rick. *Taming the Gremlins: A Surprising Simple Method for Getting Out of Your Own Way.* Quill, 2003.

Peale, Norman Vincent. *The Power of Positive Thinking.* Walker and Company, 1956.

Prochaska, James O., John C. Norcross, and Carlo C. DiClemente. *Changing for Good: A Revolutionary Six-Stage Program for Overcoming Bad Habits and Moving Your Life Positively Forward.* William Morrow, 1994.

Chapter 2

Aminov, Rustam I. "A Brief History of the Antibiotics Era: Lessons Learned and Challenges for the Future." *Frontiers in Microbiology* 1, 8 December 2010, https://www.ncbi.nlm.nih.gov/pmc/articles/PMC3109405/. *Accessed 17 April 2020.*

Crook, William G. *The Yeast Connection: A Medical Breakthrough.* Vintage, 1986.

Gates, Donna, with Linda Schatz. *The Body Ecology Diet: Recovering Your Health and Rebuilding Your Immunity.* Hay House, 2012.

"Glycemic Index for 60+ Foods." *Harvard Health Publishing,* 14 March 2018, http://www.health.harvard.edu/diseases-and-conditions/glycemic-index-and-glycemic-load-for-100-foods. Accessed 17 April 2020.

Gottfried, Sarah. *The Hormone Cure.* Scribner, 2013

Hyman, Mark. *The Blood Sugar Solution 10-Day Detox Diet.* Little, Brown, and Company, 2014.

Komaroff, Anthony L. *"Should I drop calories or boost exercise?"* Harvard Health Letter, https://www.health.harvard.edu/staying-healthy/should-i-drop-calories-or-boost-exercise. *Accessed 18 April 2020.*

"Know Your Brain: Nucleus Accumbens." 13 June 2014, https://neuroscientificallychallenged.com/blog/2014/6/11/know-your-brain-nucleus-accumbens. *Accessed 17 April 2020.*

Mullin, Gerard E., and Kathie Madonna Swift. *The Inside Tract: Your Good Gut Guide to Great Digestive Health.* Rodale, 2011.

Perlmutter, David, with Kristin Loberg. *Grain Brain: The Surprising Truth About Wheat, Carbs, and Sugar – Your Brain's Silent Killers.* Little, Brown and Company, 2013.

Pescatore, Fred and Karolyn A. Gazella. *Boost Your Health with Bacteria.* Active Interest Media, 2009.

Pesce, Nicole Lyn. *"'10-Day Detox Diet' author Mark Hyman tells how to end sugar addiction and clean up your diet."* New York Daily News, 11 February, 2014, https://www.nydailynews.com/life-style/health/dr-mark-hyman-shows-deadly-sugar-addiction-article-1.1608553. *Accessed 17 April 2020.*

"Pineapple, raw, all varieties nutrition facts and calories." Self Nutrition Data, https://nutritiondata.self.com/facts/fruits-and-fruit-juices/2019/2. *Accessed 8 May 2020.*

Rubin, Jordan with Bernard Bulwer, *Perfect Weight: Change Your Diet. Change Your Life. Change Your World.* Siloam, 2008.

Sanders, Francis W. B. and Julian L. Griffin. *"De novo lipogenesis in the liver in health and disease: more than a shunting yard for glucose."* National Institutes of Health, 4 March 2015, https://www.ncbi.nlm.nih.gov/pmc/articles/PMC4832395/. *Accessed 8 May 2020.*

Taubes, Gary. *Why We Get Fat and What to Do About It.* Anchor Books, 2011.

"Tropicana orange juice w/pulp nutrition facts and calories." Self Nutrition Data, https://nutritiondata.self.com/facts/custom/710703/2. *Accessed 8 May 2020.*

Willett, Walter C. *Eat, Drink, and Be Healthy.* Fireside, 2001.

Wszelaki, Magdalena. *Cooking for Hormonal Balance.* Harper One, 2018.

Chapter 3

Atkins, Robert C., M.D. Dr. Atkins Diet Revolution: The High Calorie Way to Stay Thin Forever. 1st Edition. D. McKay Co., 1972.

Atkins, Robert C., with Mary C. Vernon and Jacqueline A. Eberstein. Atkins Diabetes Revolution. William Morrow, 2004.

Jeremy M. Berg, John L. Tymoczko, and Lubert Stryer. Biochemistry. 5th Edition. W.H. Freeman, 2002, https://www.ncbi.nlm.nih.gov/books/NBK21190/. Accessed 17 April 2020.

Burani, Johanna, and Linda Rao. Good Carbs Bad Carbs: An Indispensable Guide to Eating the Right Carbs for Losing Weight and Optimum Health. Marlow and Company, 2002.

Eades, Mary Dan and Michael R. Eades. Protein Power: You Can Now Eat Your Way to Dynamic Weight Loss with the Clinically Proven Breakthrough Plan that Defies the Food Myths. Bantam, 1996.

Eades, Mary Dan and Michael R. Eades. The 6 Week Cure for the Middle-Aged Middle. The Simple Plan to Flatten Your Belly Fast! Random House, Inc., 2009.

Furman, Joel. Eat to Live: The Revolutionary Formula for Fast and Sustained Weight Loss. Little, Brown and Company, 2003.

"Glycemic Index for 60+ Foods." Harvard Health Publishing, 14 March 2018, http://www.health.harvard.edu/diseases-and-conditions/glycemic-index-and-glycemic-load-for-100-foods. Accessed 17 April 2020. Accessed 8 May 2020.

Groth, Leah. "The One Food Scientifically Proven to Boost Metabolism." 16 May 2018, https://www.livestrong.com/article/1012814-one-food-scientifically-proven-boost-metabolism/. Accessed 17 April 2020.

Gunnars, Kris. "How Many Carbs Should You Eat per Day to Lose Weight." 9 January 2018, https://www.healthline.com/nutrition/how-many-carbs-per-day-to-lose-weight. Accessed 17 April 2020.

Heller, Rachel F., and Richard F. Heller. The Carbohydrate Addict's Diet. Signet, 1991.

Heller, Richard F., Rachel F. Heller, and Frederic J. Vagnini. *The Carbohydrate Addict's Healthy Heart Program: Break Your Carbo-Insulin Connection to Heart Disease.* Ballantine, 1999.

"How to Eat 37 Grams of Fiber in a Day." *WebMD*, 1 June 2018, https://www.webmd.com/diet/eat-this-fiber-chart. Accessed 8 May 2020.

Hyman, Mark. *The Blood Sugar Solution 10-Day Detox Diet: Activate Your Body's Ability to Burn Fat and Lose Weight Fast.* Little, Brown and Company, 2014.

Mercola, Joseph. *"The Longevity Paradox: How to Die Young at a Ripe Old Age."* https://articles.mercola.com/sites/articles/archive/2019/08/11/longevity-paradox.aspx?utm_source=dnl&utm_medium=email&utm_content=art1&utm_campaign=20190811Z1&et_cid=DM309995&et_rid=683971589 *Accessed 17 April 2020. [Interview with Dr. Stephen Gundry, author of The Longevity Paradox]*

Mercola, Joseph. *"Top 6 Tips to Prevent Constipation." 23 January 2019,* https://articles.mercola.com/sites/articles/archive/2019/01/23/effective-way-to-improve-constipation.aspx?utm_source=dnl&utm_medium=email&utm_content=art1&utm_campaign=20190123Z1_B_UCM&et_cid=DM262252&et_rid=526734829. *Accessed 17 April 2020.*

SELFNutritionData. https://nutritiondata.self.com/foods-glycemic%20index0000000000000000000.html. *Accessed 8 May 2020.*

Taubes, Gary. *Why We Get Fat and What to Do About It.* Anchor Books, 2011.

The University of Rhode Island. *"What Counts as 1 Ounce of Grains."* https://web.uri.edu/snaped/files/What-Counts-as-1-Ounce-of-Grains-ENG.pdf. *Accessed 6 May 2020.*

Tourney, Anne. *"The Glycemic Index of Pumpkin." 14 August 2017,* https://www.livestrong.com/article/332065-the-glycemic-index-of-pumpkin/. *Accessed 17 April 2020.*

Willett, Walter C. *Eat, Drink, and Be Healthy.* Fireside, 2001.

World Health Organization. *"Micronutrients."* https://www.who.int/nutrition/topics/micronutrients/en/. Accessed 8 May 2020.

Wszelaki, Magdalena. *Cooking for Hormonal Balance.* Harper One, 2018.

Yang, Sarah. "New gene found that turns carbs into fat, could be target for future drugs." *UC Berkeley Online News*, https://news.berkeley.edu/2012/12/06/gene-converts-carbs-to-fat/. Accessed 17 April 2020.

Zeratsky, Katherine. "What's an easy way to see how much fat I eat each day?" *Mayo Clinic*, https://www.mayoclinic.org/healthy-lifestyle/nutrition-and-healthy-eating/expert-answers/fat grams/faq-20058496. Accessed 17 April 2020.

Chapter 4

Alba-Lois, L. and Segal-Kischinevzky, C. "Yeast Fermentation and the Making of Beer and Wine." *Nature Education 3(9):17*, https://www.nature.com/scitable/topicpage/yeast-fermentation-and-the-making-of-beer-14372813/. Accessed 18 April 2020.

Axe, Josh. *Eat Dirt: Why Leaky Gut May Be the Root Cause of Your Health Problems and 5 Surprising Steps to Cure It.* Harper Wave, 2016.

Berg, Eric. *The 7 Principles of Fat Burning: Get Healthy, Lose Weight and Keep It Off.* KB Publishing, 2010.

Carrasco, Alejandra. "Why Chewing Your Food Can Change Your Life." *MBG Health*, https://www.mindbodygreen.com/0-7775/why-chewing-your-food-can-change-your-life.html. Accessed 18 April 2020.

Christianson, Alan Glen. "4 Surprising Reasons to Never Soak Your Beans Again." *Huffington Post*, 8 September 2017, https://www.huffingtonpost.com/entry/4-surprising-reasons-to-never-soak-your-beans-again_us_59663823e4b0911162fc303d. Accessed 18 April 2020.

Crook, William G. *The Yeast Connection: A Medical Breakthrough.* Vintage, 1986.

Finlay, B. Brett and Marie-Claire Arrieta. *Let Them Eat Dirt: Saving Your Child from an Oversanitized World.* Algonquin, 2016.

Gál, Kat. "Benefits of oil pulling with coconut oil." *MedicalNewsToday*, 21 November 2018, https://www.medicalnewstoday.com/articles/323757.php. Accessed 18 April 2020.

Ganjhu, Lisa. "Your Gut Feeling: A Healthier Digestive System Means a Healthier You." *New York University School of Medicine*, https://med.

nyu.edu/medicine/gastro/about-us/Gastroenterology-news-archive/ your-gut-feeling-healthier-digestive-system-means-healthier. *Accessed 18 April 2020.*

Gates, Donna, with Linda Schatz. *The Body Ecology Diet: Recovering Your Health and Rebuilding Your Immunity. Hay House, 2012.*

Mercola, Joseph. *"Fermented Foods Top the Superfoods List." 4 February 2019,* https://articles.mercola.com/sites/articles/archive/2019/02/04/ fermented-foods-tops-superfoods-list.aspx?utm_source=dnl&utm_ medium=email&utm_content=art2&utm_campaign=20190204Z1_ UCM&et_cid=DM265574&et_rid=536453126. *Accessed 18 April 2020.*

Mullin, Gerard E., and Kathie Madonna Swift. *The Inside Tract: Your Good Gut Guide to Great Digestive Health. Rodale, 2011.*

Pescatore, Fred and Karolyn A. Gazella. *Boost Your Health with Bacteria. Active Interest Media, 2009.*

Shi, L., K. Mu, S.D. Amtfield and M.T. Nickerson. *"Changes in the levels of enzyme inhibitors during soaking and cooking for pulses available in Canada." Journal of Food Science Technology. 54 (4): 1014-1022,* https://www.ncbi. nlm.nih.gov/pubmed/28303052. Accessed 18 April 2020.

Shockey, Kirsten K. and Christopher Shockey. *Fermented Vegetables: Creative Recipes for Fermenting 64 Vegetables and Herbs in Krauts, Kimchis, Brined Pickles, Chutneys, Relishes and Pastes. Storey, 2015.*

Smith, Lindsey. *Junk Foods, Junk Moods. Incredible Messages Press, 2012.*

University of Pennsylvania. *"9,000-year History of Chinese Fermented Beverages Confirmed." Science Daily, 7 December 2004,* https://www.sciencedaily. com/releases/2004/12/041206205817.htm. *Accessed 18 April 2020.*

WebMD. *"What Is SIBO?"* https://www.webmd.com/digestive-disorders/ sibo-overview-what-is-it#1. *Accessed 18 April 2020.*

Chapter 5

Boyles, Salynn. *"Incredible, Edible, and Good for Your Brain? Research Links Nutrient in Eggs to Improved Memory." 12 March, 2004,* https://www.

webmd.com/baby/news/20040312/incredible-edible-good-for-your-brain#1. *Accessed 3 April 2020.*

Caporuscio, Jessia. *"What are the most healthful oils?", 30 March 2019,* https://www.medicalnewstoday.com/articles/324844. *Accessed 2 April 2020.*

Castelli, William P., and Glen C. Griffin. *The New Good Fat Bad Fat: Lower Your Cholesterol and Reduce Your Odds of a Heart Attack. Fisher Books, 1997.*

Clower, Will. *The Fat Fallacy. Three Rivers, 2003.*

Crosby, Guy. *"Ask the Expert: Concern About Canola Oil", 13 April 2015 (updated December 2018),* https://www.hsph.harvard.edu/nutritionsource/2015/04/13/ask-the-expert-concerns-about-canola-oil/. *Accessed 2 April 2020.*

Douillard, John. *Eat Wheat. Morgan James, 2017.*

Eades, Mary Dan and Michael R. Eades. *The 6 Week Cure for the Middle-Aged Middle. The Simple Plan to Flatten Your Belly Fast! Random House, Inc., 2009.*

Fuhrman, Joel. *Eat to Live: The Amazing Nutrient-Rich Program for Fast and Sustained Weight Loss. Little, Brown and Company, 2011.*

Fung, Jason. *"The Shocking Origin of Vegetable Oil - Garbage!" 22 August 2018,* https://medium.com/@drjasonfung/the-shocking-origin-of-vegetable-oil-garbage-1c2ce14ae513. *Accessed 2 April 2020.*

Gates, Donna, with Linda Schatz. *The Body Ecology Diet: Recovering Your Health and Rebuilding Your Immunity. Hay House, 2012.*

Gottfried, Sarah. *The Hormone Cure. Scribner, 2013.*

Harvard Health Publishing. *"The Truth About Fats: the Good, the Bad, and the In-between." February 2015 (updated 11 December 2019),* https://www.health.harvard.edu/staying-healthy/the-truth-about-fats-bad-and-good. *Accessed 2 April 2020.*

Healthline. *"Antibiotics in Your Food: Should You Be Concerned?" 17 June 2017,* https://www.healthline.com/nutrition/antibiotics-in-your-food. *Accessed 2 April 2020.*

Hyman, Mark. *"How Do I Know If I'm Eating Enough Healthy Fat?", 28 December 2016,* https://www.drhyman.com/blog/2016/12/28/know-im-eating-enough-healthy-fat/. *Accessed 2 April 2020.*

Leech, Joe. "11 Proven Benefits of Olive Oil." 14 Sep. 2018, https://www.
healthline.com/nutrition/11-proven-benefits-of-olive-oil. Accessed 3
April 2020.

Leech, Joe. "What are Trans Fats, and Are They Bad for You?" 30 July 2019,
https://www.healthline.com/nutrition/why-trans-fats-are-bad. Accessed
2 April 2020.

Levy, Jillian. "MCT Oil Health Benefits, Dosage Recommendations and Recipes."
3 September 2019, https://www.draxe.com/nutrition/fats-and-oils/
mct-oil/. Accessed 3 April 2020.

Malekinejad, Hassan and Aysa Rezabakhsh. "Hormones in Dairy Foods and
Their Impact on "Public Health - A Narrative Review Article." Iranian Journal
of Public Health, vol., 44, 2015, pp. 742-758, https://www.ncbi.nlm.nih.
gov/pmc/articles/PMC4524299. Accessed 2 April 2020.

Mercola, Joseph. "Choline is Crucial for Liver Health." 19 November 2018,
https://articles.mercola.com/sites/articles/archive/2018/11/19/
choline-fatty-liver.aspx?utm_source=dnl&utm_medium=email&utm_
content=secon&utm_campaign=20181202Z1_UCM&et_cid=D-
M251381&et_rid=484408545. Accessed 3 April 2020.

Mercola, Joseph. "Choline is Essential for Your Brain, Heart, Liver, and Nervous
System." https://articles.mercola.com/vitamins-supplements/choline.
aspx. Accessed 19 April 2020.

Mercola, Joseph. "Cottonseed Oil: America's Original Vegetable Oil." 18 April,
2019, https://articles.mercola.com/herbal-oils/cottonseed-oil.aspx.
Accessed 2 April 2020.

Mercola, Joseph. "The Secret Sauce in Grass-fed Beef." https://www.mercola.
com/beef/cla.htm. Accessed 2 April 2020.

Noonan, Michael. "Are There Really Vegetables in Vegetable Oil?" 3 October
2013, https://bangordailynews.com/2013/10/03/health/are-there-re-
ally-vegetables-in-vegetable-oil. Accessed 2 April 2020.

Perlmutter, David, with Kristin Loberg. Grain Brain: The Surprising Truth About
Wheat, Carbs, and Sugar – Your Brain's Silent Killers. Little, Brown and
Company, 2013.

Price, Annie. "What is Butyric Acid? 6 Benefits You Need to Know About." 15 June 2017, https://www.draxe.com/nutrition/supplements/butyric-acid/. Accessed 19 April 2020.

Rosenthal, Joshua. *Integrative Nutrition: A Whole-Life Approach to Health and Happiness.* Integrative Nutrition, 2018.

Rosenthal, Joshua. *Integrative Nutrition: Feed Your Hunger for Health and Happiness.* Integrative Nutrition, 2011.

Sheriff L. Jill, Therese A O'Sullivan, Catherine Properzi, Josephine-Lee Oddo, and Leon A Adams. "Choline: Its Potential Role in Nonalcoholic Fatty Liver Disease, and the Case for Human and Bacterial Genes." *Advanced Nutrition,* vol. 7, no. 1, pp. 5-13, https://www.ncbi.nlm.nih.gov/pmc/articles/PMC4717871/. Accessed 3 April 2020.

United States Department of Agriculture (USDA). *Food Guide Pyramid - Graphic Resources 30 November 2014,* https://www.fns.usda.gov/food-guide-pyramid-graphic-resources. Accessed 3 April 2020.

Vanderhaeghe, Lorna R., and Karlene Karst. *Health Fats For Life: Preventing and Treating Common Health Problems With Essential Fatty Acids.* John Wiley and Sons Canada, 2004.

Wake Forest University Baptist Medical Center. "Trans Fat Leads to Weight Gain Even on Same Total Calories, Animal Study Shows." 19 June 2006, https://sciencedaily.com/releases/2006/06/060619133024.htm. Accessed 2 April 2020.

Ware, Meghan. "12 Health Benefits of Avocadoes." 12 September 2017, https://www.medicalnewstoday.com/articles/270406.php. Accessed 3 April 2020.

WebMD. "Palm Oil." https://www.webmd.com/vitamins/ai/ingredient-mono-1139/palm-oil. Accessed 3 April 2020.

Wylde, Bryce. "Why You Should Give Red Palm Oil A Try." https://www.doctoroz.com/article/why-you-should-give-red-palm-oil-try. Accessed 3 April 2020.

Chapter 6

Berg, Eric. *The 7 Principles of Fat Burning: Get Healthy, Lose Weight and Keep It Off.* KB Publishing, 2010.

Braverman, Eric. "Dopamine and Cortisol." 22 January 2018, https://www. medium.com/@EricBravermanMD/dopamine-and-cortisol-6662cd-5cac7f. *Accessed 20 April 2020.*

Gottfried, Sara. The Hormone Cure. Scribner, 2013.

Harvard Medical School. "5 surprising benefits of walking." Harvard Health Publishing, https://www.health.harvard.edu/staying-healthy/5-sur-prising-benefits-of-walking. *Accessed 25 April 2020.*

Harvard Medical School. "Natural 'exercise' hormone transforms fat cells." Harvard Health Publishing, https://www.health.harvard.edu/healthbeat/natural-exercise-hormone-transforms-fat-cells. *Accessed 20 April 2020.*

Harvard Medical School. "The secret to better health – exercise." Harvard Health Publishing, https://www.health.harvard.edu/healthbeat/the-secret-to-better-health-exercise. *Accessed 20 April 2020.*

Laskowski, Edward R. "What are the risks of sitting too much?" Mayo Clinic, https://www.mayoclinic.org/healthy-lifestyle/adult-health/expert-an-swers/sitting/faq-20058005. *Accessed 20 April 2020.*

Lee, John with Victoria Hopkins. What your doctor may not tell you about menopause. The breakthrough book about natural progesterone. Warner Books, 1996.

Mercola, Joseph. "Strengthening Your Body Strengthens Your Mind." 27 November 2015, https://fitness.mercola.com/sites/fitness/archive/2015/11/27/strength-training-brain-health.aspx. *Accessed 20 April 2020.*

Mercola, Joseph. "The Many Health Benefits of Sweating." 24 July 2015, https://fitness.mercola.com/sites/fitness/archive/2015/07/24/benefits-of-sweating.aspx. *Accessed 20 April 2020.*

Mercola, Joseph. "The Most Effective Forms of Exercise for Diabetes: Strength Training and High-Intensity Exercise." 29 March 2019, https://fitness.mercola.com/sites/fitness/archive/2019/03/29/best-exercise-for-di-abetes.aspx. *Accessed 20 April 2020.*

Mercola, Joseph. "The secret sauce in grass-fed beef - on health benefits of conjugated linoleic acid (CLA)." https://www.mercola.com/beef/cla.htm. *Accessed 20 April 2020.*

Prevention. *Walk Off Weight.* Rodale, n.d.

Spillner, Maggie. *Prevention's Complete Book of Walking: Everything You Need to Know to Walk Your Way to Better Health.* Rodale, n.d.

Stevenson, Shawn. *Sleep Smarter: 21 Essential Strategies to Sleep Your Way to a Better Body, Better Health, and Bigger Success.* Rodale, 2016.

Steward, H. Leighton, Morrison G. Bethea, Sam S. Andrews, and Luis A. Balart. *Sugar Busters: Cut Sugar to Trim Fat.* Ballantine, 1995.

Walker, Jesse. *"7 unexpected reasons why you're not losing weight." 19 January 2018,* https://www.livestrong.com/slideshow/13708846-7-reasons-why-youre-not-losing-weight/?slide=3. *Accessed 20 April 2020.*

"Yoga with Erica." Morning Yoga for Weight Loss - 20 Minute Workout Fat Burning Yoga Meltdown Beginner & Intermediate. https://www.youtube.com/watch?v=7UpWgS7WtGg. *Accessed 20 April 2020.*

Zalis, Shelly. *"Why Self-Care Isn't Selfish: Equality Starts with Taking Care of Yourself." Forbes, 18 April 2017,* https://www.forbes.com/sites/shelleyzalis/2017/04/18/why-self-care-isnt-selfish-equality-starts-with-taking-care-of-yourself/#43fc10c362fd. *Accessed 20 April 2020.*

"10 min Morning Yoga Full Body Stretch with Kassandra." https://www.youtube.com/watch?v=4pKly2JojMw. *Accessed 20 April 2020.*

"15 Yoga Poses That'll Change your Body in Less Than a Month." https://www.bing.com/videos/search?q=%e2%80%9c15+Yoga+Poses+That%27ll+Change+your+Body+in+Less+Than+a+Month.&docid=608003601631805596&mid=3E976F90505E163AA1233E-976F90505E163AA123&view=detail&FORM=VIRE. *Accessed 20 April 2020.*

Chapter 7

Berg, Eric. *The 7 Principles of Fat Burning: Get Healthy, Lose Weight and Keep It Off.* KB Publishing, 2010.

Blonna, Richard. *Stress Less Live More: How Acceptance and Commitment Therapy Can Help You Live a Busy Yet Balanced Life.* New Harbinger, 2010.

Braverman, Eric R. *"Dopamine and Cortisol."* www.pathmed.com/blog/dopamine-and-cortisol. Accessed 25 April 2020.

Dolan, Eric W. "Listening to the music you love will make your brain release more dopamine, study finds." https://www.psypost.org/2019/02/listening-to-the-music-you-love-will-make-your-brain-release-more-dopamine-study-finds-53059. Accessed 25 April 2020.

Gottfried, Sara. The Hormone Cure. Scribner, 2013.

Gupta, Sanjay. "One Nation Under Stress: Deaths of Despair in the United States." HBO Documentary, 8 April 2019, https://www.youtube.com/results?search_query=one+nation+under+stress+dr+sanjay+gupta. Accessed 25 April 2020.

McQuade, Walter and Ann Aikman. Stress: What It Is, What It Can Do to Your Health, How to Handle It. Signet, Penguin Books, 1993.

National Institutes of Health. "About Adrenal Gland Disorders." 31 January 2017, https://www.nichd.nih.gov/health/topics/adrenalgland/conditioninfo. Accessed 25 April 2020.

Osnato, Jaime. "8 Ways to Beat Stress-Induced Belly Fat." 16 October 2019, https://www.livestrong.com/article/13716923-stress-cortisol-and-belly-fat. Accessed 25 April 2020.

Talbott, Shawn. The Cortisol Connection: Why Stress Makes You Fat – and What You Can Do About It. Hunter House Publishers, 2002.

Tello, Monique. "Intensive lifestyle change: it works, and it's more than diet and exercise." Health.harvard.edu. Harvard Health Publishing, 21 August 2017 (updated 3 May 2018), https://www.health.harvard.edu/blog/intensive-lifestyle-change-it-works-and-its-more-than-diet-and-exercise-2017082112287. Accessed 25 April 2020.

Tolle, Eckhart. The Power of Now: A Guide to Spiritual Enlightenment. Namaste Publishing, 1999.

Walker, Jesse. "7 Unexpected Reasons Why You're Not Losing Weight." 19 January 2018, https://www.livestrong.com/slideshow/13708846-7-unexpected-reasons-why-youre-not-losing-weight/. Accessed 25 April 2020.

Wilson, James L. Adrenal Fatigue: The 21st Century Stress Syndrome. Smart Publications, 2001.

Wood-Moen, Robin. "Dopamine and Stress Response." https://www.livestrong. com/article/366013-dopamine-and-stress-response/. Accessed 25 April 2020.

Chapter 8

American Academy of Sleep Medicine. "Study suggests that what you eat can influence how you sleep." 14 January 2016, https://aasm.org/study-suggests-that-what-you-eat-can-influence-how-you-sleep/. Accessed 29 March 2020.

Berg, Eric. The 7 Principles of Fat Burning: Get Healthy, Lose Weight and Keep It Off. KB Publishing, 2010.

Breus, Michael. "Ideal Home Sleep Environment." 14 March 2017, https:// thesleepdoctor.com/2017/03/14/ideal-home-sleep-environment/. Accessed 29 March 2020.

Breus, Michael. "5 Vitamin Deficiencies that Can Affect Your Sleep." 12 February 2019, https://thesleepdoctor.com/2019/02/12/5-vitamin-deficiencies-that-can-affect-your-sleep/. Accessed 29 March 2020.

Breus, Michael, with Debra Fulghum Bruce. The Sleep Doctor's Diet Plan: Lose Weight Through Better Sleep. Rodale, 2011.

Galic, Bojana. "Do You Really Need to Drink 8 Glasses of Water a Day?" 13 July 2020, https://www.livestrong.com/article/534298-how-much-water-to-drink-per-day-by-body-weight/?reload=1. Accessed 17 July 2020.

Garrard, Cathy. "10 Ways to Beat Menopausal Belly Fat." 6 September 2018, https://www.everydayhealth.com/menopause-pictures/ways-to-beat-menopausal-belly-fat.aspx. Accessed 28 March 2020.

Gates, Donna and Linda Schatz. The Body Ecology Diet. Hay House: Carlsbad, California, 2011.

Hall, Martica H., Christopher E. Kline, and Sara Nowakowski. "Insomnia and Sleep Apnea in Midlife Women: Prevalence and Consequences to Health and Functioning." 26 March 2015. https://www.ncbi.nlm.nih.gov/pmc/articles/PMC4447062/. Accessed 28 March 2020.

Healthline. "7 Health Benefits of Kiwi." https://www.healthline.com/health/7-best-things-about-kiwi. *Accessed 29 March 2020.*

Idzikowski, Chris. *Learn to Sleep Well: A Practical Guide to Getting a Good Night's Rest. Chronicle, 2000.*

Jabr, Ferris. "Blue LEDs Light Up Your Brain: Why Electronic Screens Keep You Awake at Night and What You Can Do About It." *Scientific American, 1 November 2016,* https://www.scientificamerican.com/article/blue-leds-light-up-your-brain/?redirect=1. *Accessed 29 March 2020.*

McKenna, Paul. *I Can Make You Sleep: Overcome Insomnia Forever and Get the Best Rest of Your Life! Sterling, 2009.*

Morrone, Lisa. *Sleep Well Again. Harvest House, 2012.*

National Sleep Foundation. "The Connection Between Hydration and Sleep." https://www.sleepfoundation.org/articles/connection-between-hy-dration-and-sleep. *Accessed 29 March 2020.*

National Sleep Foundation. ""Women and Sleep." https://www.sleepfounda-tion.org/articles/women-and-sleep. *Accessed 28 March 2020.*

O'Connor, Anahad. "Really? Using a Computer Before Bed Can Disrupt Sleep." *New York Times, 10 September, 2012,* https://well.blogs.nytimes.com/2012/09/10/really-using-a-computer-before-bed-can-disrupt-sleep/. *Accessed 29 March 2020.*

Ortner, Nick. *The Tapping Solution: A Revolutionary System for Stress-Free Living. Hay House, 2013.*

Osnato, Jaime. "How to Prevent Stress from Making You Fat." *16 October 2019,* https://www.livestrong.com/article/13716923-stress-cortisol-and-bel-ly-fat/. *Accessed 28 March 2020.*

Steen, Juliette. "8 Easy Ways to Boost Nutrient Absorption." *21 August 2017 (Updated 23 August 2018),* https://www.huffingtonpost.com.au/2017/08/20/8-easy-ways-to-boost-nutrient-absorp-tion_a_23079874/. *Accessed 28 March 2020.*

Stevenson, Shawn. "4 Hidden Things that Could Be Destroying Your Sleep Quality." *6 March 2019 podcast,* https://www.youtube.com/watch?v=W78LRPCPXkQ. *Accessed 28 March 2020.*

Stevenson, Shawn. *Sleep Smarter: 21 Essential Strategies to Sleep Your Way to a Better Body, Better Health, and Bigger Success.* Rodale, 2016.

UCLA Sleep Disorder Center. "Sleep and Health." https://www.uclahealth.org/sleepcenter/sleep-and-health. *Accessed 28 March 2020.*

Vitti, Alisa. *Woman Code: Perfect Your Cycle, Amplify Your Fertility, Supercharge Your Sex Drive, and Become a Power Source.* HarperOne, 2014.

WebMD. "An Overview of Insomnia." https://www.webmd.com/sleep-disorders/insomnia-causes#. *Accessed 28 March 2020.*

WebMD. "What Are REM and Non-REM Sleep?" *26 October 2018,* https://www.webmd.com/sleep-disorders/guide/sleep-101. *Accessed 29 March 2020.*

Weil, Andrew. *Spontaneous Happiness.* New York: Little, Brown and Company, 2011.

Wszelaki, Magdalena. "11 Sleep Strategies to Help the Hormones, Waistline, Mood and Cravings." *19 March 2020,* https://hormonesbalance.com/articles/11-sleep-strategies-help-hormones-waistline-mood-cravings-part-1/?inf_contact_key=35021faede7c243109c79789b6d-5123709c74070ac2bf3cfa7869e3cfd4ff832&utm_source=newsletter&utm_medium=email. *Accessed 29 March 2020.*

Final Thoughts

Berg, Eric. *The 7 Principles of Fat Burning: Get Healthy, Lose Weight and Keep It Off.* KB Publishing, 2010.

"How to Measure Your Waist." *WebMD,* https://www.webmd.com/diet/guide/calculating-your-waist-circumference. *Accessed 26 April 2020.*

Vaccariello, Liz, with Cynthia Sass. *Flat Belly Diet!* Rodale, 2008.

Walker, Alice. *We Are the Ones We Have Been Waiting For: Inner Light in a Time of Darkness.* The New Press, 2006.

INDEX

124, 153, 166, 187, 199, 200, 240, 291, 338
and preferences 43
false assumptions 180
healthy 20
neglecting 146
organic 72
processed 72, 86, 114
quality 94
Food combinations 139
Food elimination 138, 140
Food group 4, 25, 85, 89, 90, 93, 99, 100, 111, 198, 338
Food intake 90, 201
Food intolerance 139
Food poisoning 200
Food production 86, 124
Food pyramid 92
Food safety 206
Food sensitivities 109, 117, 138
Forgiveness 265, 282, 283
France 87
Francina, Suza 246
Free radicals 189, 208
Friendly bacteria 58, 62, 65, 77, 78, 82, 132, 134, 149, 166
Friendly germs 136
Frozen dough balls 84
Fructosamine 185
Fructose 47, 52, 64, 74, 141, 205
and NAFLD 51
Fruit juices
concentrate 74
giving up 70
Fruits consumption 74
Fuhrman, Joel 121, 204, 335
Fungal infections 77
Fungal skin infection 56
Fungal skin rash 81
Fungicides 144
Fung, Jason 183
Fungus 59, 60, 66, 67, 69, 72, 167

G

Galactose 74

Gál, Kat 136
Ganjhu, Lisa 129
Gardening
gut-healing journey through 142
spiritual journey through 157
Garrard, Cathy 293, 296
Gastrointestinal function 253
Gastrointestinal system 128, 129
Gates, Donna 7, 50, 56, 76, 77, 109, 121, 127, 146, 305
Gazella, Karolyn A. 53, 65
Genes 54, 229, 293
Genetically Modified Organisms (GMOs) 94, 191, 195
Genetic factors 206
Genetic makeup 44, 135, 265
Genetic predisposition 33, 48
to diabetes 65, 75, 99
Geneva Global 260
Ghee 118, 202
Ghrelin 301
Gittleman, Anne Louise 41
GLA 201
Glucagon 118, 241
Glucocorticoids 254
Glucose 46, 52, 88, 89, 104, 141, 153, 193, 243, 255, 256
control 243
excess 269
fasting 7
glycogen 254
raised blood 254
Gluten 90, 138, 141, 291
food sources 141
Gluten-free 72, 109, 110, 114, 115
Glycemic Index
and carbohydrates 106
Glycemic load 108, 116
and Glycemic Index 108
Glycogen 88
storage 255
GMOs. See Genetically Modified Organisms
Golden berries 74, 150
Good bacteria 53, 76, 77, 121, 122, 130, 133, 135, 144, 153, 164

P

Trans fats 178, 183, 184, 185, 186,
187, 188, 189, 205
Treadmill 234, 241, 242, 243, 335
Triiodothyronine (T3) 232
Tropical fats
and oils 207
Tropical oils 181, 182, 194, 205, 208
Tropicana orange juice 70
Tuck, Fiona 304
Tums 164
Turner, Natasha 297
TV curfew 325
Tymoczko, John L 88
Type 2 diabetes 44, 45, 47, 119, 124,
125, 189, 229, 235, 344
Types of exercises 4, 5, 25, 226, 228,
233, 236, 238, 247

U

Ugali 83
Underweight 170, 203
Undigested foods 130, 137, 141
Unfriendly organisms 136
Unhealthy fats 205
United Kingdom
slimming regimes 92
United Soybean Board 183
United States 87, 92, 95, 113, 154,
177, 207
carbs availability 101
comfort living 171
cottonseed oil 172
DDT banned insecticide 145
food groups 101
GMOs 195
life at 198
olive oil 183
RDA for sugar 70
sleep disorders 293
slimming regimes 92
unsafe trans fats 186
Universe 160, 161, 341, 342
Unprocessed carbs 51, 113
Unprocessed foods 51, 95, 114, 129,
190

Unrealistic goals 284
Unrefined plant products 204
Unripe bananas 76, 77, 115
Unripe tropical fruits 122
Unsaturated fats 202
USDA 91
Food Guide Pyramid 181

V

Vaccariello, Liz 335
Vaginal birth 64, 65
Vaginal walls 60
Vaginal yeast infections 165
Vanderhaeghe, Lorna R. 201
Varicose veins 229
Vegan 119, 138
Vegan diet 29, 192
Vegan-friendly 138
Veganism 192
Vegetable oil 179
Vegetarian diet 174, 192
Velasquez-Manoff, Moises 148
Ventral Tegmented Area (VTA) 49
Vinegar and salt 154
Vision loss 322
Vital organs 10, 321
Vitamin A 208, 210
Vitamin B 132
Vitamin B6 69
Vitamin C 284
Vitamin D3 323
Vitamin D deficiency 316, 317
Vitamin Deficiencies 321, 323
Vitamin E 195, 207, 208, 210
Vitamins 72, 104, 115, 121, 129, 132,
146, 209, 305, 321, 322
Vitti, Alissa 298
VTA. *See* Ventral Tegmented Area

W

Wake Forest University Baptist Medical Center 185
Walker, Alice 336
Walker, Jesse 234, 243, 252

Made in the USA
Las Vegas, NV
02 September 2021

29444423R00226